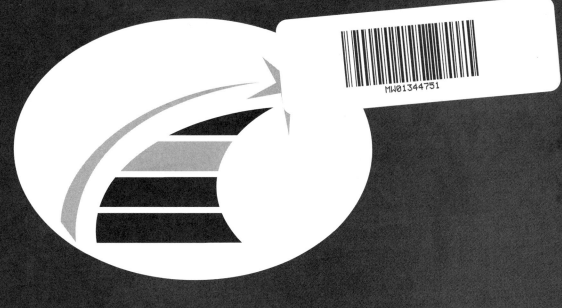

Step 3: Certify

"The average salary across the board is 17% higher for a certified coder."
— AAPC Salary Survey, 2007

Congratulations on reaching the certification step in your career! As you know, certified coders are in top demand in today's marketplace. That's why, as a lifelong coder and educator, I have dedicated myself to providing the most up-to-date, comprehensive, and user-friendly certification review books on the market. I update this book every year so you will have the best tool possible when studying for your certification exam. It's time to hit the books. ***You can do it! I know you can!***

— Carol J. Buck, MS, CPC-I, CPC, CPC-H, CCS-P

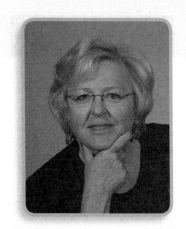

Track your progress!

See the checklist in the back of this book to learn more about your next step toward coding success!

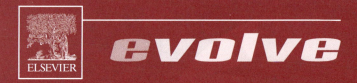

❖ *To access your Student Resources, visit:*

http://evolve.elsevier.com/Buck/cpc/

Evolve® Student Resources for **Buck: CPC® Coding Exam Review 2009: The Certification Step** offer the following features:

Student Resources

- **Study Tips**
  Thoughts and advice from the author to help medical coding students.

- **Content Updates**
  The latest content updates from the author to keep you current with recent developments in this area.

- **WebLinks**
  Links to places of interest on the web specific to your needs.

- **HCPCS and ICD-9-CM Updates**
  The latest developments and rules for these coding sets.

http://evolve.elsevier.com/Buck/cpc/

CPC CODING EXAM REVIEW
The Certification Step

2009 CPC CODING EXAM REVIEW

The Certification Step

CAROL J. BUCK
MS, CPC-I, CPC, CPC-H, CCS-P
Program Director, Retired
Medical Secretary Programs
Northwest Technical College
East Grand Forks, Minnesota

Karla R. Lovaasen, RHIA, CCS, CCS-P
Coding and Consulting Services
Abingdon, Maryland

Judith Neppel, RN, MS
Executive Director
Minnesota Rural Health Association
University of Minnesota, Crookston
Crookston, Minnesota

Marilyn Rasmussen, RHIA, CPC
Coding, Reimbursement, Compliance Specialist
Albert Lea, Minnesota

Keith Russell, CPC, CPC-H
Senior Compliance Analyst
Baylor College of Medicine
Houston, Texas

Cynthia Stahl, CPC, CCS-P, CPC-H
Reimbursement and Coding Specialist
Lebanon, Indiana

SAUNDERS
ELSEVIER

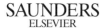

11830 Westline Industrial Drive
St. Louis, Missouri 63146

CPC® CODING EXAM REVIEW 2009: ISBN: 978-1-4160-3713-2
THE CERTIFICATION STEP

Copyright © 2009, 2008, 2007, 2006, 2005, 2004 by Saunders, an imprint of Elsevier Inc.

All rights reserved. No part of this publication may be reproduced or transmitted in any form or by any means, electronic or mechanical, including photocopying, recording, or any information storage and retrieval system, without permission in writing from the publisher.

Notice

Neither the Publisher nor the Author assumes any responsibility for any loss or injury and/or damage to persons or property arising out of or related to any use of the material contained in this book. It is the responsibility of the treating practitioner, relying on independent expertise and knowledge of the patient, to determine the best treatment and method of application for the patient.

The Publisher

NOTE: *Current Procedural Terminology, 2009,* was used in updating this text.

Current Procedural Terminology (CPT) is copyright 2008 American Medical Association. All Rights Reserved. No fee schedules, basic units, relative values, or related listings are included in CPT. The AMA assumes no liability for the data contained herein. Applicable FARS/DFARS restrictions apply to government use.

Library of Congress Cataloging-in-Publication Data

CPC coding exam review : the certification step / Carol J. Buck . . . [et al.]. — 2009 ed.
    p. ; cm.
    Includes index.
    IISBN 978-1-4160-3713-2 (pbk. : alk. paper)   1. Nosology—Code numbers—Examinations, questions, etc.   2. Medical records—Management—Examinations, questions, etc.   3. Medical transcription—Examinations, questions, etc.   I. Buck, Carol J.
    [DNLM: 1. Classification—Problems and Exercises.   2. Terminology as Topic—Problems and Exercises.   3. Forms and Records Control—methods—Problems and Exercises.   WB 18.2 C882 2009]
    RB115.C77 2009
    651.5'04261076—dc22

2008035907

Publisher: Michael S. Ledbetter
Developmental Editor: Joshua S. Rapplean
Publishing Services Manager: Melissa Lastarria
Publishing Services Manager: Pat Joiner-Myers
Senior Designer: Renee Duenow
Senior Designer: Amy Buxton

Printed in Canada

Last digit is the print number: 9 8 7 6 5 4 3 2 1

Working together to grow libraries in developing countries

www.elsevier.com | www.bookaid.org | www.sabre.org

ELSEVIER   BOOK AID International   Sabre Foundation

Dedication

*To coding instructors,
who each day strive to enhance the lives
of their students and provide the next generation
of knowledgeable medical coders.*

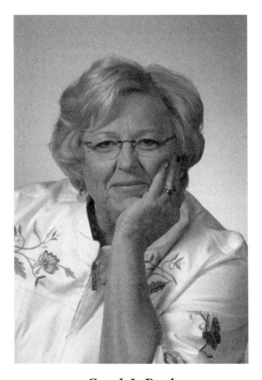

Carol J. Buck

Acknowledgments

There are so many, many people who participated in the development of this text, and only through the effort of all of the team members has it been possible to publish this text. **Cynthia Stahl,** who has taken this text into her expert hands and lifted it higher each year. **Karla R. Lovaasen, Marilyn Rasmussen,** and **Keith Russell,** who lent their technical coding knowledge and enthusiasm to this project. **Judith Neppel,** whose exceptional knowledge of medical terminology improved the terminology material.

    Sally Schrefer, Executive Vice President, Nursing and Health Professions, who possesses great listening skills and the ability to ensure the publication of high-quality educational materials. **Andrew Allen,** Vice President and Publisher, Health Professions, who sees the bigger picture and shares the vision. **Michael Ledbetter,** Publisher, who maintains an excellent sense of humor and is a valued member of the team who can always be depended upon for reasoned judgment. **Josh Rapplean,** Developmental Editor, who has taken over the developmental duties of this text with calm, confidence, and tremendous efficiency. **Laura Slown Sullivan,** Production Editor, Graphic World, who assumed responsibility for many projects while maintaining a high degree of professionalism. The employees of Elsevier have participated in the publication of this text and demonstrated exceptional professionalism and competence.

Preface

Thank you for purchasing *CPC® Coding Exam Review 2009: The Certification Step,* the latest guide to the outpatient physician coding certification exam. This 2009 edition has been carefully reviewed and updated with the latest content, making it the most current guide for your review. The author and publishers have made every effort to equip you with skills and tools you will need to succeed on the exam. To this end, this review guide presents essential information about all health care coding systems, anatomy, terminology, and pathophysiology, as well as practice and final examinations in print and on CD-ROM. No other review guide on the market brings together such thorough coverage of all necessary examination material in one source.

ORGANIZATION OF THIS TEXTBOOK

Following a basic outline approach, *CPC Coding Exam Review 2009* takes a practical approach to assisting you with your examination preparations. The text is divided into four units—Anatomy, Terminology, and Pathophysiology; Reimbursement Issues; Overview of CPT, ICD-9-CM, and HCPCS Coding; and Coding Challenge—and there are several appendices for your reference. Additionally, there is a bound-in CD-ROM with examinations to help your progress.

Preface

Unit I, Anatomy, Terminology, and Pathophysiology
Covers all the essential body systems and terms you'll need to get certified. Organized by body systems to follow the CPT codes, the sections also include illustrations to review each major anatomical area and quizzes to check your understanding and recall.

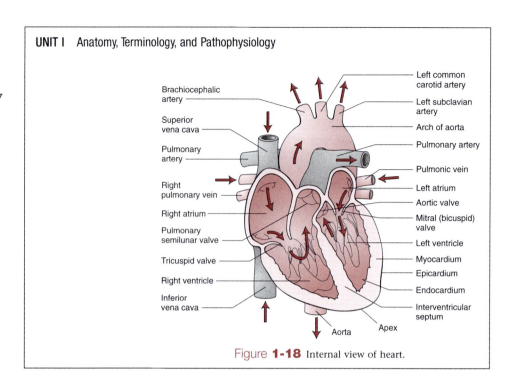

Figure **1-18** Internal view of heart.

Unit II, Reimbursement Issues
Provides a review of important insurance and billing information to help you review the connections between medical coding, insurance, billing, and reimbursement.

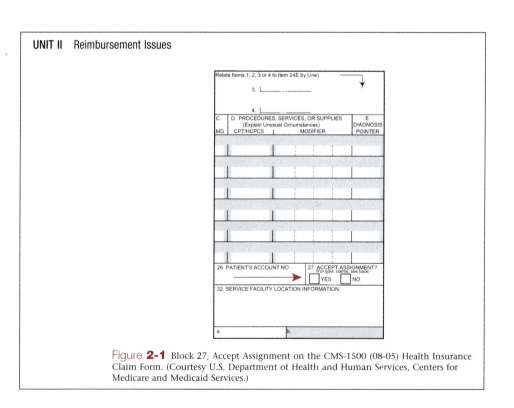

Figure **2-1** Block 27, Accept Assignment on the CMS-1500 (08-05) Health Insurance Claim Form. (Courtesy U.S. Department of Health and Human Services, Centers for Medicare and Medicaid Services.)

Preface

Unit III, Overview of CPT, ICD-9-CM, and HCPCS Coding
Contains comprehensive coverage of the different coding systems and their applications, making other references unnecessary! Simplified text and clear examples are the highlights of this unit, and illustrations are included to clarify difficult concepts.

UNIT III Overview of CPT, ICD-9-CM, and HCPCS Coding

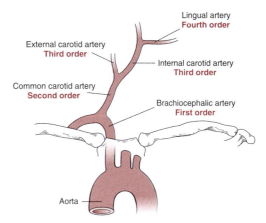

Figure **3-12** Brachiocephalic vascular family with first-, second-, third-, and fourth-order vessels.

Balloon: Threaded into vessel, inflated under mass, pulled out with mass
- Codes are divided by site of incision and whether artery or vein

Venous Reconstruction—CV Repairs (34501-34530)
Types of repairs
- Valve of the femoral vein
- Vena Cava
- Saphenopopliteal vein anastomosis

Unit IV, Coding Challenge
Contains a Final Examination modeled after the actual CPC examination, to be taken at the end of your complete program of study. To help you quantify the examination, this is meant to be taken using paper and pencil.

Final Examination

■ FINAL EXAMINATION
SECTION 1

QUESTIONS 1-43

Medical Terminology

1. This term means the surgical removal of the fallopian tube:
   A. ligation
   B. hysterectomy
   C. salpingostomy
   D. salpingectomy

2. This combining form means thirst:
   A. dips/o
   B. acr/o
   C. cortic/o
   D. somat/o

Preface

ABOUT THE CD-ROM

The companion CD-ROM included in the back of this review guide contains valuable software to assist you with your preparation for the CPC coding certification examination. It includes two timed and scored 150-question practice examinations (the same examination is taken twice) modeled after the actual format of the CPC examination, which contains three major sections. The Pre-Examination on the CD-ROM should be completed at the start of your study, and the Post-Examination, also on the CD-ROM, should be taken after your study is complete. By comparing the results of these examinations, you can see your improvement after using the review guide! Once you check your scores, your are ready to take the Final Examination in Unit IV of the text.

Summary Screen

When using the program, the Summary screen serves as home base. Here you can find information relating to your progress and performance in different examination sections and subject areas. From this screen, you can choose an examination mode, submit an examination section, check your progress, review your results, and access the Final Examination scoresheet and answers.

In addition to displaying your scores for completed sections and tracking the total elapsed time, this screen also shows the answered, unanswered, and flagged questions in each subsection. You can return to the Summary screen at any point while taking or reviewing an examination, and all information related to your answers and position is saved.

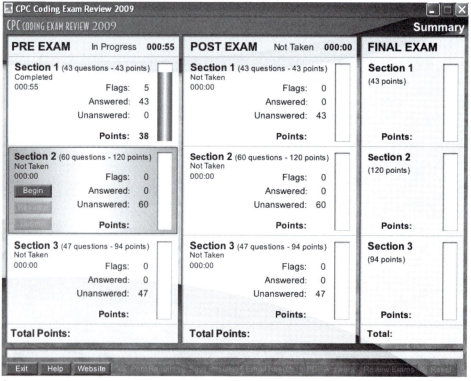

Summary screen.

Taking the Examination

While taking the examination, click on the letter of your answer choice, and the answer will be highlighted in red. You can also use the corresponding letter keys and arrows on the keyboard to answer and navigate. The Question screen displays the current question number, which doubles as a pull-down menu that allows you jump to any question in the current section. Additionally, the Flag button at the bottom of the screen allows you to mark questions for later reference.

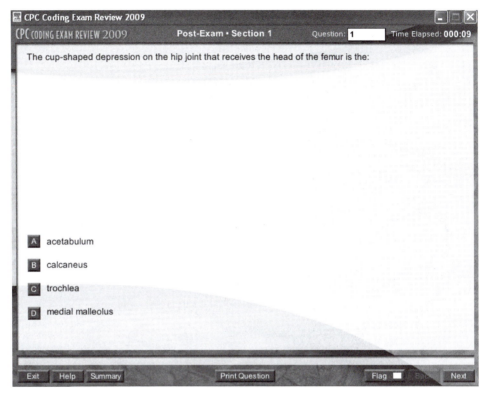

Question screen.

Reviewing Your Results

Once you have taken the Post-Examination on the CD-ROM, you have the option to review all the examination questions with rationales, even the ones you answered correctly. The correct answer is shown for each question, and a rationale is given for each answer option. You can also compare your results on the Pre- and Post-Examinations by viewing the bar graphs on the Summary screen or printing out a score sheet.

Once you have completed the Final Examination in Unit IV, you will access the electronic score sheet on the CD-ROM and enter your answers. The software will then provide you with the answers and rationales, as well as the option to compare your scores to the previous examinations.

Additional instructions and help files are included on the CD-ROM to assist you in using the software.

SUPPLEMENTAL RESOURCES

However you decide to prepare for the certification examination, we have developed supplements designed to complement the *CPC Coding Exam Review 2009*. Each of these supplements has been developed with the needs of both students and instructors in mind.

Instructor's Electronic Resource

No matter what your level of teaching experience, this total-teaching solution will help you plan your lessons with ease, and the author has developed all the curriculum materials necessary to use the textbook in the classroom. This CD-ROM includes additional unit quizzes, a course calendar and syllabus, lesson plans, ready-made tests for easy assessment, and PDF files with the questions and answers for the Pre-/Post- and Final Examinations. Also included is a comprehensive PowerPoint collection for the entire text, and ExamView test banks. The PowerPoint slides can be easily customized to support your lectures or formatted as overhead transparencies or handouts for student note-taking. The ExamView test generator will help you quickly and easily prepare quizzes and exams from the ready-made test questions, and can be customized to your specific teaching methods.

Evolve Resources

The Evolve companion website offers many resources that will extend your studies beyond the classroom. Related WebLinks offer you the opportunity to expand your knowledge base and stay current with this ever-changing field, and additional material is available for help and practice. Instructors can also download all materials from the Instructor's Electronic Resource, as well as content updates.

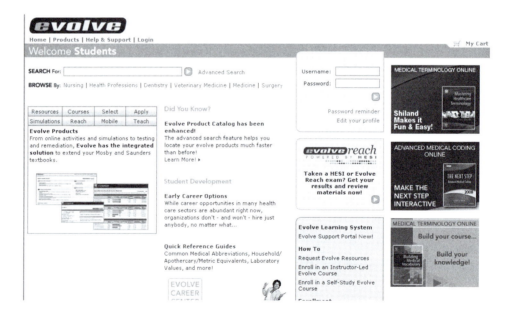

A Course Management System (CMS) is also available free to instructors who adopt this textbook. This web-based platform gives instructors yet another resource to facilitate learning and to make medical coding content accessible to students. In addition to the Evolve Resources available to both faculty and students, there is an entire suite of tools available that allows for communication between instructors and students. Students can log on through the Evolve portal to take online quizzes, participate in threaded discussions, post assignments to instructors, or chat with other classmates, while instructors can use the online grade book to follow class progress.

To access this comprehensive online resource, simply go to the Evolve home page at http://evolve.elsevier.com and enter the user name and password provided by your instructor. If your instructor has not set up a Course Management System, you can still access the free Evolve resources at http://evolve.elsevier.com/Buck/cpc/.

Development of This Edition

This book would not have been possible without a team of educators and professionals, including practicing coders and technical consultants. The combined efforts of the team members have made this text an incredible learning tool.

SENIOR ICD-9-CM CODING REVIEWER

Karla R. Lovaasen, RHIA, CCS, CCS-P*
Coding and Consulting Services
Abingdon, Maryland

*Co-author of: *ICD-9-CM Coding: Theory and Practice, 2009 Edition*, St. Louis, 2009, Saunders.

CODING SPECIALISTS

Patricia Cordy Henricksen, CPC, CCP
Approved PMCC Instructor
President, Lexington Local Chapter of AAPC
Bluegrass Medical Managers Association
Lexington, Kentucky

Jody Klitz, CPC
Coding Reimbursement Specialist
Cancer Center of North Dakota
Grand Forks, North Dakota

Nancy Maguire, ACS, CRT, PCS, FCS, CPC, CPC-H, HCS-D, APC, AFC
Physician Consultant for Auditing and Education
Universal City, Texas

Keith Quigley, CCS-P
Patient Record Abstractor 4
Instructor
University of California, Davis Health System
Sacramento, California

Marilyn Rasmussen, RHIA, CPC
Coding, Reimbursement, Compliance Specialist
Albert Lea, Minnesota

Keith Russell, CPC, CPC-H
Senior Compliance Analyst
Baylor College of Medicine
Houston, Texas

Patricia Harrison Skibbe
Welcoming Officer
AAPC Richardson, Texas, Chapter
Richardson, Texas

Cynthia Stahl, CPC, CCS-P, CPC-H
Reimbursement and Coding Specialist
Lebanon, Indiana

Jane Tuttle, CPC-I, CCS-P
Coding Education Endeavors
Westford, Massachusetts

TERMINOLOGY SPECIALIST

Judith Neppel, RN, MS
Executive Director
Minnesota Rural Health Association
University of Minnesota, Crookston
Crookston, Minnesota

Contents

Success Strategies, S-1

Course Syllabus and Student Calendar, C-1

Unit I **Anatomy, Terminology, and Pathophysiology, 1**

1 **Integumentary System**
Integumentary System—Anatomy and Terminology, 2
Integumentary System Anatomy and Terminology Quiz, 7
Integumentary System—Pathophysiology, 9
Integumentary System Pathophysiology Quiz, 27

2 **Musculoskeletal System**
Musculoskeletal System—Anatomy and Terminology, 29
Musculoskeletal System Anatomy and Terminology Quiz, 45
Musculoskeletal System—Pathophysiology, 47
Musculoskeletal System Pathophysiology Quiz, 53

3 **Respiratory System**
Respiratory System—Anatomy and Terminology, 55
Respiratory System Anatomy and Terminology Quiz, 63
Respiratory System—Pathophysiology, 65
Respiratory System Pathophysiology Quiz, 71

4 **Cardiovascular System**
Cardiovascular System—Anatomy and Terminology, 73
Cardiovascular System Anatomy and Terminology Quiz, 83
Cardiovascular System—Pathophysiology, 85
Cardiovascular System Pathophysiology Quiz, 95

5 **Female Genital System and Pregnancy**
Female Genital System and Pregnancy—Anatomy and Terminology, 97
Female Genital System and Pregnancy Anatomy and Terminology Quiz, 105
Female Genital System and Pregnancy—Pathophysiology, 107
Female Genital System and Pregnancy Pathophysiology Quiz, 121

6 **Male Genital System**
Male Genital System—Anatomy and Terminology, 123
Male Genital System Anatomy and Terminology Quiz, 127

Male Genital System—Pathophysiology, 129
Male Genital System Pathophysiology Quiz, 139

7 Urinary System
Urinary System—Anatomy and Terminology, 141
Urinary System Anatomy and Terminology Quiz, 147
Urinary System—Pathophysiology, 149
Urinary System Pathophysiology Quiz, 159

8 Digestive System
Digestive System—Anatomy and Terminology, 161
Digestive System Anatomy and Terminology Quiz, 169
Digestive System—Pathophysiology, 171
Digestive System Pathophysiology Quiz, 189

9 Mediastinum and Diaphragm
Mediastinum and Diaphragm—Anatomy and Terminology, 191
Mediastinum and Diaphragm Anatomy and Terminology Quiz, 193

10 Hemic and Lymphatic System
Hemic and Lymphatic System—Anatomy and Terminology, 195
Hemic and Lymphatic System Anatomy and Terminology Quiz, 199
Hemic and Lymphatic System—Pathophysiology, 201
Hemic and Lymphatic System Pathophysiology Quiz, 209

11 Endocrine System
Endocrine System—Anatomy and Terminology, 211
Endocrine System Anatomy and Terminology Quiz, 217
Endocrine System—Pathophysiology, 219
Endocrine System Pathophysiology Quiz, 227

12 Nervous System
Nervous System—Anatomy and Terminology, 229
Nervous System Anatomy and Terminology Quiz, 235
Nervous System—Pathophysiology, 237
Nervous System Pathophysiology Quiz, 251

13 Senses
Senses—Anatomy and Terminology, 253
Senses Anatomy and Terminology Quiz, 261
Senses—Pathophysiology, 263
Senses Pathophysiology Quiz, 269

14 Unit I Quiz Answers, 271

Unit II Reimbursement Issues, 277

1 Reimbursement Issues, 278

2 National Correct Coding Initiative, 281

3 *Federal Register*, 282

4 Quality Improvement Organizations (QIO), 282

5 Resource-Based Relative Value Scale (RBRVS), 282

6 Medicare Fraud and Abuse, 284

7	**Managed Health Care, 285**
8	**Reimbursement Terminology, 286**
9	**Reimbursement Quiz, 291**
10	**Reimbursement Quiz Answers, 293**

Unit III Overview of CPT, ICD-9-CM, and HCPCS Coding, 295

1 Introduction to Medical Coding, 296

2 CPT, 296
- A. Evaluation and Management (E/M) Section, 302
- B. Anesthesia Section, 321
- C. CPT/HCPCS Level I Modifiers, 323
- D. Surgery Section, 329
  1. General Subsection, 331
  2. Integumentary System Subsection, 331
  3. Musculoskeletal System Subsection, 340
  4. Respiratory System Subsection, 345
  5. Cardiovascular (CV) System Subsection, 349
  6. Hemic and Lymphatic System Subsection, 360
  7. Mediastinum Subsection, 361
  8. Diaphragm Subsection, 361
  9. Digestive System Subsection, 361
  10. Urinary System Subsection, 362
  11. Male Genital System Subsection, 364
  12. Reproductive System Procedures, 365
  13. Intersex Surgery Subsection, 365
  14. Female Genital System Subsection, 365
  15. Maternity Care & Delivery Subsection, 369
  16. Endocrine System Subsection, 371
  17. Nervous System Subsection, 372
  18. Eye and Ocular Adnexa Subsection, 374
  19. Auditory System Subsection, 375
  20. Operating Microscope Subsection, 375
- E. Radiology Section, 375
- F. Pathology and Laboratory Section, 382
- G. Medicine Section, 387

3 HCPCS Coding, 399

4 An Overview of the ICD-9-CM, 401
- A. Introduction, 401
- B. Format of ICD-9-CM, 402
- C. ICD-9-CM Conventions, 402
- D. Volume 2, Alphabetic Index, 403
- E. Sections, 404
- F. Volume 1, Tabular List, 406

5 Using the ICD-9-CM, 407
- A. General Guidelines, 407
- B. Steps to Diagnosis Coding, 407
- C. Selection of Primary Diagnosis, 408

Contents

D. V Codes, 409
E. Late Effects, 410
F. Diagnostic Coding and Reporting Guidelines for Outpatient Services, 410
G. ICD-9-CM, Chapter 1, Infectious and Parasitic Diseases, 413
H. ICD-9-CM, Chapter 2, Neoplasms, 414
I. ICD-9-CM, Chapter 3, Endocrine, Nutritional, and Metabolic Diseases and Immunity Disorders, 416
J. ICD-9-CM, Chapter 4, Diseases of Blood and Blood-Forming Organs, 416
K. ICD-9-CM, Chapter 5, Mental Disorders, 417
L. ICD-9-CM, Chapter 6, Diseases of Nervous System and Sense Organs, 417
M. ICD-9-CM, Chapter 7, Diseases of Circulatory System, 418
N. ICD-9-CM, Chapter 8, Diseases of Respiratory System, 420
O. ICD-9-CM, Chapter 9, Diseases of Digestive System, 420
P. ICD-9-CM, Chapter 10, Diseases of Genitourinary System, 420
Q. ICD-9-CM, Chapter 11, Complications of Pregnancy, Childbirth, and Puerperium, 421
R. ICD-9-CM, Chapter 12, Diseases of Skin and Subcutaneous Tissue, 423
S. ICD-9-CM, Chapter 13, Diseases of Musculoskeletal System and Connective Tissue, 423
T. ICD-9-CM, Chapters 14 and 15, Congenital Anomalies and Conditions Originating in Perinatal Period, 424
U. ICD-9-CM, Chapter 16, Symptoms, Signs, and Ill-Defined Conditions, 424
V. ICD-9-CM, Chapter 17, Injury and Poisoning, 424

Unit IV Coding Challenge, 429

1 Examinations, 430
A. Pre-Examination and Post-Examination, 430
B. Final Examination, 431
C. Answer Sheet, 433

2 Final Examination, 435
A. Section 1, 435
B. Section 2, 440
C. Section 3, 459

APPENDIX A ICD-9-CM Official Guidelines for Coding and Reporting, A-1

APPENDIX B Medical Terminology, A-94

APPENDIX C Combining Forms, A-114

APPENDIX D Prefixes, A-123

APPENDIX E Suffixes, A-125

APPENDIX F Abbreviations, A-128

APPENDIX G Further Text Resources, A-134

Index, I-1

CPC CODING EXAM REVIEW
The Certification Step

Success Strategies

This review was developed to help you as you prepare for your certification examination. First, congratulations on your initiative. Preparing for a certification examination can seem like a daunting and formidable task. You have already taken the first and hardest step: you have made a commitment. Your steely determination and organizational skills are your best tools as you prepare to complete this exciting journey successfully.

How do you prepare for a certification examination? The answers to that question are as varied as the persons preparing for it. Each person comes to the preparation with different educational, coding, and personal experiences. Therefore, each must develop a plan that meets his or her individual needs and preferences. Success Strategies will help you to develop your individual plan.

THE CERTIFICATION EXAMINATION

This text has been developed to serve as a tool in your preparation for the outpatient (physician-based) **CPC** (Certified Professional Coder) certification examination offered by the American Academy of Professional Coders (AAPC). The CPC certification examination consists of Sections 1, 2, and 3 covering medical terminology, anatomy, pathophysiology, CPT, ICD-9-CM, HCPCS, and coding concepts. You have $5^1/_2$ hours to complete the examination. Visit the AAPC website (www.aapc.com) for the latest information on the CPC examination.

To be successful on the CPC certification examination, you will have to know how to assign medical codes to patient services and diagnoses. This textbook focuses on providing you with that coding practice as well as anatomy, terminology, pathophysiology, reimbursement, and coding concepts in preparation for the CPC examination.

Date and Location

Although every journey begins with the first step, you have to know where you are going to make a plan to get there.

- Choose the **date and location** for taking the certification examination. The AAPC's website contains detailed information about the examination sites and dates.

- The American Academy of Professional Coders has information that can be downloaded from their website at www.aapc.com or sent for by contacting:

  American Academy of Professional Coders
  2480 South 3850 West, Suite B
  Salt Lake City, UT 84120
  Telephone: 800-626-2633

- After you have obtained the examination materials, read all the information carefully. Review all competencies outlined in the material to ensure that your study plan contains strategies to address each of these competencies.

- The questions within this textbook are not the same questions that are in the certification examination, but the skill and knowledge that you gain through analysis, coding, and recall will increase your ability to be successful on examination day.

- The AAPC's examination information will indicate the coding specifics. For example, the levels of the evaluation and management key components (history, examination, and medical decision making complexity) are stated in the certification questions. Do not challenge the levels.

MANAGING YOUR TIME

Role strain! That is what you get when you have so many different roles in your life and you cannot find time for all of them! Know that feeling? Are you a daughter/son, mother/father, wife/husband, student, friend, worker, volunteer, hobbyist—the list is endless. Each takes time from your schedule, and somehow you now need to fit into the role of successful learner. Because you have only 24 hours in your day, being a successful learner requires a time-balancing act. Maybe you will have to be satisfied with dust bunnies under your bed, dishes in your kitchen sink, or fewer visits with your friends. Whatever you have to do to juggle the time around to give yourself ample time to devote to this important task of examination preparation, you must do and make a plan for in advance; otherwise, life just takes over and you find you do not have adequate study time.

If you are planning a big event in your life—moving, a trip, and so on, think about postponing it until after the examination. Your focus right now has to be on yourself. Make your motto **"It's All About Me!"** Sounds self-centered, I know, and most likely very different from who you are, but just this once, you need to carve out the time you need to accomplish this important goal. This time is for yourself. Make it happen for yourself. Move everything you can out of the way, focus on this preparation, and give this preparation your best effort.

SCHEDULE

Each person has an individual learning style. The coding profession seems to attract those most influenced by logic and facts. The best way for a logical and factual person to learn is to problem-solve and apply the information. Hands-on practice is how you will build your skill and confidence for the examination.

- Choose a location to be your Study Central.

- Gather into Study Central the following study resources:

  - Certification packet or handbook from the certifying organization

  - CPT, current edition

- ICD-9-CM, current edition
- HCPCS, current edition
- ICD-9-CM Official Guidelines for Coding and Reporting (Appendix A of this text)
- Medical dictionary
- Coding textbooks, professional journals, and magazines
- Terminology, anatomy, or pathology text, as needed
- See Appendix G for Further Text Resources

Make Study Central your special place where you can get away from all other responsibilities. Make it a quiet, calm getaway, even if it is a corner of your bedroom. In this quiet place have a comfortable chair, adequate lighting, supplies, and sufficient desktop surface to use all your coding books. This is your place to focus all your attention on preparation for the examination, without distractions.

- Plan your **schedule** from now until the certification examination using a calendar. Make weekly goals so that you have definite tasks to accomplish each week and you can check the tasks off—a great feeling of accomplishment comes from being able to check off a task. In this way, you can see your progress on your countdown to success.

- Choose a specific **time** each day or several times a week when you are going to study and mark them on your calendar. Make this commitment in writing. After each study session, you should check off that date on the calendar as a visual reminder that you are sticking to your plan and are one step closer to your goal.

- You should plan your study time in advance, know what you are going to be studying the next session, and **be prepared** for that upcoming study session. This will greatly increase the amount of material you are able to cover during the session. At the end of each session, decide what you are going to study next session and ensure that you have all the material and references you will need readily available. At the end of each session, you should be ready for the next study session.

- Your plan should include those areas where you know you will need improvement. For example, when is the last time you read, not referenced or reviewed, but really read, the CPT Anesthesia Guidelines? You probably do not code anesthesia services often, if ever, and as such are not familiar with the information in these guidelines. That is an area of improvement, and your plan should include a thorough reading of all the CPT section guidelines.

- **DO THIS BEFORE YOU BEGIN YOUR STUDY: Assess** your strengths and weaknesses. By making this assessment, you will know where to concentrate your efforts and where to focus your study schedule. You know those areas where you already have strong skills and knowledge and will not need to spend as much time preparing in these areas. The **Pre-Examination,** found on the CD-ROM, is an examination that you can use as a tool to assess your current skill level. This examination should be taken before you begin your study and then again immediately after you have completed your entire study schedule. Do not analyze the questions by reviewing the rationales (located on the CD-ROM); rather, wait until after you have completed your studies and have taken this same examination a second time. If you review the rationales after the first time you take the examination, you will know the answers too

Success Strategies

well to provide a valid comparison between examinations. See Unit IV of this textbook for further information.

- After you have completed your course of study, take the **Post-Examination** on CD. You should plan to cover the examination in the same amount of time as will be given for the certification examination you are going to take. Compare your scores to those from the first time you took this examination. Note the areas where you did not demonstrate sufficient skills and knowledge.

- Develop a **second plan** to improve the specific areas where you believe you need further study.

- You are now ready to take the **Final Examination** that is located in Unit IV of this text. Take the examination in the same amount of time that will be allocated for the certification examination. It is best if you do this final in one sitting, thereby mimicking the actual examination. If your schedule does not allow for taking the examination in one sitting, plan to take it in several sessions, but always keep track of the time used to ensure that you take the examination in the same amount of time allowed for the official examination. Learning to work within the time allocated is part of the skill you are developing. Remember the certification examinations assess not only your coding knowledge but also your efficiency in completing the examination within the allocated time.

USING THIS TEXT

This text is divided into:

- Success Strategies
- Unit I, Anatomy, Terminology, and Pathophysiology
- Unit II, Reimbursement Issues
- Unit III, Overview of CPT, ICD-9-CM, and HCPCS Coding
- Unit IV, Coding Challenge
- Appendix A, ICD-9-CM Official Guidelines for Coding and Reporting
- Appendix B, Medical Terminology
- Appendix C, Combining Forms
- Appendix D, Prefixes
- Appendix E, Suffixes
- Appendix F, Abbreviations
- Appendix G, Further Text Resources

Appendices B-F are combined lists of Medical Terminology, Combining Forms, Prefixes, Suffixes, and Abbreviations used within Unit I, Anatomy, Terminology, and Pathophysiology.

The material in this review features the following:

- Comprehensive guide in outline format
- Photos and drawings to illustrate key points
- Pre-/Post-Examination (on CD-ROM)—150 questions

Success Strategies

- Final Examination (in Unit IV of this text)—150 questions
- **Unit I** is a review of the anatomy, terminology, and pathophysiology by organ systems designed to provide you with a quick review of that organ system. In addition, there is a list of combining forms, prefixes, suffixes, and abbreviations that are often used in that organ system. At the end of each organ system, there is a quiz that will give you an opportunity to assess your knowledge.
- **Unit II** is a review of reimbursement issues and terminology. A quiz is located at the end of the unit to assess your knowledge.
- **Unit III** is a review of CPT, HCPCS, and ICD-9-CM. The CPT and ICD-9-CM material follows the order of the manuals. There is no quiz at the end of this unit because you will be applying this material in the practice examinations and in the Final Examination.
- **Unit IV** contains the examinations. The Pre-/Post-Examination is a 150-question examination located on the **CD-ROM.** This same exam should be taken twice—once before you begin your study and the second time after you have completed your study. You should allow $5\frac{1}{2}$ hours (330 minutes) to complete each examination because this is the amount of time you will have for the CPC examination. The computer software stores your scores and compares the results from the first and second time you took the examination; so you can see not only your score on each section but also the improvement from the first to the second examination. The Final Examination is also a 150-question examination, but located in the text with answers on the CD-ROM. All examinations are divided into the following sections:

- **Section 1—43 questions**
  - Medical Terminology (13)
  - Anatomy (9)
  - ICD-9-CM (11)
  - HCPCS (5)
  - Practice Management (5)

- **Section 2—60 questions**
  - Integumentary System (10000 range) (9)
  - Musculoskeletal System (20000 range) (10)
  - Respiratory and Cardiovascular Systems (30000 range) (10)
  - Digestive System (40000 range) (10)
  - Urinary, Male Genital System, Female Genital System, and Maternity Care and Delivery (50000 range) (11)
  - Endocrine and Nervous Systems, and Eye/Ocular Adnexa (60000 range) (10)

- **Section 3—47 questions**
  - Evaluation and Management (99201-99499 range) (12)
  - Anesthesia (00100-01999, 99100-99140 range) (6)

- Radiology (70000 range) (9)
- Pathology and Laboratory (80000 range) (10)
- Medicine (90281-99199, 99500-99602 range) (10)

> NOTE: To enable the learner to calculate an examination score, minimums have been identified as "passing" within this text; however, this may or may not be the percentage identified by the American Academy of Professional Coders as a "passing" grade. It is your responsibility to review all certification information published by the American Academy of Professional Coders as they are the definitive source for information regarding the CPC certification examination.

A passing score for this test is as follows:

- **Section I 63% or 27 of the 43 questions correct**
- **Section II 72% or 44 of the 60 questions correct**
- **Section III 60% or 28 of the 47 questions correct**

There are many ways you could use this text. However you decide to prepare, you should take the examination before you begin your study to ensure that you develop a study plan that includes time and activities that will increase your knowledge in those areas where your test scores indicate areas of weakness. You could then take the units in the order they are presented, or you may want to review the anatomy, terminology, and pathophysiology for a body system and then review the CPT material for that body system. There is no one best way to approach the use of this text because each individual will have a personal learning style and preferences that will direct how the material is used. Your skills may be very strong in one or more coding or knowledge areas, and you will want to delete those areas from your individual study plan.

This text is not meant to be the only study source, but only one tool of many that you will use. For example, if your terminology skills need a complete overhaul, the brief overview in this text may not meet your needs. You may want to supplement this text with a terminology text and an in-depth study of terminology.

- **Appendices** are a resource for you as you prepare your study plan.
  - **Appendix A,** ICD-9-CM Official Guidelines for Coding and Reporting, is the rules for use of ICD-9-CM codes and will be referenced in Unit III when reviewing the use of ICD-9-CM codes.
  - **Appendix B,** Medical Terminology, is a complete alphabetic list of all the medical terms listed in the Medical Terminology portion of the organ system reviews used in Unit I.
  - **Appendix C,** Combining Forms, is a complete alphabetic list of the combining forms used in Unit I.
  - **Appendix D,** Prefixes, is a complete alphabetic list of the prefixes used in Unit I.
  - **Appendix E,** Suffixes, is a complete alphabetic list of the suffixes used in Unit I.
  - **Appendix F,** Abbreviations, is a complete list of the abbreviations referenced in Unit I.
  - **Appendix G,** Further Text Resources, is a list of texts that you may want to obtain to supplement your study plan.

DAY BEFORE THE EXAMINATION

- No cramming! Your study time is now over, and cramming the day before the test is not a good idea because it just increases your anxiety level. This day is your day to prepare yourself. Do some things you enjoy this day. Take your mind off the examination. Pamper yourself: you deserve it.

- Prepare pencils (no. 2), erasers, picture identification, CPT (AMA standard or professional version only), ICD-9-CM (Vols. 1 and 2), HCPCS code manuals, and examination admission card. For a paper/pencil examination, take a ruler so that if you skip a question and want to mark that question to return to later, you can use the ruler to make certain you return to the correct question.

- You cannot have excessive writing, sticky notes, labels, etc. in your code books. Check the AAPC examination information to ensure that your books meet the specifications identified by the testing organization.

- Review the certification packet information one last time to ensure that you have all the required material.

- Pack snacks and bottled water sufficient for $5\frac{1}{2}$ hours.

- Listen to the weather and traffic reports. Plan your route to the examination site. If it is in a new location, drive to the location before the big day.

- Eat a light supper and get to bed early. Set the alarm in plenty of time to arrive at the site early. It is a good idea to have a friend or family member give you an early wake-up call to ensure that you do not oversleep.

DAY OF THE EXAMINATION

- Wear comfortable clothes and be prepared for any room temperature. A short-sleeved shirt with a sweater is a good plan. Dress in layers so you can ensure that you will be comfortable in any environment.

- Take a watch with you.

- Eat a good breakfast. Avoid caffeine because it initially stimulates you, but in the long run will decrease your concentration.

- Arrive early. The doors are locked to those who arrive late. This is a day to be early.

- Ensure that you have the correct room for your examination. Often there are several examinations being administered at one time, so be certain you are in the correct room for your examination.

THE CERTIFICATION EXAMINATION

You are ready for this! You have planned your work and have worked your plan. Now it is time to reap the rewards for all that hard work.

- Choose a good location in which to sit. Choose a location that will not get a lot of traffic from those leaving the room.

- Place all your supplies on the table.

- Take several deep breaths before you begin to help relax you.

- Some prefer to take the parts of the examination out of order, taking those questions they are most confident of first. Others prefer to start at the beginning and work through all questions in order. The approach that you use will depend on your individual test-taking style.

Success Strategies

- When you come to a question for which you are unsure of the answer, you may wish to skip over and come back to all those ones you were unsure of at the end of the examination, depending on the time available. Or you may want to attempt each question and note those you are unsure of to return to when you have finished the exam section. Again, the approach you will use depends on your individual style.

- Read the directions. This may sound too simple, but many persons do not completely read the directions, only to find that the directions gave specific directions about what or what not to code on a certain case (for example, "code only this certain portion of the procedure"). Yet the choices for answers included the full coding of the case as a selection; if you did not read all the directions, you would choose the response with codes for all the items listed in the report. For example, the question may have directed you to code the service only, not the diagnosis, and yet one of the choices would be the correct service and diagnosis codes, which of course would be an incorrect answer based on the directions. So read all of the directions.

- Your speed and accuracy are being tested. You do not have time to labor over each question for a long time if you intend to complete all the questions. Read the directions, read the question, put down your best assessment of the answer, and then move on to the next question.

- Words such as *always, every, never,* and *all* generally indicate broad terms that, with true/false questions, usually indicate a false question.

- If you do not know the answer to the question, try eliminating those that you know are incorrect first and then select that answer that seems more likely to be correct.

- Judge the time as you are moving through the examination. Keep assessing whether you are making sufficient progress or whether you can slow down or need to speed up.

- Answer all questions. Even if you have to guess quickly, at least fill in an answer. The best situation is that you answer all questions and have time left over to go back over the questions about which you are in doubt.

- Be certain to carefully complete the information sheet that accompanies the examination. This sheet will include your name, address, and other information that ensures that your test results are accurately recorded.

- Use every minute of the test time, but it is not a good idea to begin second-guessing yourself. Do not return to those questions for which you did not have serious doubts about the correct answer. Usually, your first answer is the best.

- When the time is finished, hand in your examination, and pat yourself on the back! You have done an excellent job. Now it is time to go get a good supper and a good night's sleep.

DAYS AFTER THE EXAMINATION

- You will miss the preparation! Okay, maybe not miss it exactly, but your life will be different now without that constant preparation.

- Relax and await the results in confidence. You have done your best. That is always good enough!

- Be proud of yourself; this was no small undertaking, and you did it.

My personal best wishes to you as you prepare for your certification. You can do this!

Best regards
Carol J. Buck, MS, CPC-I, CPC, CPC-H, CCS-P

Our goals can only be reached through a vehicle of a plan, in which we must fervently believe, and upon which we must vigorously act. There is no other route to success.

Stephen A. Brennen

Course Syllabus and Student Calendar

The following documents are the syllabus and the course calendar that would be used in a classroom setting. It is suggested that these documents be used in development of your personal educational plan.

COURSE SYLLABUS

Course Description

The focus of this class is a review of terminology, anatomy, pathophysiology, and reimbursement as a preparation to take the coding certification examination. A review of CPT, ICD-9-CM, and HCPCS coding will be an integral part of this review course. Two practice certification review examinations will be taken under timed conditions. The course assists the learner in establishing a personal plan for continued development in preparation for a certification examination.

Texts

CPC Coding Exam Review 2009: The Certification Step, by Carol J. Buck, Elsevier

The Extra Step: Physician-Based Coding Practice, 2009 edition, by Carol J. Buck, Elsevier

2009 ICD-9-CM, Volumes 1 & 2, by Carol J. Buck, Elsevier

2009 HCPCS Level II, by Carol J. Buck, Elsevier

2009 CPT, American Medical Association

Medical dictionary

Performance Objectives

1. Write a personal plan for preparation for a certification examination.
2. Review the structure, function, terminology, pathophysiology, and abbreviations of the integumentary system.
3. Review the structure, function, terminology, pathophysiology, and abbreviations of the musculoskeletal system.

4. Review the structure, function, terminology, pathophysiology, and abbreviations of the respiratory system.

5. Review the structure, function, terminology, pathophysiology, and abbreviations of the cardiovascular system.

6. Review the structure, function, terminology, pathophysiology, and abbreviations of the female genital system and pregnancy.

7. Review the structure, function, terminology, pathophysiology, and abbreviations of the male genital system.

8. Review the structure, function, terminology, pathophysiology, and abbreviations of the urinary system.

9. Review the structure, function, terminology, pathophysiology, and abbreviations of the digestive system.

10. Review the structure, function, terminology, pathophysiology, and abbreviations of the mediastinum and diaphragm.

11. Review the structure, function, terminology, pathophysiology, and abbreviations of the hemic and lymphatic systems.

12. Review the structure, function, terminology, pathophysiology, and abbreviations of the endocrine system.

13. Review the structure, function, terminology, pathophysiology, and abbreviations of the nervous system.

14. Review the structure, function, terminology, pathophysiology, and abbreviations of the senses of the body.

15. Demonstrate knowledge of organ system structure, function, terminology, pathophysiology, and abbreviations.

16. Review medical reimbursement issues.

17. Demonstrate knowledge of medical reimbursement issues.

18. Review CPT E/M section.

19. Review CPT Anesthesia section.

20. Review CPT Surgery section.

21. Review CPT Radiology section.

22. Review CPT Pathology and Laboratory section.

23. Review CPT Medicine section.

24. Review HCPCS.

25. Review format and conventions of ICD-9-CM.

26. Review assignment of ICD-9-CM codes.

27. Review ICD-9-CM Official Guidelines for Coding and Reporting.

28. Demonstrate coding ability by assigning CPT codes.

29. Demonstrate coding ability by assigning HCPCS codes.

30. Demonstrate coding ability by assigning ICD-9-CM codes.

Personal Objectives

The student will:

- Attend class sessions.
- Prepare for class sessions.
- Complete assignments in a timely manner.
- Demonstrate a high level of responsibility.
- Display respect for other members of the class.
- Participate in class discussions.

Evaluation and Grading

- Evaluation is directly related to the performance objectives.
- Performance is measured by examination, assignments, and/or quizzes.
- The letter grade is based on the percentage of the total points earned throughout the semester based on the following scale:
  - A = 93% to 100%
  - B = 85% to 92%
  - C = 79% to 84%
  - D = 70% to 78%
  - F = 69% and below
- Examinations are scheduled in advance. To qualify for the total points on the examinations, the student must take the examination at the scheduled time. Five points will be deducted from each examination if the examination is not taken at the scheduled time. This rule reinforces the need for on-time performance. Any make-up examination must be completed within 3 days of the scheduled examination or no points will be awarded for the examination.
- Assignments are scheduled in advance. To qualify for the total points on the assignment, the student must submit the completed assignment at the scheduled time. Five points are deducted from each assignment if the assignment is not submitted at the scheduled time. This rule reinforces the need for on-time performance. Any late assignment must be completed within 3 days from the date the assignment was due or no points will be awarded for the assignment.
- Quizzes are scheduled in advance. Quizzes cannot be made up, and no points are awarded for missed quizzes.

Methods of Instruction

The instructional methods used include lecture, class discussion, and assignments.

COURSE CALENDAR

Lesson 1

Reading assignment(s): Success Strategies, pages S1-S10

Assignment(s): Complete the Pre-Examination located on the CD-ROM, and at Lesson 3 class period, hand in your summary sheet with your scores calculated on the three sections for 128.5 points. The Pre-Examination is NOT graded if each question has been attempted. 2 points will be deducted for each question not attempted.
Download certification examination information at http://www.aapc.com/
Print one page to hand in at **Lesson 2** to demonstrate successful access to certification information from web (10 points—nongraded)
The Extra Step: Physician-Based Coding Practice, 2009 edition, Integumentary, Cases 1-4 (8 points)

Lesson 2

Student hand in: One printed page to demonstrate successful access to certifying organization's information from web (10 points—nongraded)
The Extra Step: Physician-Based Coding Practice, 2009 edition, Integumentary, Cases 1-4 (8 points)

Reading assignment(s): Unit 1, pages 1-54 (through Musculoskeletal System)

Assignment(s): Develop a personal plan for preparation for Certification Review (20 points—graded) to be submitted at **Lesson 6** class period
Integumentary Anatomy/Terminology (12 points) and Pathophysiology Quizzes (12 points)
Musculoskeletal Anatomy/Terminology (12 points) and Pathophysiology Quizzes (12 points)
The Extra Step: Physician-Based Coding Practice, 2009 edition, Orthopedics, Cases 1-4 (8 points)

Lesson 3

Student hand in: Integumentary System Quizzes (24 points)
Musculoskeletal Quizzes (24 points)
Pre-Examination (128.5 points, nongraded if each question attempted, deduct 2 points for each question not attempted)
The Extra Step: Physician-Based Coding Practice, 2009 edition, Orthopedics, Cases 1-4 (8 points)

Reading assignment(s): Unit 1, pages 55-116 (through Female Genital System and Pregnancy)

Assignment(s): Respiratory Anatomy/Terminology (12 points) and Pathophysiology Quizzes (12 points)
Cardiovascular Anatomy/Terminology (12 points) and Pathophysiology Quizzes (12 points)

Female Genital System and Pregnancy Anatomy/
  Terminology (12 points) and Pathophysiology
  Quizzes (12 points)
The Extra Step: Physician-Based Coding Practice,
  2009 edition, Emergency Medicine, Cases 11-12
  (4 points)
  Cardiology, Cases 1-6 (12 points)
  Obstetrics and Gynecology, Cases 1-4 (8 points)
  Pediatrics, Neonatology, and Adolescent Medicine,
  Cases 1-4 (8 points)

Lesson 4

Student hand in: Respiratory Quizzes (24 points)
Cardiovascular Quizzes (24 points)
Female Genital System and Pregnancy Quizzes (24
  points)
The Extra Step: Physician-Based Coding Practice,
  2009 edition, Emergency Medicine, Cases 11-12
  (4 points)
  Cardiology, Cases 1-6 (12 points)
  Obstetrics and Gynecology, Cases 1-4 (8 points)
  Pediatrics, Neonatology, and Adolescent Medicine,
  Cases 1-4 (8 points)

Reading assignment(s): Unit 1, pages 117-186 (through Mediastinum and
Diaphragm)

Assignment(s): Male Genital System Anatomy/Terminology (12
  points) and Pathophysiology Quizzes (12 points)
Urinary System Anatomy/Terminology (12 points) and
  Pathophysiology Quizzes (12 points)
Digestive System Anatomy/Terminology (12 points)
  and Pathophysiology Quizzes (12 points)
Mediastinum and Diaphragm Quiz (12 points) (There
  is NO pathophysiology quiz for Mediastinum and
  Diaphragm.)
The Extra Step: Physician-Based Coding Practice, 2009
  edition, Urology, Cases 1-4 (8 points)
  Gastroenterology, Cases 1-4 (8 points)
  Nephrology, Cases 1-4 (8 points)
  Pediatrics, Neonatology, and Adolescent Medicine,
  Cases 5-6 (4 points)

Lesson 5

Student hand in: Male Genital System Quizzes (24 points)
Urinary System Quizzes (24 points)
Digestive System Quizzes (24 points)
Mediastinum and Diaphragm Quiz (12 points)
(There is no pathophysiology quiz for Mediastinum
  and Diaphragm.)
The Extra Step: Physician-Based Coding Practice, 2009
  edition, Urology, Cases 1-4 (8 points)
  Gastroenterology, Cases 1-4 (8 points)
  Nephrology, Cases 1-4 (8 points)

Course Syllabus and Student Calendar

	Pediatrics, Neonatology, and Adolescent Medicine, Cases 5-6 (4 points)
Reading assignment(s):	Unit 1, pages 187-214 (through Endocrine System)
Assignment(s):	Hemic and Lymphatic Anatomy/Terminology (12 points) and Pathophysiology Quizzes (12 points)
	Endocrine Anatomy/Terminology (12 points) and Pathophysiology Quizzes (12 points)
	Prepare to submit Personal Plan for Preparation for Certification Examination (20 points—graded)
	The Extra Step: Physician-Based Coding Practice, 2009 edition, Nephrology, Cases 5-8 (8 points)

Lesson 6

Student hand in:	Hemic and Lymphatic Quizzes (24 points)
	Endocrine Quizzes (24 points)
	Submit Personal Plan for Preparation for Certification Examination
	The Extra Step: Physician-Based Coding Practice, 2009 edition, Nephrology, Cases 5-8 (8 points)
Reading assignment(s):	Unit 1, pages 215-262 (through end of Unit 1)
Assignment(s):	Nervous System Anatomy/Terminology (12 points) and Pathophysiology Quizzes (12 points)
	Senses Anatomy/Terminology (12 points) and Pathophysiology Quizzes (12 points)
	Prepare for Unit 1, Anatomy, Terminology, and Pathophysiology, Test 1 (50 points, 25 questions, 15 minutes)
	The Extra Step: Physician-Based Coding Practice, 2009 edition, Neurology and Ophthalmology, Cases 1-4 (8 points)

Lesson 7

	UNIT 1: ANATOMY, TERMINOLOGY, AND PATHOPHYSIOLOGY, TEST 1 **Timed Test: 15 Minutes**
Student hand in:	Nervous System Quizzes (24 points)
	Senses Quizzes (24 points)
	The Extra Step: Physician-Based Coding Practice, 2009 edition, Neurology and Ophthalmology, Cases 1-4 (8 points)
Reading assignment(s):	Unit 2, pages 263-278 (through end of Unit 2)
Assignment(s):	None

Lesson 8

Student hand in:	Reimbursement Quiz (10 points)
Reading assignment(s):	Unit 3, pages 279-285 (up to E/M section)
Assignment(s):	Prepare for Reimbursement, Test 2 (20 points, 10 questions, 10 minutes)

Lesson 9

UNIT 2: REIMBURSEMENT, TEST 2
Timed Test: 10 Minutes

Student hand in: None

Reading assignment(s): Unit 3, pages 286-295 (up to Contributory Factors)
Read E/M Guidelines

Assignment(s): *The Extra Step: Physician-Based Coding Practice,* 2009 edition, Evaluation and Management, Cases 1-8 (16 points)
Emergency Medicine, Cases 1-6 (12 points)

Lesson 10

Student hand in: *The Extra Step: Physician-Based Coding Practice,* 2009 edition, Evaluation and Management, Cases 1-8 (16 points)
Emergency Medicine, Cases 1-6 (12 points)

Reading assignment(s): Unit 3, pages 295-302 (up to Anesthesia section)

Assignment(s): *The Extra Step: Physician-Based Coding Practice,* 2009 edition, Evaluation and Management, Cases 9-19 (22 points)
Emergency Medicine, Cases 7-10 (8 points)

Lesson 11

Student hand in: *The Extra Step: Physician-Based Coding Practice,* 2009 edition, Evaluation and Management, Cases 9-19 (22 points)
Emergency Medicine, Cases 7-10 (8 points)

Reading assignment(s): Unit 3, pages 302-304 (up to CPT/HCPCS Level I Modifiers)

Read Anesthesia Guidelines

Assignment(s): Prepare for E/M, Test 3 (25 points, 5 Guidelines questions [10 points] and 3 cases [15 points], 15 minutes)
The Extra Step: Physician-Based Coding Practice, 2009 edition, Anesthesiology, Cases 1-6 (12 points)

Lesson 12

E/M, TEST 3
Timed Test: 15 Minutes

Student hand in: *The Extra Step: Physician-Based Coding Practice,* 2009 edition, Anesthesiology, Cases 1-16 (12 points)

Reading assignment(s): Unit 3, pages 304-311 (up to Surgery section)

Assignment(s): Prepare for Anesthesia, Test 4 (20 points, 5 Guidelines questions [10 points], 2 cases [10 points], 15 minutes)
The Extra Step: Physician-Based Coding Practice, 2009 edition, Anesthesiology, Cases 7-11 (10 points)

Lesson 13

	ANESTHESIA, TEST 4 **Timed Test: 15 Minutes**
Student hand in:	*The Extra Step: Physician-Based Coding Practice,* 2009 edition, Anesthesiology, Cases 7-11 (10 points)
Reading assignment(s):	Unit 3, pages 311-313 (up to Integumentary System Subsection) Read Surgery Guidelines
Assignment(s):	None

Lesson 14

Student hand in:	None
Reading assignment(s):	Unit 3, pages 313-322 (up to Musculoskeletal System Subsection)
Assignment(s):	*The Extra Step: Physician-Based Coding Practice,* 2009 edition, Integumentary, Cases 5-9 (10 points)

Lesson 15

Student hand in:	*The Extra Step: Physician-Based Coding Practice,* 2009 edition, Integumentary, Cases 5-9 (10 points)
Reading assignment(s):	Unit 3, pages 322-327 (up to Respiratory System Subsection)
Assignment(s):	*The Extra Step: Physician-Based Coding Practice,* 2009 edition, Orthopedics, Cases 5-13 (18 points)

Lesson 16

Student hand in:	*The Extra Step: Physician-Based Coding Practice,* 2009 edition, Orthopedics, Cases 5-13 (18 points)
Reading assignment(s):	Unit 3, pages 327-331 (up to Cardiovascular [CV] System Subsection)
Assignment(s):	*The Extra Step: Physician-Based Coding Practice,* 2009 edition, Cardiology, Case 7 (Respiratory case) (2 points) Otorhinolaryngology, Cases 2, 8, 11-13 (10 points)

Lesson 17

Student hand in:	*The Extra Step: Physician-Based Coding Practice,* 2009 edition, Cardiology, Case 7 (Respiratory case) (2 points) Otorhinolaryngology, Cases 2, 8, 11-13 (10 points)
Reading assignment(s):	Unit 3, pages 331-336 (up to Venous Reconstruction—CV Repairs)
Assignment(s):	*The Extra Step: Physician-Based Coding Practice,* 2009 edition, Cardiology, Cases 8-10 (Cardiology cases) (6 points)

Lesson 18

Student hand in: *The Extra Step: Physician-Based Coding Practice,* 2009 edition, Cardiology, Cases 8-10 (Cardiology cases) (6 points)

Reading assignment(s): Unit 3, pages 336-342 (up to Hemic and Lymphatic System Subsection)

Assignment(s): None

Lesson 19

Student hand in: None

Reading assignment(s): Unit 3, pages 342-347 (up to Female Genital System Subsection)

Assignment(s): *The Extra Step: Physician-Based Coding Practice,* 2009 edition, Gastroenterology, Cases 5-6 (4 points) Urology, Cases 5-10 (12 points)

Lesson 20

Student hand in: *The Extra Step: Physician-Based Coding Practice,* 2009 edition, Gastroenterology, Cases 5-6 (4 points) Urology, Cases 5-10 (12 points)

Reading assignment(s): Unit 3, pages 347-357 (through Auditory System Subsection)

Assignment(s): *The Extra Step: Physician-Based Coding Practice,* 2009 edition, Obstetrics and Gynecology, Cases 5-11 (14 points)
General Surgery, Cases 1-11 (22 points)

Lesson 21

Student hand in: *The Extra Step: Physician-Based Coding Practice,* 2009 edition, Obstetrics and Gynecology, Cases 5-11 (14 points)
General Surgery, Cases 1-11 (22 points)

Reading assignment(s): None

Assignment(s): *The Extra Step: Physician-Based Coding Practice,* 2009 edition, Neurology and Ophthalmology, Cases 5-10 (12 points)
Otorhinolaryngology, Cases 1, 3-7, 9, and 10 (16 points)
Diagnostic Radiology, Cases 1-13 (26 points)

Lesson 22

Student hand in: *The Extra Step: Physician-Based Coding Practice,* 2009 edition, Neurology and Ophthalmology, Cases 5-10 (12 points)
Otorhinolaryngology, Cases 1, 3-7, 9, and 10 (16 points)
Diagnostic Radiology, Cases 1-13 (26 points)

Reading assignment(s):	Unit 3, pages 357-369 (through Nuclear Medicine Subsection)
Assignment(s):	Prepare for Surgery, Test 5 (30 points, 9 questions, 5 Guidelines questions [10 points], 4 cases [20 points], 20 minutes) *The Extra Step: Physician-Based Coding Practice,* 2009 edition, Interventional Radiology and Radiation Oncology, Cases 1-7 (14 points)

Lesson 23

SURGERY, TEST 5
Timed Test: 20 Minutes

Student hand in:	*The Extra Step: Physician-Based Coding Practice,* 2009 edition, Interventional Radiology and Radiation Oncology, Cases 1-7 (14 points)
Reading assignment(s):	Unit 3, pages 364-369 (up to Medicine Section)
Assignment(s):	Prepare for Radiology, Test 6 (22 points, 5 Guidelines questions, 1 non-Guidelines question [12 points], 2 cases [10 points], 15 minutes) *The Extra Step: Physician-Based Coding Practice,* 2009 edition, Interventional Radiology and Radiation Oncology, Cases 8-14 (14 points)

Lesson 24

RADIOLOGY, TEST 6
Timed Test: 15 Minutes

Student hand in:	*The Extra Step: Physician-Based Coding Practice,* 2009 edition, Interventional Radiology and Radiation Oncology, Cases 8-14 (14 points)
Reading assignment(s):	Unit 3, pages 369-375 (up to Ophthalmology)
Assignment(s):	Prepare for Pathology and Laboratory, Test 7 (47 points, 5 Guidelines questions, 1 non-Guidelines question [12 points], 7 cases [35 points], 20 minutes) *The Extra Step: Physician-Based Coding Practice,* 2009 edition, Pathology, Cases 1-10 (20 points)

Lesson 25

PATHOLOGY AND LABORATORY, TEST 7
Timed Test: 20 Minutes

Student hand in:	*The Extra Step: Physician-Based Coding Practice,* 2009 edition, Pathology, Cases 1-10 (20 points)
Reading assignment(s):	Unit 3, pages 375-380 (up to HCPCS Coding)
Assignment(s):	*The Extra Step: Physician-Based Coding Practice,* 2009 edition, Medicine, Cases 1-5 (10 points)

Lesson 26

Student hand in:	*The Extra Step: Physician-Based Coding Practice*, 2009 edition, Medicine, Cases 1-5 (10 points)
Reading assignment(s):	Unit 3, pages 380-388 (up to Using the ICD-9-CM)
Assignment(s):	Prepare for Medicine/HCPCS, Test 8 (36 points, 5 Guidelines questions, 3 non-Guidelines questions [16 points], 4 cases [20 points], 10 minutes) *The Extra Step: Physician-Based Coding Practice*, 2009 edition, Medicine, Cases 6-10 (10 points)

Lesson 27

MEDICINE/HCPCS, TEST 8
Timed Test: 10 Minutes

Student hand in:	*The Extra Step: Physician-Based Coding Practice*, 2009 edition, Medicine, Cases 6-10 (10 points)
Reading assignment(s):	Unit 3, pages 388-389 (up to Selection of Primary Diagnosis)
Assignment(s):	None

Lesson 28

Student hand in:	None
Reading assignment(s):	Unit 3, pages 389-400 (up to Chapter 8, Diseases of Respiratory System)
Assignment(s):	Post-Examination (to hand in results at Lesson 30 class period)

Lesson 29

Student hand in:	None
Reading assignment(s):	Unit 3, pages 400-408 (through end of Unit 3)
Assignment(s):	None

Lesson 30

Student hand in:	Post-Examination results (128.5 points, nongraded if each question attempted, deduct 2 points for each question not attempted; hand in printed copy of summary of your score)
Reading assignment(s):	None
Assignment(s):	Prepare for ICD-9-CM, Test 9 (25 points, 5 cases, 20 minutes) Bring ICD-9-CM, CPT, and HCPCS to class to begin Final Examination

Lesson 31

ICD-9-CM, TEST 9
Timed Test: 20 Minutes

Final Examination beginning

Student hand in: None
Reading assignment(s): None
Assignment(s): Complete Final Examination

Lesson 32

Final grade calculation
Course evaluation

UNIT I

Anatomy, Terminology, and Pathophysiology

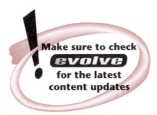

INTEGUMENTARY SYSTEM

INTEGUMENTARY SYSTEM—ANATOMY AND TERMINOLOGY

The skin and accessory organs (nails, hair, and glands)

Layers (Fig. 1–1)

Two layers make up skin: epidermis and dermis

Epidermis. Outermost layer; containing keratin

Stratum corneum, most superficial layer of four layers called stratum

Basal layer, deepest region of epidermis (stratum germinativum or stratum basale), is growth layer

Dermis. The second layer of skin

Two layers are papillare and reticulare and contain:
- Fibrous connective tissue or skin appendages
- Blood vessels
- Nerves
- Hair
- Nails
- Glands

Subcutaneous Tissue or Hypodermis. Not considered a layer of skin

Contains fat tissue and fibrous connective tissue

AKA: superficial fascia

Connects skin to underlying muscle

Nails

Keratin plates covering dorsal surface of each finger and toe

Lunula—semilunar or half-moon
- White area at base of nail plate is growth area
- Thickens and lengthens nail
- Eponychium or Cuticle: narrow band of epidermis at base and sides of nail

Paronychium: soft tissue around nail border

Glands

Sebaceous glands located in dermal layer

Secrete sebum that lubricates skin/hair

Influenced by sex hormones so they hypertrophy in adolescence and atrophy in old age

Sudoriferous glands originate in dermis. See Fig. 1–1.

AKA: sweat glands

Extend up through epidermis opening as pores

Secrete mostly water and salts to cool body

Integumentary System—Anatomy and Terminology

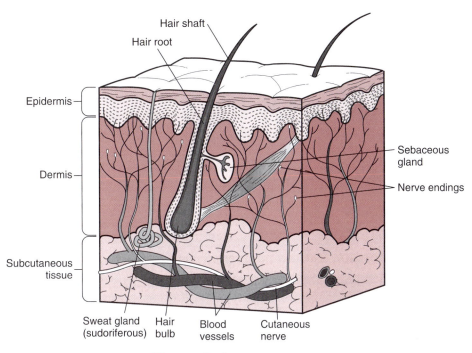

Figure **1-1** Integumentary system.

COMBINING FORMS

1.	aden/o	in relationship to a gland
2.	adip/o	fat
3.	albin/o	white
4.	aut/o	self
5.	bi/o	life
6.	caus/o	burning sensation
7.	cauter/o	burn
8.	crypt/o	hidden
9.	cutane/o	skin
10.	cyan/o	blue
11.	derm/o, dermat/o	skin
12.	diaphor/o	profuse sweating
13.	eosin/o	rosy
14.	erythem/o	red
15.	erythr/o	red
16.	heter/o	different
17.	hidr/o	sweat
18.	ichthy/o	dry/scaly
19.	jaund/o	yellow
20.	kerat/o	hard

UNIT I Anatomy, Terminology, and Pathophysiology

21.	leuk/o	white
22.	lip/o	fat
23.	lute/o	yellow
24.	melan/o	black
25.	myc/o	fungus
26.	necr/o	death
27.	onych/o	nail
28.	pachy/o	thick
29.	pht/o	plant
30.	pil/o	hair
31.	poli/o	gray matter
32.	py/o	pus
33.	rhytid/o	wrinkle
34.	rube/o	red
35.	seb/o	sebum/oil
36.	staphyl/o	clusters
37.	steat/o	fat
38.	strept/o	twisted chain
39.	steat/o	fat
40.	squam/o	flat/scalelike
41.	trich/o	hair
42.	ungu/o	nail
43.	xanth/o	yellow
44.	xer/o	dry

PREFIXES

1.	epi-	on/upon
2.	hyper-	over
3.	hypo-	under
4.	intra-	within
5.	para-	beside
6.	per-	through
7.	peri-	surrounding
8.	sub-	under

Integumentary System—Anatomy and Terminology

SUFFIXES

1. -coccus — spherical bacterium
2. -ectomy — removal
3. -ia — condition
4. -malacia — softening
5. -opsy — view of
6. -plasty — surgical repair
7. -rrhea — discharge
8. -tome — an instrument to cut
9. -tomy — to cut

MEDICAL ABBREVIATIONS

1. bx — biopsy
2. ca — cancer
3. derm — dermatology
4. I&D — incision and drainage
5. subcu, subq, SC, SQ — subcutaneous
6. PPD — tuberculin skin test

MEDICAL TERMS

Absence	Without
Adipose	Fatty
Albinism	Lack of color pigment
Allograft	Homograft, same species graft
Alopecia	Condition in which hair falls out
Anhidrosis	Deficiency of sweat
Autograft	From patient's own body
Avulsion	Ripping or tearing away of part either surgically or accidentally
Biopsy	Removal of a small piece of living tissue for diagnostic purposes
Causalgia	Burning pain
Collagen	Protein substance of skin
Debridement	Cleansing of or removal of dead tissue from a wound
Delayed flap	Pedicle of skin with blood supply that is separated from origin over time
Dermabrasion	Planing of skin by means of sander, brush, or sandpaper
Dermatologist	Physician who treats conditions of skin
Dermatoplasty	Surgical repair of skin
Electrocautery	Cauterization by means of heated instrument
Epidermolysis	Loosening of epidermis

UNIT I Anatomy, Terminology, and Pathophysiology

Epidermomycosis	Superficial fungal infection
Epithelium	Surface covering of internal and external organs of body
Erythema	Redness of skin
Escharotomy	Surgical incision into necrotic (dead) tissue
Fissure	Cleft or groove
Free full-thickness graft	Graft of epidermis and dermis that is completely removed from donor area
Furuncle	Nodule in skin caused by *Staphylococci* entering through hair follicle
Hematoma	A localized collection of blood, usually result of a break in a blood vessel
Hemograft	Allograft, same species graft
Ichthyosis	Skin disorder characterized by scaling
Incise	To cut into
Island pedicle flap	Contains a single artery and vein that remains attached to origin temporarily or permanently
Leukoderma	Depigmentation of skin
Leukoplakia	White patch on mucous membrane
Lipocyte	Fat cell
Lipoma	Fatty tumor
Melanin	Dark pigment of skin
Melanoma	Tumor of epidermis, malignant and black in color
Mohs' surgery or Mohs' micrographic surgery	Removal of skin cancer in layers by a surgeon who also acts as a pathologist during surgery
Muscle flap	Transfer of muscle from origin to recipient site
Neurovascular flap	Contains artery, vein, and nerve
Pedicle	Growth attached with a stem
Pilosebaceous	Pertains to hair follicles and sebaceous glands
Sebaceous gland	Secretes sebum
Seborrhea	Excess sebum secretion
Sebum	Oily substance
Split-thickness graft	All epidermis and some of dermis
Steatoma	Fat mass in sebaceous gland
Stratified	Layered
Stratum (strata)	Layer
Subungual	Beneath nail
Xanthoma	Tumor composed of cells containing lipid material, yellow in color
Xenograft	Different species graft
Xeroderma	Dry, discolored, scaly skin

INTEGUMENTARY SYSTEM ANATOMY AND TERMINOLOGY QUIZ

1. This is the outermost layer of skin:
   a. basal
   b. dermis
   c. epidermis
   d. subcutaneous

2. Which of the following is NOT a part of skin or accessory organs:
   a. sudoriferous glands
   b. sebaceous gland
   c. nail
   d. arterioles

3. This prefix means beside:
   a. para-
   b. intra-
   c. per-
   d. epi-

4. This combining form means hair:
   a. xanth/o
   b. trich/o
   c. ichthy/o
   d. kerat/o

5. Lunula is the:
   a. narrow band of epidermis at base of nail
   b. opening of pores
   c. outermost layer of epidermis
   d. white area at base of nail plate

6. Subcutaneous tissue is also known as:
   a. dermal
   b. adipose
   c. hypodermis
   d. stratum corneum

7. Which of the following combining forms does not refer to a color?
   a. cyan/o
   b. jaund/o
   c. eosin/o
   d. pachy/o

8. This medical term means surgical incision into dead tissue:
   a. onychomycosis
   b. escharotomy
   c. keratotomy
   d. curettage

UNIT I Anatomy, Terminology, and Pathophysiology

9. This suffix means surgical repair:
   a. -opsy
   b. -rrhea
   c. -plasty
   d. -tome

10. Soft tissue around nail border is the:
    a. cuticle
    b. lunula
    c. paronychium
    d. corium

INTEGUMENTARY SYSTEM—PATHOPHYSIOLOGY

Lesions and Other Abnormalities (Fig. 1-2)

Macule
Flat area of color change (mostly reddened)

No elevation or depression

> *Example:* flat moles, freckles

Papule
Solid elevation

Less than 1.0 cm in diameter

May run together and form plaques

> *Example:* warts, lichen planus, elevated mole

Nodule
Solid elevation 1-2 cm in diameter

Extends deeper into dermis than papule

> *Example:* lipoma, erythema nodosum, enlarged lymph nodes

Pustule
Elevated area

Filled with purulent fluid

> *Example:* pimple, impetigo, abscess

Tumor
Solid mass

Uncontrolled, progressive growth of cells

> *Example:* hemangioma, neoplasm, lipoma

Plaque
Flat, elevated surface

Equal or greater than 1.0 cm

> *Example:* psoriasis, seborrheic keratosis

Wheal
Temporary localized elevation of skin

Results in transient edema in dermis

> *Example:* insect bite, allergic reaction

Vesicle
Small blister

Less than 1 cm in diameter

Filled with serous fluid in epidermis

> *Example:* herpes zoster (shingles), varicella (chickenpox)

Bulla
Large blister

Greater than 1.0 cm in diameter

> *Example:* blister

UNIT I Anatomy, Terminology, and Pathophysiology

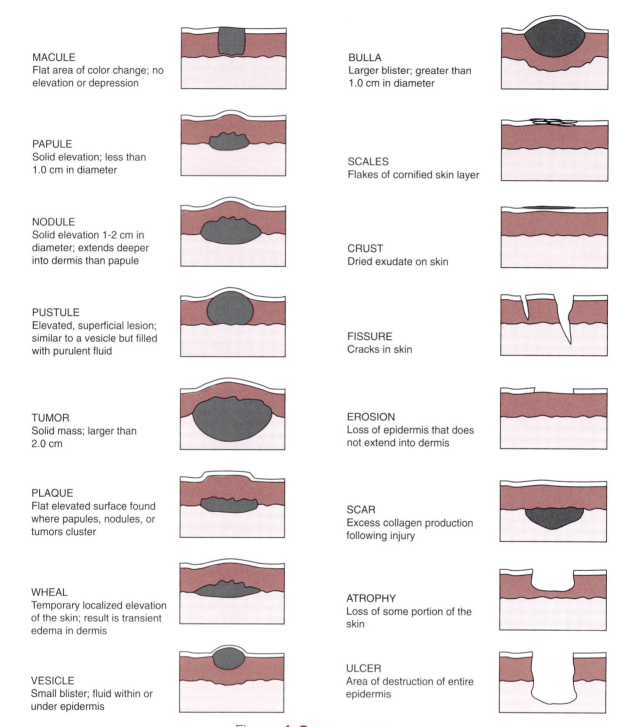

Figure 1-2 Lesions of skin.

Scales
Flakes of cornified skin layer

Example: dry skin

Crust
Dried exudate on skin

Example: scab

Fissure
Cracks in skin

Example: athlete's foot, openings in corners of mouth

Erosion
Loss of epidermis

Does not extend into dermis

Example: blisters

Scar
Excess collagen production following surgery or trauma

Example: healed surgical wound

Atrophy
Loss of some portion of skin and appears translucent

Example: aged skin

- Not a lesion, but a physiologic response in aging process

Ulcer
Area of destruction of entire epidermis

Example: missing tissue on heel, decubitus bedsore (pressure sore)

Pressure Ulcer (Decubitis Ulcer) (Fig. 1-3)
Result of pressure or force
Occludes blood flow, causing ischemia and tissue death

Develops over bony prominence

Locations
- Coccygeal (end of spine)
- Sacral (between hips)
- Heel
- Elbow
- Ischial (lower hip)
- Trochanteric (outer hip)

Staging or classification system
- Stage I: erythema (redness) of skin
- Stage II: partial loss of skin (epidermis or dermis)

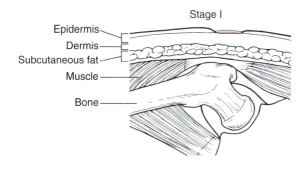
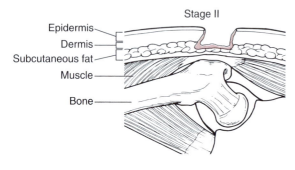

Figure 1-3 Stage I, II, III, and IV of pressure ulcers.

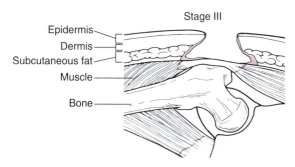
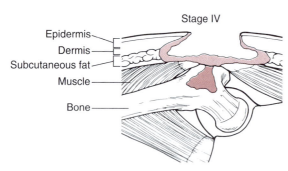

- Stage III: full thickness loss of skin (up to but not through fascia)
- Stage IV: full thickness loss (extensive destruction and necrosis)
  Deep ulcers may require surgical debridement

Keloids
Sharply elevated, irregularly shaped scars that progressively enlarge

Due to excessive collagen in corneum during connective tissue repair

Result of tissue repair or trauma

Familial tendency for formation

Cicatrix
Normal scar left after wound healing

Inflammatory Disorders

Atopic Dermatitis
Unknown etiology

Exogenous (external causes) include
    Irritant dermatitis

    Allergic contact dermatitis

Endogenous (internal cause) includes
    Seborrheic dermatitis

Results in activation of
- Mast cells
- Eosinophils
- T lymphocytes
- Monocytes

Greater in those with family history of
- Asthma
- Dry skin
- Eczema
- Allergic rhinitis

Common in
- Children
- Infants

Results in
- Chronic inflammation
- Scratching
- Erythema
- Thickened, leathery skin (lichenification)
- Secondary *Staphylococcus aureus* infection

Treatment
- Topical steroid
- Antibiotic for secondary infection
- Antihistamines

Allergic Contact Dermatitis
Most common in infants and children

Potential causes
- Hypersensitivity to allergens
  - Microorganisms
  - Drugs

- Foreign proteins
- Chemicals
- Latex
- Metals
- Plants

Manifestations
- Scaling
- Lichenification (leathery, thickened skin)
- Erythema
- Itching (pruritus)
- Vesicular lesions
- Edema

Diagnosis and treatment
- Check medical history
- Patch test
- Avoidance of irritant
- Skin lubrication and hydration
- Steroids
  - Topical
  - Systemic
- Topical tacrolimus (immunosuppressive agent)

Irritant Contact Dermatitis
Response to
- Chemical
- Exposure to irritant

Treatment
- Removal of irritant
- Topical agents

Stasis Dermatitis
Usually on the legs from venous stasis

Associated with
- Phlebitis
- Vascular trauma
- Varicosities

Progress
- Begins with erythema and pruritus
- Progresses to scaling, hyperpigmentation, petechia (small hemorrhagic areas)
- Lesion becomes ulcerated

Treatment
- Elevate legs
- Reduce standing
- No constricting clothes
- Eliminate external compression
- Antibiotics for acute lesions
- Silver nitrate or Burow's solution dressings for chronic lesions

Seborrheic Dermatitis
Common chronic inflammation of sebaceous glands—cause unknown

Periods of remission and exacerbation

Commonly occurs on
- Scalp (cradle cap in infants)
- Ear canals
- Eyelids
- Eyebrow
- Nose
- Axillae
- Chest
- Groin

Lesions are
- Scaly (dry or greasy)
- White or yellowish
- Mildly pruritic

Treatment of mild cases
- Soap/shampoo of
  - Coal tar
  - Sulfur
  - Salicylic acid

Treatment of more severe cases
- Corticosteroid

Papulosquamous Disorders
Conditions associated with
- Scales
- Papules
- Plaque
- Erythema

Three types
- Psoriasis
- Pityriasis
- Lichen planus

Psoriasis
Chronic, relapsing, proliferating skin disorder

Usually begins by age 20

Cause unknown, suggested to be
- Exacerbated by anxiety, appears to run in families
- Immunologic
- Biochemical alterations
- Triggering agent

Commonly occurs on
- Face
- Scalp
- Forearms and elbows
- Knees and legs

Results in
- Thickened dermis and epidermis
- Well-demarcated plaque
- Cell hyperproliferation/scaly
- Inflammation (pruritus)
- Lesions are deep red color

Treatment
- Only palliative (treatment of symptoms)

Mild cases
- Keratolytic agents
- Corticosteroids
- Emollients

Moderate cases
- Interleukin-2 inhibitors
- Psoralens and ultraviolet A (PUVA) light therapy
- Coal tar
- Cyclosporin
- Vitamin D analogs

Severe cases
- Topical agents
- Systemic corticosteroids

- Antimetabolic
- Hospitalization

Pityriasis Rosea
Unknown cause

Self-limiting inflammatory disorder

Occurs most often in young adults

Primary lesion
- Begins with herald patch 3 to 4 cm
- Salmon-pink colored
- Circular and well-defined lesions

Secondary lesions
- 14 to 21 days

Trunk and upper extremities
- Oval lesions
- Severe pruritus

Diagnosis
May be confused with
- Secondary syphilis
- Seborrheic dermatitis
- Psoriasis

Treatment
- Antipruritics
- Antihistamines
- Corticosteroids
- Ultraviolet light
- Sunlight

Lichen Planus
Occurs on skin and mucous membranes

Unknown cause (idiopathic)

Autoimmune inflammatory disorder

Onset ages 30 to 70

Lesions
- Begin as pink lesions that turn into violet-colored pruritic papules
- Results in hyperpigmentation
- 2- to 10-mm flat lesions with central depression
- Last 12 to 18 months
- Tend to reoccur

Treatment
- Antihistamines
- Corticosteroids
  Topical
  Systemic

Acne Vulgaris

Site of lesion is sebaceous (pilosebaceous) follicles

Primarily on face and upper trunk

Occurs in 85% of the population between the ages of 12 and 25

Exact cause: unknown

Causative factor: sebum accumulation/inflammation in pores of skin

Types
Noninflammatory acne
- Whiteheads
- Blackheads

Inflammatory acne
- Follicle walls rupture
- Sebum expels into dermis
- Inflammation begins
  - Pustules, cysts, and papules result

Cause
Unknown

Treatment
Topical
- Antibiotics
- Salicylic acid
- Benzoyl peroxide
- Tretinoin

Systemic
- Antibiotic
- Hormones
- Corticosteroids
- Isotretinoin

Diaper Dermatitis

Variety of disorders

Causes
Urine

Feces

Plastic diaper cover

Allergic reaction

Secondary *Candida albicans* infection

Treatment
    Clean, dry area

    Expose to air

    Topical antifungal medications

    Topical steroids

Pruritus (Itching)
Symptom of skin disorder/dermatitis

Can be localized or generalized and is a condition not an inflammation

Results from stimulation of nerves of skin reacting to an allergen or irritation from substances in blood or foreign bodies

Causes
Primary skin disorder

    Example: eczema or lice

Systemic disease

    Example: chronic renal failure

Opiates

Allergic reaction

Treatment is for underlying condition
    Antihistamines

    Minor tranquilizers

    Application of emollients (lotions)

    Topical steroids

Skin Infections

■ Bacterial
Impetigo
Most common in infants and children

    Usually on face and begins as small vesicles

    Caused primarily by *Staphylococcus*

- Sometimes by group A beta-hemolytic *Streptococcus*

It is a highly contagious pyoderma

Treatment in mild cases
    Topical antibiotics

    Topical antiseptics

Treatment in moderate cases
    Systemic antibiotics

    Local compresses

    Analgesics

Cellulitis
Caused primarily by *Staphylococcus*

Often secondary to an injury

Results in
 Erythema, usually of lower trunk and legs
 Fever
 Localized pain
 Lymphangitis

Treatment
 Systemic antibiotics
 Burow's soaks for pain relief

Furuncles (Boils)
Infected hair follicle

Usually caused by *Staphylococcus*

Developed boil drains pus and necrotic tissue

Squeezing spreads infection

Collection of furuncles that have merged is a carbuncle

Folliculitis
Infection of hair follicles

Results in
 Erythema
 Pustules

Causes
 Skin trauma, such as irritation or friction
 Poor hygiene
 Excessive skin moisture

Treatment
 Cleansing of area
 Topical antibiotics

Erysipelas
Infection of skin

Cause
 Group A beta-hemolytic *Streptococci*
 Common occurrence: face, ears, lower legs

Prior to outbreak, presents with
- Fever
- Malaise
- Chills

Lesions appear as
Bright red and hot

- Develops raised borders
- Itching
- Burning
- Tenderness

Acute Necrotizing Fasciitis
Flesh-eating disease
Virulent strain of gram-positive, group A beta-hemolytic *Streptococcus*

Mortality rate of over 40%

Causes
   Skin trauma

   Skin infection

Areas secrete tissue-destroying enzyme, proteases
Extreme inflammation and pain

Rapidly increasing

Dermal gangrene develops

Systemic toxicity may develop with
   Fever

   Disorientation

   Hypotension

   Tachycardia (fast heart rate)

May lead to organ failure

Treatment
   Antimicrobial therapy

   Fluid replacement

   Removal of areas of infection

■ Viral
Herpes Simplex (Cold Sores)
Causes
Herpes simplex virus type 1 (HSV-1)

- Most common type
- Results in fever blisters or cold sores on or near lips or canker sores of the mouth

Herpes simplex virus type 2 (HSV-2)

- Genital and oral type
- Prominent sexually transmitted disease

Primary infections may show no symptoms (asymptomatic)

Virus remains in nerve tissue to later reactivate

Reactivation may be triggered by
    Stress

    Common cold

    Exposure to sun

Presents with
    Burning or tingling

Develops painful vesicles that rupture
Causes spreading

May cause secondary infection of eye

- Episode lasts several weeks
- Treatment may include antiviral medication
  - No permanent cure exists

Herpes Zoster (Shingles)
Usually older adult

Caused by varicella-zoster virus (VZV)
Virus was dormant and then reactivates

Result of varicella or chickenpox, usually in childhood

Affects
    One cranial nerve or one dermatome (an area of skin supplied with afferent nerve fibers by a posterior spinal root)

Results in
    Pain

    Rash (unilateral)

    Paresthesia (abnormal touch sensation, such as burning)

Course
    Several weeks

    Pain may continue even after lesion disappears

Treatment
    Clears spontaneously

    Antiviral medications provide symptomatic relief

    Sedatives

    Analgesic

    Antipruritics

Warts (Verrucae)
Verruca vulgaris (common wart)

Caused by human papillomavirus (HPV)

- Numerous types of HPV

Spread by contact

Appear anywhere on body

Present with a grayish appearance

Integumentary System—Pathophysiology

Variety of shapes and sizes

Transmitted by touch

Plantar warts (verrucae) are located on pressure points of body (such as feet; *plantar* means the bottom surface of foot)

Painful when pressure is applied

Juvenile warts occur on feet and hands of children

Venereal warts occur on genitals/anus

Treatment
- Liquid nitrogen
- Topical keratolytics
- Laser
- Electrocautery
- Often persist even with treatment

Fungal (Mycoses)
Usually superficial dermatophytes (fungus)

Fungus lives off dead cells

Tinea
Superficial skin infections

Tinea capitis
- Infection of scalp
- Common in children
- Treatment with oral antifungal medication

Tinea corporis (ringworm)
- Infection of body
- Presents as a red ring
- Produces burning sensation and pruritus
- Treatment with topical antifungal medication

Tinea pedis (athlete's foot)
- Involves feet and toes
- Produces pain, inflammation, fissures, and foul odor
- Treatment with topical antifungal medication

Tinea unguium (onychomycosis)
- Nail infection
  - Usually toenails
- Nail turns white then brown, thickens and cracks
- Spreads to other nails

Candidiasis
Caused by *Candida albicans*

Normally on mucous membranes of gastrointestinal tract and vagina

Poor health and certain conditions predispose individuals to overarching infection by candidiasis

- Antibiotic therapy, which changes the balance of the normal flora in the body

Treatment is topical or oral antifungal medications

Tumors of Skin

■ Benign Tumors
Keratosis(es)
Seborrheic keratosis
    Proliferation of basal cells

    Dark colored lesion

    Found on trunk and face

Actinic keratosis
    Pigmented, scaly patch

    Often caused by exposure to sun

    Often in fair-skinned individuals

    Premalignant lesion

    May develop into squamous cell carcinoma

Treatment with cryosurgery (freezing area) or excision

Keratoacanthoma
    Occurs in hair follicles

    Usually in those over 60

    Often of face, neck, back of hands, and other locations exposed to the sun

    Resolve spontaneously or are excised

Moles (Nevi)
    Located on any body part

    Various shapes and sizes

    May become malignant

    - Especially if located in area of continual irritation

■ Malignant Tumors
Squamous Cell Carcinoma
Similar to basal cell carcinoma

Grows wherever squamous epithelium is located (mouth, pharynx, esophagus, lungs, bladder)

Most often appears in areas exposed to sun (actinic keratosis—precancerous)

Scaly appearance

Rarely metastatic (spreading)

Easily treated with good prognosis

    Surgical excision

Cryotherapy

Curettage

Electrodesiccation

Radiotherapy

Basal Cell Carcinoma

Common type of skin cancer

Developed in deeper skin layers (basal cells) than squamous cell carcinoma

Often occurs with sun exposure in fair-skinned individuals

Shiny appearance and slow growing

Easily treated with good prognosis

Malignant Melanoma

Originates in cells that produce pigment (melanocytes) or nevi

Increased incidence with
Sun exposure

Fair hair and skin/freckles

Genetic predisposition

Skin nevus (mole) often brown and evenly colored with irregular borders

Grow downward into tissues

- Metastasize quickly

Treatment is removal with extensive border excision

- Depending on extent, chemotherapy or radiation therapy may be used

Kaposi's Sarcoma

Rare form of vascular skin cancer

Associated with
Human immunodeficiency virus (HIV)

Acquired immunodeficiency syndrome (AIDS)

Herpes virus may be found in lesions

Cells originate from endothelium in small blood vessels

Painful lesions develop rapidly, appearing as purple papules; spreads quickly to lymph nodes and internal organs

Treatment

Radiation

Chemotherapy

INTEGUMENTARY SYSTEM PATHOPHYSIOLOGY QUIZ

1. A pimple is an example of a:
   a. papule
   b. vesicle
   c. pustule
   d. nodule

2. A Stage III pressure ulcer involves:
   a. erythema of skin
   b. partial loss of epidermis and dermis
   c. full thickness loss of skin up to but not through fascia
   d. full thickness loss of skin with extensive destruction and necrosis

3. This type of dermatitis may be exogenous or endogenous and is common in children and infants:
   a. atopic
   b. irritant contact
   c. stasis
   d. seborrheic

4. Psoriasis, pityriasis, and lichen planus are three types of this disorder:
   a. dermatitis
   b. inflammatory
   c. acne
   d. papulosquamous

5. This condition begins with a herald spot:
   a. psoriasis
   b. pityriasis
   c. lichen planus
   d. dermatitis

6. This skin infection is caused by group A beta-hemolytic *Streptococci*, and the lesions appear as firm red spots with itching, burning, and tenderness:
   a. furuncles
   b. folliculitis
   c. erysipelas
   d. fasciitis

7. This type of herpes produces cold sores:
   a. herpes zoster
   b. shingles
   c. VZV
   d. herpes simplex

8. This condition is caused by human papillomavirus:
   a. mycoses
   b. verrucae
   c. shingles
   d. folliculitis

UNIT I   Anatomy, Terminology, and Pathophysiology

9. This type of tumor occurs in hair follicles:
   a. keratoses
   b. nevi
   c. Kaposi's sarcoma
   d. keratoacanthoma

10. This type of superficial carcinoma is rarely metastatic:
    a. squamous cell
    b. basal cell
    c. melanoma
    d. Kaposi's sarcoma

MUSCULOSKELETAL SYSTEM
MUSCULOSKELETAL SYSTEM—ANATOMY AND TERMINOLOGY

Skeletal System

Comprises 206 bones, cartilage, and ligaments

Provides organ protection, movement, framework, stores calcium, hematopoiesis (formation of blood cells)

Classification of Bones

Long bones (tubular)
Length exceeds width of bone

Broad at ends, such as thigh, lower leg, upper arm, and lower arm

Short bones (cuboidal)
Cubelike bones, such as carpals (wrist) and tarsals (ankle)

Flat
Thin—flattened with curved surfaces

Cover body parts, such as skull, scapula, sternum, ribs

Irregular
Varied shapes, such as zygoma of face or vertebrae

Sesamoid
Rounded

Found near joint, such as patella (kneecap)

Patella is largest sesamoid bone in body.

Structure

Long Bones (Fig. 1–4)
Diaphysis: shaft

Epiphysis: both ends of long bones—bulbular shape with muscle attachments

- Articular cartilage covers epiphyses and serves as a cushion

Epiphyseal line or plate: growth plate that disappears when fully grown

Metaphysis: flared portion of bone near epiphyseal plate

Periosteum: dense, white outer covering (fibrous)

Cortical or compact bone: hard bone beneath periosteum mainly found in shaft

- Medullary cavity contains yellow marrow (fatty bone marrow)

Cancellous bones: spongy or trabecular

- Contains red bone marrow (blood cell development)

Endosteum is thin epithelial membrane lining medullary cavity of long bone

UNIT I Anatomy, Terminology, and Pathophysiology

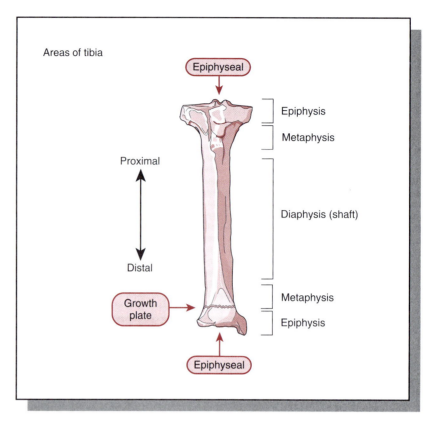

Figure **1-4** Structure of bones.

Two Skeletal Divisions
Axial (trunk)

Appendicular (appendages)

Axial Skeleton, comprised of 80 bones
Skull, hyoid bone, vertebral column, sacrum, ribs, and sternum

Skull (Fig. 1–5)
Cranial
Frontal (forehead)

Parietal (sides and top)

Temporal (lower sides)

Occipital (posterior of cranium)

Sphenoid (floor of cranium)

Ethmoid (area between orbits and nasal cavity)

Styloid process (below ear)

Zygomatic process (cheek)

Middle ear bones (Fig. 1–6)
Malleus (hammer)

Incus (anvil)

Stapes (stirrup)

Musculoskeletal System—Anatomy and Terminology

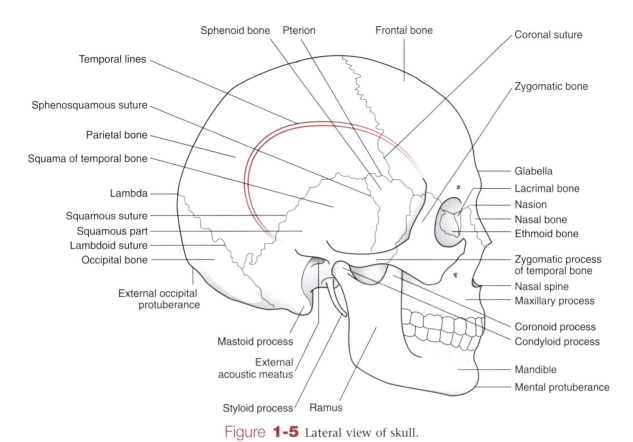

Figure **1-5** Lateral view of skull.

Figure **1-6** Structure of ear and three divisions of external, middle, and inner ear.

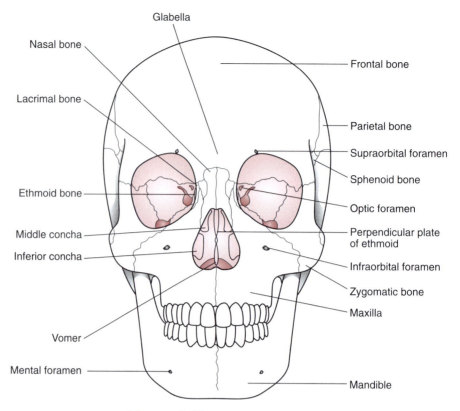

Figure **1-7** Frontal view of skull.

Face (Fig. 1–7)
Nasal (bridge of nose)
Maxilla (upper jaw)
Zygomatic (arch of cheekbone)
Mandible (lower jawbone)
Lacrimal (near orbits)
Palate (separates oral and nasal cavities)
Vomer (base, nasal septum)
Nasal conchae (turbinates)
    Interior
    Middle
    Superior

Hyoid
Supports tongue
U shaped
Attached by ligaments and muscles to larynx and skull

Spine (33 vertebrae) (Fig. 1–8)
Cervical vertebrae (7)
- C1-7
- (C1)-atlas
- (C2)-axis

Musculoskeletal System—Anatomy and Terminology

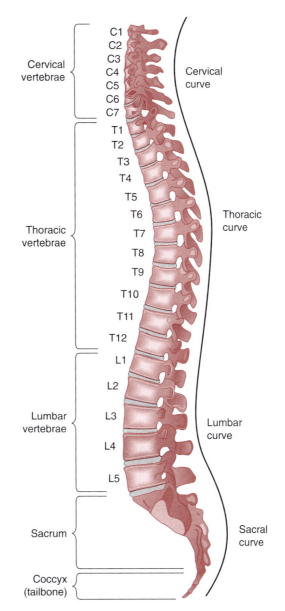

Figure 1-8 Anterior view of vertebral column.

Thoracic vertebrae (12) (T1-12)

Lumbar vertebrae (5) (L1-5)

Sacrum (5)—fused in adults

Coccyx (4)—fused in adults

Thorax (Fig. 1–9)
Ribs, 12 pairs

- True ribs, 1-7
- False ribs, 8-10
- Floating ribs, 11 and 12

Sternum

UNIT I Anatomy, Terminology, and Pathophysiology

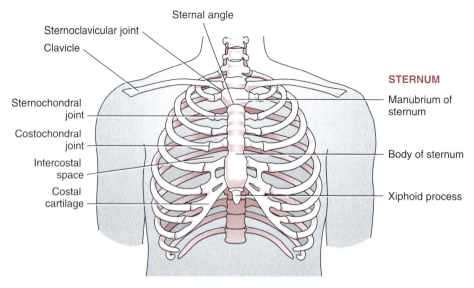

Figure **1-9** The thoracic cage.

Appendicular Skeleton, comprised of 126 bones (Fig. 1-10)
Shoulder, girdle, pelvic girdle, and extremities
Pelvis
Ilium (uppermost part) wing shaped

- Acetabulum, depression on lateral hip surface into which head of femur fits

Ischium (posterior part)

Pubis (anterior part)

Pubis symphysis (cartilage between pubic bones)

Lower extremities
Femur (thighbone)
Trochanter (processes at neck of femur)

Head fits into acetabulum

Patella (kneecap)

Tibia (shinbone)

Fibula (smaller lateral bone in lower leg)

Talus (ankle bone)

Calcaneus (heel bone)

Metatarsals (foot instep)

Phalanges (toes)

Lateral malleolus (lower part of fibula)

Medial malleolus (lower part of tibia)

Upper extremities
Clavicle (collarbone)

Scapula (shoulder blade)

Musculoskeletal System—Anatomy and Terminology

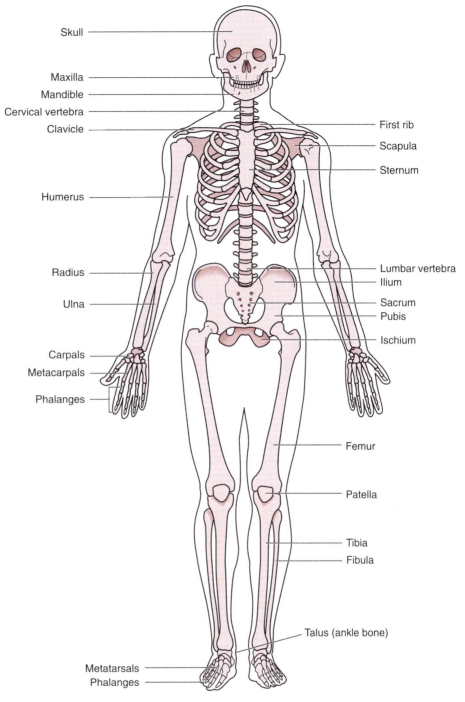

Figure **1-10** Skeletal system.

Humerus (upper arm)

Radius (forearm, thumb side)

Ulna (forearm, little finger side)

Olecranon (projection of ulna at elbow)

Carpals (wrist)—eight bones bound by ligaments in two rows with 4 bones in each

Metacarpals (hand)—framework or palm of hand (5 bones)

Phalanges (finger)

Olecranon (tip of elbow)

Joints (Articulations)
Condyle, rounded end of bone

Classified by degree of movement

- Synarthrosis (immovable and fibrous)

    Example: joint between cranial bones

- Amphiarthrosis (slightly movable and cartilaginous)

    Example: intervertebral (joint between bodies of vertebra)

- Diarthrosis (considerably movable and synovial)

Types

- Uniaxial—hinge and pivot joints

    Example—elbow (hinge and pivot) and cervical 2 (axis) (pivot)

- Biaxial—saddle and condyloid joints

    Example—thumb and joints between radius and carpal bones

- Multiaxial—ball and socket and gliding

    Example—shoulder and hip/joints between articular surfaces of vertebrae

Example: elbow, hip

- Bursa, sac of synovial fluid located in the tissues to prevent friction

Muscular System
Functions
Heat production

Movement

Posture

Protection

Shape

Muscle Tissue Types
Skeletal—600 muscles constituting 40% to 50% of body weight
Striated (cross stripes) (Figs. 1–11 and 1–12)

Move body

Voluntary

Attaches to bones

- Most attach to two bones with a joint in between

- Origin, point where muscle attaches to stationary bone

- Insertion, where muscle attaches to movable bone

- Body of muscle, main part of muscle

Musculoskeletal System—Anatomy and Terminology

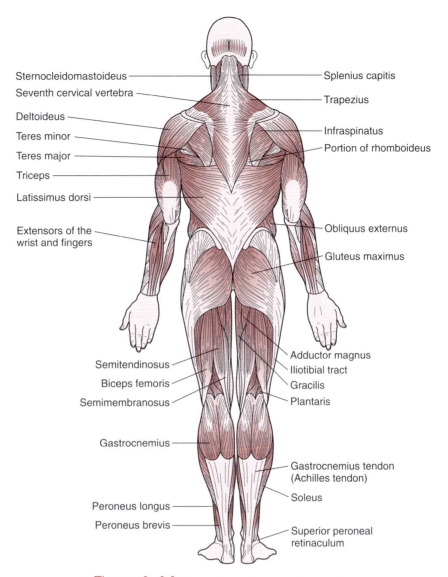

Figure **1-11** Muscular system, posterior view.

Cardiac/Heart Muscle
Striated and smooth muscle

Specialized cells which interlock so that muscle cells contract together

Involuntary

Moves blood by means of contractions

Smooth/Visceral
Linings such as bowel, urethra, blood vessels

Nonstriated

Involuntary

Tendons Anchor Muscle to Bone
Ligaments Anchor Bones to Bones

UNIT I Anatomy, Terminology, and Pathophysiology

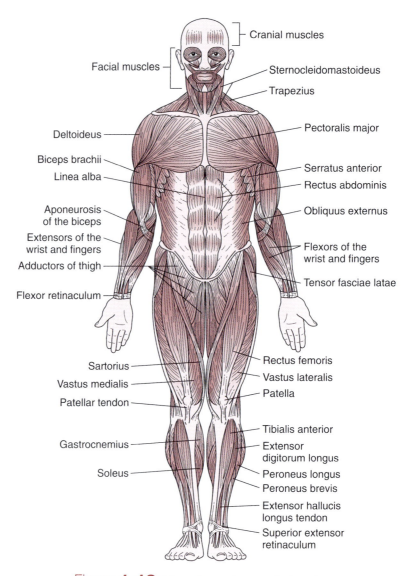

Figure **1-12** Muscular system, anterior view.

Muscle Action

Muscle Capabilities
Stretches

Contracts

Receives and responds to stimulus

Returns to original shape and length

Muscle Movement
Prime mover, responsible for movement (agonist)

Synergist, assists prime mover

Antagonist, relaxes as prime mover and synergists contract, resulting in movement

Fixator, acts as joint stabilizer

Musculoskeletal System—Anatomy and Terminology

Terms of Movement—from midline of body

Flexion (bend)

Extension (straighten)

Abduction (away)

Adduction (toward)

Rotation (turn on axis)

Circumduction (circular)

Supination (turning palm upward or forward [anteriorly] or lying down with face upward)

Pronation (turning palm downward or backward or act of lying face down)

Hyperextension (overextension)

Inversion (inward)

Eversion (outward)

Names of Muscles

Head and neck
Facial expression

- Occipitofrontalis (raises eyebrows and wrinkles forehead horizontally)
- Corrugator supercilii (wrinkles forehead vertically)
- Orbicularis oris (opens mouth)
- Zygomaticus (elevates corners of mouth)
- Orbicularis oculi (opens and closes eyelid)
- Buccinator (smiling and blowing)

Mastication (chewing)

- Masseter (used to chew closing jaw)
- Temporalis (closes jaw)
- Pterygoids (grates teeth)

Muscles moving head

- Sternocleidomastoid (flexes head)
- Semispinalis capitis (complexus) (extends head)
- Splenius capitis (extends head, bends and rotates head to side where muscle is contracting)
- Longissimus capitis (trachelomastoid muscle) (extends head, bends and rotates to contracting side)

Trapezius (extends head)

Upper extremities
Biceps brachii (flexes elbow)

Triceps brachii and anconeus (extends elbow)

Brachialis (flexes prone forearm)

Brachioradialis (flexes semi-prone/supinated forearm)

Deltoid (abducts upper arm)

Latissimus dorsi (extends upper arm)

Pectoralis major (flexes upper arm)

Trapezius (raises/lowers shoulder)

Trunk
External oblique (compresses abdomen)

Internal oblique (compresses abdomen)

Transversus abdominis (compresses abdomen)

Rectus abdominis (flexes trunk)

Quadratus lumborum (flexes vertebral column laterally)

Respiratory
Diaphragm (enlarges thorax/inspiration)

External intercostals (raise ribs)

Internal intercostal (depress ribs)

Lower extremities
Thigh

- Gluteus group, maximus, medius, minimus (abducts thigh)
- Tensor fasciae latae (abducts thigh)
- Abductor group, brevis, longus, magnus (adducts thigh)
- Gracilis (adducts thigh)
- Iliopsoas (flexes thigh)
- Rectus femoris (flexes thigh)

Hamstring group, biceps femoris, semitendinosus, semimembranosus (extends thigh)

Quadriceps group, rectus femoris, vastus lateralis, vastus medialis, vastus intermedius (extends lower leg)

Sartorius (flexes, abducts, and rotates leg)

Lower leg

Tibialis anterior (dorsiflexes foot)

Peroneus group, longus, brevis, tertius (everts foot)

Gastrocnemius (calf, with soleus extends foot, also flexes knee)

Soleus (calf, extends foot)

Extensor digitorum longus (extends toes, flexes foot)

Achilles tendon (largest tendon, extending from gastrocnemius to calcaneus)

COMBINING FORMS

1.	acetabul/o	hip socket
2.	ankyl/o	bent, fused

Musculoskeletal System—Anatomy and Terminology

3. aponeur/o — tendon type
4. arthr/o — joint
5. articul/o — joint
6. burs/o — fluid-filled sac in a joint
7. calc/o, calci/o — calcium
8. calcane/o — calcaneus (heel)
9. carp/o — carpals (wrist bones)
10. chondr/o — cartilage
11. clavic/o, clavicul/o — clavicle (collar bone)
12. cost/o — rib
13. crani/o — cranium (skull)
14. disk/o — intervertebral disk
15. femor/o — thighbone
16. fibul/o — fibula
17. humer/o — humerus (upper arm bone)
18. ili/o — ilium (upper pelvic bone)
19. ischi/o — ischium (posterior pelvic bone)
20. kinesi/o — movement
21. kyph/o — hump
22. lamin/o — lamina
23. lord/o — curve
24. lumb/o — lower back
25. malleol/o — malleolus (process on lateral ankle)
26. mandibul/o — mandible (lower jawbone)
27. maxill/o — maxilla (upper jawbone)
28. menisc/o — meniscus
29. menisci/o — meniscus
30. metacarp/o — metacarpals (hand)
31. metatars/o — metatarsals (foot)
32. myel/o — bone marrow
33. my/o, muscul/o — muscle
34. olecran/o — olecranon (elbow)
35. orth/o — straight
36. oste/o — bone
37. patell/o — patella (kneecap)
38. pelv/i — pelvis (hip)
39. perone/o — fibula

40.	petr/o	stone
41.	phalang/o	phalanges (finger or toe)
42.	plant/o	sole of foot
43.	pub/o	pubis
44.	rachi/o	spine
45.	radi/o	radius (lower arm)
46.	rhabdomy/o	skeletal (striated muscle)
47.	rheumat/o	watery flow (collection of fluids in joints)
48.	sacr/o	sacrum
49.	scapul/o	scapula (shoulder)
50.	scoli/o	bent
51.	spondyl/o	vertebra
52.	stern/o	sternum (breast bone)
53.	synovi/o	synovial joint membrane
54.	tars/o	tarsal (ankle/foot)
55.	ten/o	tendon
56.	tend/o	tendon (connective tissue)
57.	tendin/o	tendon (connective tissue)
58.	tibi/o	shin bone
59.	uln/o	ulna (lower arm bone)
60.	vertebr/o	vertebra

PREFIXES

1.	inter-	between
2.	supra-	above
3.	sym-	together
4.	syn-	together

SUFFIXES

1.	-asthenia	weakness
2.	-blast	embryonic
3.	-clast, -clasia, -clasis	break
4.	-desis	bind together
5.	-listhesia	slipping
6.	-malacia	softening
7.	-physis	to grow
8.	-porosis	passage, cavity formation
9.	-schisis	split
10.	-stenosis	narrowing

11. -tome   instrument that cuts
12. -tomy   incision

MEDICAL ABBREVIATIONS

1. ACL — anterior cruciate ligament
2. AKA — above-knee amputation
3. BKA — below-knee amputation
4. C1-C7 — cervical vertebrae
5. CTS — carpal tunnel syndrome
6. fx — fracture
7. L1-L5 — lumbar vertebrae
8. OA — osteoarthritis
9. RA — rheumatoid arthritis
10. T1-T12 — thoracic vertebrae
11. TMJ — temporomandibular joint

MEDICAL TERMS

Arthrocentesis	Injection and/or aspiration of joint
Arthrodesis	Surgical immobilization of a joint
Arthrography	Radiography of joint
Arthroplasty	Reshaping or reconstruction of a joint
Arthroscopy	Use of scope to view inside joint
Arthrotomy	Incision into a joint
Articular	Pertains to a joint
Aspiration	Use of a needle and a syringe to withdraw fluid
Atrophy	Wasting away
Bunion	Hallux valgus, abnormal increase in size of metatarsal head that results in displacement of great toe
Bursitis	Inflammation of bursa (joint sac)
Chondral	Referring to the cartilage
Carpal tunnel syndrome	Compression of medial nerve
Closed fracture repair	Not surgically opened with/without manipulation and with/without traction
Closed treatment	Fracture site that is not surgically opened and visualized
Colles' fracture	Fracture at lower end of radius that displaces bone posteriorly
Dislocation	Placement in a location other than original location
Endoscopy	Inspection of body organs or cavities using a lighted scope that may be inserted through an existing opening or through a small incision

Fasciectomy	Removal of band of fibrous tissue
Fissure	Groove
Fracture	Break in a bone
Ganglion	Knot or knotlike mass
Internal/External fixation	Application of pins, wires, screws, placed externally or internally to immobilize a body part
Kyphosis	Humpback
Lamina	Flat plate
Ligament	Fibrous band of tissue that connects cartilage or bone
Lordosis	Anterior curve of spine
Lumbodynia	Pain in lumbar area
Lysis	Releasing
Manipulation or reduction	Alignment of a fracture or joint dislocation to normal position
Open fracture repair	Surgical opening (incision) over or remote opening as access to a fracture site
Osteoarthritis	Degenerative condition of articular cartilage
Osteoclast	Absorbs or removes bone
Osteotomy	Cutting into bone
Percutaneous	Through skin
Percutaneous fracture repair	Repair of a fracture by means of pins and wires inserted through the fracture site
Percutaneous skeletal fixation	Considered neither open nor closed; fracture is not visualized, but fixation is placed across fracture site under x-ray imaging
Reduction	Replacement to normal position
Scoliosis	Lateral curve of spine
Skeletal traction	Application of pressure to bone by means of pins and/or wires inserted into bone
Skin traction	Application of pressure to bone by means of tape applied to the skin
Spondylitis	Inflammation of vertebrae
Subluxation	Partial dislocation
Supination	Supine position—lying on back, face upward
Synchondrosis	Union between two bones (connected by cartilage)
Tendon	Attaches a muscle to a bone
Tenodesis	Suturing of a tendon to a bone
Tenorrhaphy	Suture repair of tendon
Traction	Application of pressure to maintain normal alignment
Trocar needle	Needle with a cannula that can be removed; used to puncture and withdraw fluid from a cavity

MUSCULOSKELETAL SYSTEM ANATOMY AND TERMINOLOGY QUIZ

1. Tubular is another name for these bones:
   a. short
   b. long
   c. flat
   d. irregular

2. These bones are found near joints:
   a. irregular
   b. flat
   c. sesamoid
   d. broad

3. Zygoma is an example of this type of bone:
   a. irregular
   b. flat
   c. sesamoid
   d. broad

4. Diaphysis is this part of bone:
   a. end
   b. surface
   c. shaft
   d. marrow

5. Which is NOT a part of cranium?
   a. condyle
   b. sphenoid
   c. ethmoid
   d. parietal

6. This is NOT an ear bone:
   a. malleus
   b. stapes
   c. incus
   d. styloid

7. This term describes growth plate:
   a. endosteum
   b. epiphyseal
   c. metaphysis
   d. periosteum

8. This is a depression on lateral hip surface into which head of femur fits:
   a. ilium
   b. ischium
   c. patella
   d. acetabulum

UNIT I Anatomy, Terminology, and Pathophysiology

9. Tip of elbow is the:
   a. olecranon
   b. trapezium
   c. humerus
   d. tarsal

10. This term describes an immovable joint:
    a. amphiarthrosis
    b. diarthrosis
    c. synarthrosis
    d. ischium

MUSCULOSKELETAL SYSTEM—PATHOPHYSIOLOGY

Injuries

■ Fractures

Classification of fractures

Open/closed
Open (compound): broken bone penetrates skin

Closed (simple): broken bone does not penetrate skin

Complete/incomplete
Complete: bone is broken all way through

Example: oblique, linear, spiral, and transverse

Incomplete: bone is not broken all way through

Example: greenstick, bowing, torus, stress, and transchondral

Treatment
Closed reduction (realignment of bone fragments by manipulation)

Reduction (the returning of the bone to normal alignment)

Immobilization (returns to normal alignment and holds in place)

Traction (application of pulling force to hold bone in alignment)

- Skeletal traction uses internal devices (pins, screws, wires, etc.) inserted into bone with ends sticking out through skin for attachment of traction device (Fig. 1-13)

- Skin traction is use of strapping, elastic wrap, or tape attached to skin to which weights are attached (Fig. 1-14)

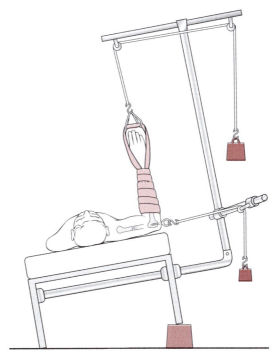

Figure **1-13** Skeletal traction uses patient's bones to secure internal devices to which traction is attached.

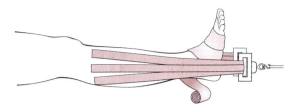

Figure **1-14** Skin traction utilizes strapping, wraps, or tape to which traction is attached.

Improper union
    Nonunion: failure of bone ends to grow together

    Malunion: incorrect alignment of bone ends

    Delayed union: delay of bone union 8 or 9 months

Dislocations
    Bone and soft tissue damage usually caused by trauma

    Any part of bone is displaced

    Can result in nerve and tissue damage

Treatment
    Reduction

    Immobilization

Sprains and strains
    Soft tissue damage usually caused by trauma to tendons and ligaments

Strain: partial tear of a tendon

Sprain results from overuse or overextension/tearing or rupture of some part of musculature

Bone Disorders

Osteomyelitis
Bone infection

Usually caused by bacteria

- Exogenous osteomyelitis is caused by bacteria that enter from outside body

- Hematogenous osteomyelitis (endogenous) is caused from a bacterial infection within body

Osteoporosis
Common disorder in postmenopausal women and elderly and most common metabolic disease

- Malabsorption of calcium and magnesium; certain trace elements and vitamins C and D contribute to bone loss

Decreased bone mass and density

- Fractures more common due to decrease in strength of bone

Treatment

Increased intake of calcium, magnesium, and vitamin D

Increased weight-bearing activity

Osteomalacia and Rickets
Osteomalacia is softened adult bones, while rickets is softened growing bones in children

Caused by vitamin D and phosphate deficiency

Osteitis Deformans (Paget's Disease)
Abnormal bone remodeling and resorption resulting in enlarged, soft bones

Unknown cause but strong genetic considerations

Treatment
  Calcitonin and biophosphates

Spinal Curvatures
Lordosis: swayback

- Inward curvature of spine

Kyphosis: humpback

- Outward curvature of spine

Scoliosis

- Lateral curvature of spine

Spina Bifida
Congenital abnormality in which vertebrae do not close correctly around the spinal cord

Joint Disorders

Bursitis: inflammation of bursa (joint sac)

Arthritis: inflammation of joints

Osteoarthritis (OA)
This is degenerative or wear/tear arthritis

- DJD, degenerative joint disease

Chronic inflammation of joint

Increased pain on weightbearing or movement

Affects weight-bearing joints

- Loss of articular cartilage
- Sclerosis of bone—eburnation

  Turning bone into ivorylike mass—polished

- Osteophytes (bone spurs)

Symptoms
  Pain and stiffness

   Crepitation (bone on bone creates characteristic grinding sound)

Classifications
: Primary (idiopathic)
- No known cause

Secondary
- Associated with joint instability, joint stress, or congenital abnormalities

Treatment
: Symptomatic
Arthroplasty

Rheumatoid Arthritis (RA)

Inflammatory connective tissue in joints disease that is progressive

Systemic autoimmune disease

- Can invade arteries, lung, skin, and other organs with nodules

Affects small joints

- Destroys synovial membrane, articular cartilage, and surrounding tissues

Leads to loss of function due to fixation and deformity

Treatment
: Pharmaceuticals to modify autoimmune and inflammatory processes
Gene therapy and stem cell transplantation are being researched
Symptomatic
Arthroplasty

Infectious and Septic Arthritis

Infectious process

Usually affects single joint

Without antimicrobial intervention, permanent joint damage results

Example: Lyme disease

Treatment
: Antibiotics—early intervention

Gout (Gouty Arthritis)

Inflammatory arthritis

Often affects the joint of the great toe

Caused by excessive amounts of uric acid that crystallizes in connective tissue of joints

Leads to inflammation and destruction of joint

Treatment
: Pharmaceuticals—nonsteroidal antiinflammatory drugs

Ankylosing Spondylitis (AS)

Inflammatory disease that is progressive

Affects vertebral joints and insertion points of ligaments, tendons, and joint capsules

Leads to rigid spinal column and sacroiliac joints

Treatment
    Nonsteroidal anti-inflammatory drugs relieve symptoms

    Analgesics for pain

Tendon, Muscle, and Ligament Disorders

Muscular Dystrophy—Familial Disorder
Progressive degenerative muscle disorder

Multiple types of muscular dystrophy

Most often affects boys

- Genetic predisposition—Duchenne MD

Primary Fibromyalgia Syndrome
Symptoms
    Generalized aching and pain

    Tender points

    Fatigue

    Depression

Usually appears in
    Middle-aged women

Polymyositis
General muscle inflammation causing weakness

- With skin rash = dermatomyositis

Tumors

Bone Tumors
Origin of bone tumors
    Osteogenic (bone cells)

    Chondrogenic (cartilage cell)

    Collagenic (fibrous tissue cell)

    Myelogenic (marrow cell)

Osteoma
    Benign

    Abnormal outgrowth of bone

Chondroblastoma
    Rare

    Usually benign

Osteosarcoma
    Malignant tumor of long bones

    Usually in young adults

    Typically causes bone pain

Multiple myeloma
Malignant plasma cells in skeletal system and soft tissue

Progressive and generally fatal

Usually in those over 40

Chondrosarcoma
Malignant cartilage tumor

Usually in middle-aged and older individuals

In late stages, symptoms include local swelling and pain

- Worsens with time

Surgical excision is usually treatment of choice

If diagnosed in early stages, it is treatable with long-term survival possible

Muscle Tumors
Rare

Rhabdomyosarcoma

Aggressive, invasive carcinoma with widespread metastasis

MUSCULOSKELETAL SYSTEM PATHOPHYSIOLOGY QUIZ

1. A compound fracture is also known as:
   a. complete
   b. incomplete
   c. closed
   d. open

2. This is a common bone disorder in postmenopausal women resulting from lower levels of calcium and potassium:
   a. Paget's disease
   b. lordosis
   c. osteoporosis
   d. rheumatoid arthritis

3. This inflammatory disease is progressive and leads to a rigid spinal column:
   a. polymyositis
   b. ankylosing spondylitis
   c. primary fibromyalgia syndrome
   d. septic arthritis of spine

4. This type of tumor arises from bone cells:
   a. osteogenic
   b. chondrogenic
   c. collagenic
   d. myelogenic

5. This type of tumor is the most common type of malignant bone tumor that occurs in those over 40 and is progressive and generally fatal:
   a. rhabdomyosarcoma
   b. chondrosarcoma
   c. osteosarcoma
   d. multiple myeloma

6. A general muscle inflammation with an accompanying skin rash is:
   a. muscular dystrophy
   b. dermatologic arthritis
   c. ankylosing spondylitis
   d. dermatomyositis

7. A cartilage tumor that usually occurs in middle-aged and older individuals:
   a. chondrosarcoma
   b. osteosarcoma
   c. chondroblastoma
   d. rhabdomyosarcoma

8. Returning of bone to normal alignment is:
   a. immobilization
   b. traction
   c. reduction
   d. manipulation

9. Result of overuse or overextension of a ligament is:
   a. strain
   b. sprain
   c. fracture
   d. displacement

10. Primary osteoarthritis is also known as:
    a. secondary
    b. functional
    c. congenital
    d. idiopathic

RESPIRATORY SYSTEM
RESPIRATORY SYSTEM—ANATOMY AND TERMINOLOGY

Supplies oxygen to body and helps clean body of waste (carbon dioxide)

Two tracts (Fig. 1–15A)

- Upper respiratory tract (nose, naso/oro/larngo, pharynx, and larynx)
- Lower respiratory tract (trachea, bronchial tree, and lungs)

Lined with ciliated mucosa

- Purifies air by trapping irritants

Warms and humidifies air

Upper Respiratory Tract (URT)

Nose
Sense of smell (olfactory)

Moistens and warms air

Nasal septum divides interior

Sinuses (Paranasal or Accessory Sinuses) (4 pair)
Frontal

Ethmoid

Maxillary

Sphenoid

Turbinates (Conchae)
Bones on inside of nose

Divided into inferior, middle, and superior (Fig. 1–15B)

Warms and humidifies air

Pharynx (Throat)
Passageway for both food and air

Nasopharynx contains adenoids

Oropharynx contains tonsils

Laryngopharynx leads to larynx

Larynx (Voice Box) (opening to trachea)
Contains vocal cords

- Cartilages of larynx, thyroid, epiglottis, and arytenoid

Lower Respiratory Tract (LRT)

Trachea (Windpipe)—Air-Conducting Structure
Mucus-lined tube with C-shaped cartilage rings to hold windpipe open

Segmental Bronchi
Trachea divides into right and left main bronchus which further divide into lobar bronchii—3 on right, 2 on left

UNIT I   Anatomy, Terminology, and Pathophysiology

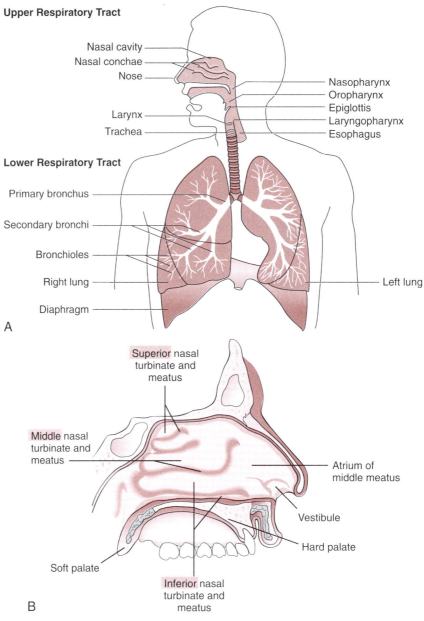

Figure **1-15** **A,** Upper and lower respiratory system. **B,** Superior, inferior, and middle nasal turbinates.

Bronchioles
Branches divide into secondary bronchi, then smaller bronchioles

Alveolar Ducts (minute branches of bronchial tree)
End in alveoli (sacs) of simple squamous cells

- Primary gas-exchange units

    Surrounded by capillaries and where exchange of oxygen and carbon dioxide takes place

Respiratory System—Anatomy and Terminology

Lungs
Covered by pleura

Cone-shaped organs filling thoracic cavity

Base rests on diaphragm and apex (top of lungs) extends to above clavicles

Hilum is medial surface of lung where pulmonary artery, pulmonary veins, nerves, lymphatics, and bronchial tubes enter and exit

Left lung contains two lobes divided by fissures

Right lung contains three lobes

Respiration
Inspiration—oxygen moves in, downward movement of lungs enlarging thoracic cavity

Expiration—carbon dioxide moves out, upward movement of diaphragm decreasing lung space

COMBINING FORMS

1. adenoid/o — adenoid
2. alveol/o — alveolus
3. atel/o — incomplete
4. bronch/o — bronchus
5. bronchi/o — bronchus
6. bronchiol/o — bronchiole
7. capn/o — carbon dioxide
8. coni/o — dust
9. cyan/o — blue
10. diaphragmat/o — diaphragm
11. epiglott/o — epiglottis
12. laryng/o — larynx
13. lob/o — lobe
14. mediastin/o — mediastinum
15. muc/o — mucus
16. nas/o — nose
17. orth/o — straight
18. ox/o — oxygen
19. oxy/o — oxygen
20. pector/o — chest
21. pharyng/o — pharynx
22. phon/o — voice

23.	phren/o	diaphragm
24.	pleur/o	pleura
25.	pneum/o	lung/air
26.	pneumat/o	air
27.	pneumon/o	lung/air
28.	pulmon/o	lung
29.	py/o	pus
30.	rhin/o	nose
31.	sept/o	septum
32.	sinus/o	sinus
33.	spir/o	breath
34.	tel/o	complete
35.	thorac/o	thorax
36.	tonsill/o	tonsil
37.	trache/o	trachea

PREFIXES

1.	a-	not
2.	an-	not
3.	endo-	within
4.	eu-	good
5.	dys-	difficult
6.	pan-	all
7.	poly-	many

SUFFIXES

1.	-algia	pain
2.	-ar	pertaining to
3.	-ary	pertaining to
4.	-capnia	carbon dioxide
5.	-centesis	puncture to remove (drain)
6.	-dynia	pain
7.	-eal	pertaining to
8.	-ectasis	stretching
9.	-emia	blood
10.	-gram	record

Respiratory System—Anatomy and Terminology

11.	-graph	recording instrument
12.	-graphy	recording process
13.	-itis	inflammation
14.	-meter	measurement or instrument that measures
15.	-metry	measurement of
16.	-osmia	smell
17.	-oxia	oxygen
18.	-pexy	fixation
19.	-phonia	sound
20.	-pnea	breathing
21.	-ptysis	spitting
22.	-rrhage, -rrhagia	abnormal, excessive flow
23.	-scopy	to examine
24.	-spasm	contraction of muscle
25.	-sphyxia	pulse
26.	-stenosis	blockage, narrowing
27.	-stomy	opening
28.	-thorax	chest
29.	-tomy	cutting, incision

MEDICAL ABBREVIATIONS

1.	ABG	arterial blood gas
2.	AFB	acid-fast bacillus
3.	ARDS	adult respiratory distress syndrome
4.	BiPAP	bi-level positive airway pressure
5.	COPD	chronic obstructive pulmonary disease
6.	CPAP	continuous positive airway pressure
7.	DLCO	diffuse capacity of lungs for carbon monoxide
8.	FEF	forced expiratory flow
9.	FEV_1	forced expiratory volume in 1 second
10.	$FEV_1:FVC$	maximum amount of forced expiratory volume in 1 second
11.	FRC	functional residual capacity
12.	FVC	forced vital capacity
13.	HHN	hand-held nebulizer
14.	IPAP	inspiratory positive airway pressure
15.	IRDS	infant respiratory distress syndrome

UNIT I Anatomy, Terminology, and Pathophysiology

16.	MDI	metered-dose inhaler
17.	MVV	maximum voluntary ventilation
18.	PAWP	pulmonary artery wedge pressure
19.	PCWP	pulmonary capillary wedge pressure
20.	PEAP	positive end-airway pressure
21.	PEEP	positive end-expiratory pressure
22.	PFT	pulmonary function test
23.	PND	paroxysmal nocturnal dyspnea
24.	RDS	respiratory distress syndrome
25.	RSV	respiratory syncytial virus
26.	RV	respiratory volume
27.	RV:TLC	ratio of respiratory volume to total lung capacity
28.	TLC	total lung capacity
29.	TLV	total lung volume
30.	URI	upper respiratory infection
31.	V/Q	ventilation/perfusion scan

MEDICAL TERMS

Ablation	Removal or destruction by cutting, chemicals, or electrocautery
Adenoidectomy	Removal of adenoids
Apnea	Cessation of breathing
Asphyxia	Lack of oxygen
Asthma	Shortage of breath caused by contraction of bronchi
Atelectasis	Incomplete expansion of lung, collapse
Auscultation	Listening to sounds, such as to lung sounds
Bacilli	Plural of bacillus, a rod-shaped bacteria
Bilobectomy	Surgical removal of two lobes of a lung
Bronchiole	Smaller division of bronchial tree
Bronchoplasty	Surgical repair of bronchi
Bronchoscopy	Inspection of bronchial tree using a bronchoscope
Catheter	Tube placed into body to put fluid in or take fluid out
Cauterization	Destruction of tissue by use of cautery
Cordectomy	Surgical removal of vocal cord(s)
Crackle	Abnormal sound when breathing (heard on auscultation)
Croup	Acute viral infection (obstruction of larynx), stridor
Cyanosis	Bluish discoloration

Respiratory System—Anatomy and Terminology

Drainage	Free flow or withdrawal of fluids from a wound or cavity
Dysphonia	Speech impairment
Dyspnea	Shortage of breath, difficult breathing
Emphysema	Air accumulated in organ or tissue
Epiglottidectomy	Excision of covering of larynx
Epistaxis	Nose bleed
Glottis	True vocal cords
Hemoptysis	Bloody sputum
Intramural	Within organ wall
Intubation	Insertion of a tube
Laryngeal web	Congenital abnormality of connective tissue between vocal cords
Laryngectomy	Surgical removal of larynx
Laryngoplasty	Surgical repair of larynx
Laryngoscope	Fiberoptic scope used to view inside of larynx
Laryngoscopy	Direct visualization and examination of interior of larynx with a laryngoscope
Laryngotomy	Incision into larynx
Lavage	Washing out
Lobectomy	Surgical excision of a lobe of lung
Nasal button	Synthetic circular disk used to cover a hole in the nasal septum
Orthopnea	Difficulty in breathing, relieved by assuming upright position
Percussion	Tapping with sharp blows as a diagnostic technique
Pertussis	Whooping cough—highly contagious bacterial infection of pharynx, larynx, and trachea
Pharyngolaryngectomy	Surgical removal of pharynx and larynx
Pleura	Covers lungs and lines thoracic cavity
Pleurectomy	Surgical excision of pleura
Pleuritis	Inflammation of pleura
Pneumocentesis/ pneumonocentesis	Surgical puncturing of a lung to withdraw fluid
Pneumonia	Inflammation of lungs with consolidation
Pneumonolysis/ pneumolysis	Surgical separation of lung from chest wall to allow lung to collapse
Pneumonotomy/ pneumotomy	Incision of lung
Pulmonary edema	Accumulation of fluid in pulmonary tissues and air spaces
Pulmonary embolism	Thrombus or other foreign material lodged in pulmonary artery or one of its branches
Rales	An abnormal respiratory sound heard in auscultation, indicating some pathologic condition

Rhinoplasty	Surgical repair of nose
Rhinorrhea	Free discharge of a thin nasal mucous
Sarcoidosis	Chronic inflammatory disease with nodules developing in lungs, lymph nodes, other organs
Segmentectomy	Surgical removal of the smaller subdivisions (segment) of lobes of a lung
Septoplasty	Surgical repair of nasal septum
Sinusotomy	Surgical incision into a sinus
Spirometry	Measuring breathing capacity
Tachypnea	Quick, shallow breathing
Thoracentesis/thoracocentesis (pleuracentesis/pleurocentesis)	Surgical puncture of thoracic cavity, usually using a needle, to remove fluids
Thoracoplasty	Surgical procedure that removes rib(s) and thereby allows collapse of a lung
Thoracoscopy	Use of a lighted endoscope to view pleural spaces and thoracic cavity or to perform surgical procedures
Thoracostomy	Surgical incision into chest wall and insertion of a chest tube
Thoracotomy	Surgical incision into chest wall
Total pneumonectomy	Surgical removal of an entire lung
Tracheostomy	Creation of an opening into trachea
Tracheotomy	Incision into trachea
Transtracheal	Across trachea
Tuberculosis	Infection of the lungs caused by bacteria (tubercle bacillus)

RESPIRATORY SYSTEM ANATOMY AND TERMINOLOGY QUIZ

1. This is NOT a part of lower respiratory tract:
   a. trachea
   b. larynx
   c. bronchi
   d. lungs

2. Another name for voice box is:
   a. oropharynx
   b. pharynx
   c. laryngopharynx
   d. larynx

3. This is the windpipe:
   a. pharynx
   b. larynx
   c. trachea
   d. sphenoid

4. Interior of nose is divided by the:
   a. septum
   b. sphenoid
   c. oropharynx
   d. apical

5. This combining form means incomplete:
   a. atel/o
   b. alveol/o
   c. ox/i
   d. pneumat/o

6. This combining form means breath:
   a. py/o
   b. lob/o
   c. spir/o
   d. pleur/o

7. This prefix means all:
   a. a-
   b. an-
   c. pan-
   d. poly-

8. This abbreviation refers to a syndrome that involves difficulty in breathing:
   a. ABG
   b. ARDS
   c. BiPAP
   d. FEF

UNIT I Anatomy, Terminology, and Pathophysiology

9. This abbreviation refers to amount of air patient can expel from the lungs in 1 second:
   a. PFT
   b. PND
   c. RDS
   d. FEV_1

10. This suffix means breathing:
    a. -stenosis
    b. -spasm
    c. -pexy
    d. -pnea

RESPIRATORY SYSTEM—PATHOPHYSIOLOGY

Signs and Symptoms of Pulmonary Disorders

Dyspnea
Difficult breathing (sense of air hunger)

Increased respiratory effort

Hypoventilation
Decreased alveolar ventilation

Hyperventilation
Increased alveolar ventilation

Hemoptysis
Bloody sputum

Hypoxia
Reduced oxygenation of tissue cells

Cough
Caused by irritant

Protective reflex

Acute cough is up to 3 weeks

Chronic cough is over 3 weeks

Tachypnea
Rapid breathing

Apnea
Lack of breathing

Orthopnea
Requiring sitting upright to facilitate breathing

Pulmonary Diseases and Disorders

Hypercapnia
Increased carbon dioxide in arterial blood

Caused by inadequate ventilation of alveoli

Can result in respiratory acidosis

Hypoxemia
Reduced oxygenation of arterial blood

Acute Respiratory Failure
Inadequate gas exchange

Hypoxemia

Can result from trauma or disease

Adult Respiratory Distress Syndrome (ARDS)
Acute injury to alveolocapillary membrane

Results in edema and atelectasis

In infants, infant respiratory distress syndrome (IRDS)

Pulmonary Edema
Accumulation of fluid in lung tissue

Most common cause is left ventricular failure

Aspiration
Passage of fluid and solid particles into lung

Can cause severe pneumonitis

- Localized inflammation of lung

Atelectasis
Collapse of lung

Three most common types are:
- Adhesive
- Compression
- Obstruction

May be chronic or acute
- Acute, such as compression as a result of an automobile accident
- Chronic from structural defect

Absorption Atelectasis
Results from absence of air in alveoli

Caused by
  Foreign body
  Tumor
  Abnormal external pressure

Bronchiectasis
Chronic, irreversible dilation of bronchi

Common types that describe severity of condition
- Cylindrical
- Varicose
- Sacular or cystic

Respiratory Acidosis
Decreased level of pH
  Due to excess retention of carbon dioxide

Bronchiolitis
Inflammation and obstruction of bronchioles

Usually in children less than 2—preceded by URI

Viral infection (respiratory syncytial virus, or RSV)

Common types
- Constrictive
- Proliferative
- Obliterative

Pneumothorax
Air collected in pleural cavity

Leads to lung collapse

Communicating pneumothorax is barometric air pressure in pleural space

Spontaneous pneumothorax is spontaneous rupture of visceral pleura

Secondary pneumothorax is a result of trauma to chest

Pneumoconiosis
Dust particles or other particulate matter in lung

Common types
- Coal
- Asbestos
- Fiberglass

Pleural Effusion-Fluid in Pleural Space
Common types
- Hemothorax—hemorrhage into pleural cavity
- Empyema—Infectious materials in pleural space
- Exudate—Fluid remaining after infection, inflammation, malignancy

Empyema
Infectious pleural effusion
Pus in pleural space

Is a complication of respiratory infection

Commonly follows pneumonia and is treated like pneumonia

Pulmonary Embolism
Air, tissue, or clot occlusion

Lodges in pulmonary artery or branch of artery

Risk with congestive heart failure

Most clots originate in leg veins

Cor Pulmonale
Hypertrophy or failure of right ventricle

Result of lung, pulmonary vessels, or chest wall disorders

Acute is secondary to pulmonary embolus

Chronic is secondary to obstructive lung disease

Pleurisy (Pleuritis)
Inflammation of pleura

Often preceded by an upper respiratory infection

Infectious Disease
Upper respiratory infection (URI)
Acute inflammatory process of mucous membranes in trachea and above

Common types
- Common cold
- Croup
- Sinusitis
- Laryngitis

Lower Respiratory Infection (LRI)

Pneumonia
Inflammation of lungs with consolidation

Categorized according to causative organism

Can be caused by

    Aspiration

    Bacteria

    Protozoa

    Fungi

    Chlamydia

    Virus

Common types
    Aspiration pneumonia

    Bacterial

    Chlamydial

    Drug resistant

    Eosinophil

    Fungal

    Hospital acquired (nosocomial)

    Legionnaire's

    Mycoplasma

    Pneumococcal

    Viral

Tuberculosis
Communicable lung disease—airborne droplet

Caused by *Mycobacterium tuberculosis (bacilli)*

Chronic Obstructive Pulmonary Disease (COPD)
Irreversible airway obstruction that decreases expiration

Includes

Chronic bronchitis

- Bronchial spasms
- Dyspnea
- Wheezing
- Productive cough
- Cyanosis
- Chronic hypoventilation
- Polycythemia
- Cor pulmonale
- Prolonged expiration

Emphysema

- Loss of elasticity and enlargement of alveoli
- Mimics symptoms of chronic bronchitis but more exaggerated

RESPIRATORY SYSTEM PATHOPHYSIOLOGY QUIZ

1. Acute injury to alveolocapillary membrane that results in edema and atelectasis:
   a. hypoxemia
   b. adult respiratory distress syndrome
   c. bronchiolitis
   d. pneumoconiosis

2. Condition in which pus is in pleural space and is often a complication of pneumonia:
   a. empyema
   b. cor pulmonale
   c. pneumothorax
   d. atelectasis

3. Which of the following is NOT one of the most common types of atelectasis?
   a. adhesive
   b. compression
   c. obstruction
   d. expansion

4. This condition is a result of accumulation of dust particles in lung:
   a. pleurisy
   b. tuberculosis
   c. chronic obstructive pulmonary disease
   d. pneumoconiosis

5. An irreversible airway obstructive disease in which symptoms are bronchial spasm, dyspnea, and wheezing:
   a. pleurisy
   b. empyema
   c. bronchiolitis
   d. COPD

6. Cylindrical, varicose, and secular/cystic are examples of:
   a. bronchiectasis
   b. cor pulmonale
   c. pneumothorax
   d. atelectasis

7. Condition in which there is a loss of elasticity and enlargement of alveoli:
   a. chronic bronchitis
   b. asthma
   c. emphysema
   d. empyema

8. Definition of a chronic cough is one that lasts for over this number of weeks:
   a. 2
   b. 3
   c. 4
   d. 5

UNIT I   Anatomy, Terminology, and Pathophysiology

9. A condition marked by an increase in carbon dioxide in arterial blood and decreased ability to breathe that can result in respiratory acidosis:
   a. hypercapnia
   b. hypoxemia
   c. acute respiratory failure
   d. pulmonary edema

10. This condition often follows a viral infection and occurs in children under 2 years of age. Examples of various types of this condition are constrictive, proliferating, and obliterative.
    a. pneumoconiosis
    b. pulmonary edema
    c. bronchiolitis
    d. bronchiectasis

CARDIOVASCULAR SYSTEM
CARDIOVASCULAR SYSTEM—ANATOMY AND TERMINOLOGY

Consists of blood, blood vessels, and heart

Blood (function is to maintain a constant environment)

Composed of cells suspended in plasma (clear, straw-colored liquid)

Carries
Oxygen and nutrients to cells

Waste and carbon dioxide to kidneys, liver, and lungs

Hormones from endocrine system

Regulates
Temperature by circulating blood

Protection
White cells (leukocytes) produce antibodies

Composed of Two Parts
Liquid part (extracellular) is plasma
- Water 91%
- Protein 1%, albumin, globulins, fibrinogen, ferritin, transferrin
- 2% ions, nutrients, waste products, gases, regulating substances

Cellular structures
Leukocytes (WBCs) granular and agranular—fight infections
- Neutrophils
- Lymphocytes
- Monocytes
- Eosinophils
- Basophils

Erythrocytes (red blood cells)—hemoglobin carries oxygen

Thrombocytes (platelets)—important for hemostasis

Blood types: A, B, AB, and O are genetically endowed
- Blood type O negative is known as universal donor (no Rh and no red cell antigens present)

Vessels—Circulatory System

Function
To carry blood delivering nutrients and oxygen (arterial system) and carry away cell waste and carbon dioxide (venous system)

Types
Arteries (Fig. 1–16) carrying oxygenated blood
Inner layer, endothelium

Lead away from heart

Branches are arterioles

UNIT I Anatomy, Terminology, and Pathophysiology

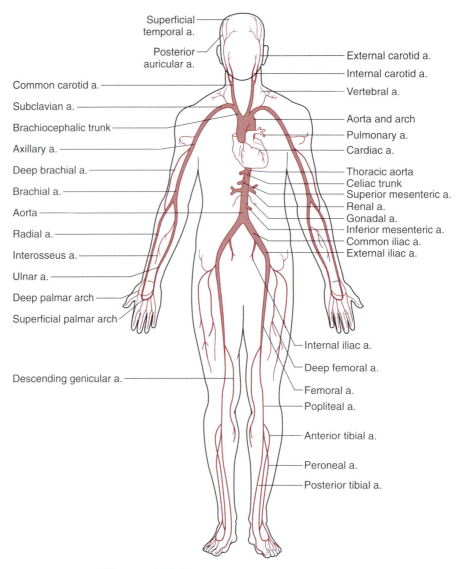

Figure **1-16** Arteries of circulatory system.

Capillaries
  Connection between arterioles and venules

  Exchange structure (oxygen and carbon dioxide, nutrients, and waste)

Veins (Fig. 1–17) carrying deoxygenated blood
Carry blood to heart

Venules are small branches

Heart

Circulates blood

Four Chambers (Fig. 1–18)
Two upper
  Right and left atria (singular: atrium) receive blood

Two lower
  Right and left ventricles discharge blood (pump)

Cardiovascular System—Anatomy and Terminology

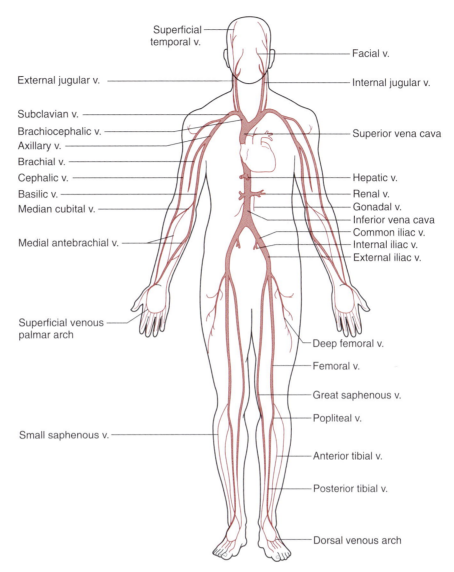

Figure **1-17** Veins of circulatory system.

Chamber Walls
Composed of three layers

- Endocardium: smooth inner layer

- Myocardium: middle muscular layer

- Epicardium: outer layer

Septa (singular: septum)
Divide chambers

- Interatrial septum

  Separates two upper chambers

- Interventricular septum

  Separates two lower chambers

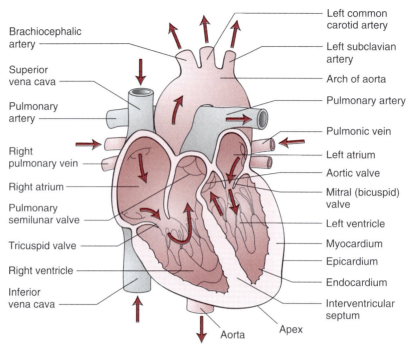

Figure **1-18** Internal view of heart.

Major Blood Vessels

Inferior vena cava—carries deoxygenated blood from lower extremities, pelvic and abdominal viscera to right atrium

Superior vena cava—drains deoxygenated blood from head, neck, upper extremities, and chest to right atrium

Pulmonary artery bifurcates and becomes right and left pulmonary artery—carries deoxygenated blood from right ventricle to lungs

Right and left pulmonary veins (4)—carry oxygenated blood from lungs to left atrium

Aorta—carries oxygenated blood from left side of heart to body

Pericardium

Sac comprised of two layers that covers heart

- Parietal pericardium: outermost covering
- Visceral pericardium: innermost (epicardium)
- Pericardial cavity: contains about 30 cc of fluid

Valves (4 in heart)

Tricuspid: between right atrium and right ventricle

Pulmonary: at entrance of pulmonary artery leading from right ventricle

Aortic: at entrance of aorta leading from left ventricle

Bicuspid (mitral): between left atrium and left ventricle

Conduction System (Fig. 1-19)

Sinoatrial node: SAN, nature's pacemaker, sends impulses to atrioventricular node

Cardiovascular System—Anatomy and Terminology

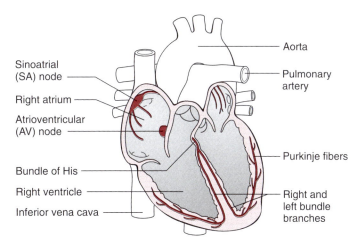

Figure **1-19** Electrical system of heart.

Atrioventricular node (AVN): located on interatrial septum and sends impulses to bundle of His

Bundle of His: divides into right bundle branch (RBB) and left bundle branch (LBB) in septum

Purkinje fibers: merge from bundle branches into specialized cells of myocardium, located at base of heart

Heartbeat

Two Phases—Correspond to Blood Pressure Readouts
Systole: contraction—top number reading

Diastole: relaxation—lower number reading

Trace a drop of blood from trunk of body (deoxygenated) to trunk of body (oxygenated)

    Inferior vena cava to right atrium

    Through tricuspid valve to right ventricle

    From right ventricle to pulmonary artery to lung capillaries

    From lung capillaries to pulmonary veins

    To left atrium through mitral (bicuspid) valve to left ventricle

    Though aortic valve to aorta

COMBINING FORMS

1.	angi/o	vessel
2.	aort/o	aorta
3.	ather/o	yellow plaque (fat)
4.	arter/o	artery
5.	arteri/o	artery
6.	atri/o	atrium
7.	brachi/o	arm

UNIT I   Anatomy, Terminology, and Pathophysiology

8.	cardi/o	heart
9.	cholesterol/o	cholesterol
10.	coron/o	heart
11.	cyan/o	blue
12.	my/o, muscul/o	muscle
13.	myx/o	mucous
14.	ox/o	oxygen
15.	pericardi/o	pericardium
16.	phleb/o	vein
17.	sphygm/o	pulse
18.	steth/o	chest
19.	thromb/o	clot
20.	valv/o	valve
21.	valvul/o	valve
22.	vascul/o	vessel
23.	vas/o	vessel
24.	ven/o	vein
25.	ventricul/o	ventricle

PREFIXES

1.	a-	not
2.	an-	not
3.	bi-	two
4.	brady-	slow
5.	de-	lack of
6.	dys-	bad, difficult, painful
7.	endo-	in
8.	hyper-	over
9.	hypo-	under
10.	inter-	between
11.	intra-	within
12.	meta-	change, after
13.	peri-	surrounding
14.	tachy-	fast
15.	tetra-	four
16.	tri-	three

SUFFIXES

1. -dilation — widening, expanding
2. -emia — blood
3. -graphy — recording process
4. -lysis — separation
5. -megaly — enlargement
6. -oma — tumor
7. -osis — condition
8. -plasty — repair
9. -sclerosis — hardening
10. -stenosis — blockage, narrowing
11. -tomy — cutting, incision

MEDICAL ABBREVIATIONS

1. ASCVD — arteriosclerotic cardiovascular disease
2. ASD — atrial septal defect
3. ASHD — arteriosclerotic heart disease
4. AV — atrioventricular
5. CABG — coronary artery bypass graft
6. CHF — congestive heart failure
7. CK — creatine kinase
8. CPK — creatine phosphokinase
9. CVI — cerebrovascular insufficiency
10. DSE — dobutamine stress echocardiography
11. HCVD — hypertensive cardiovascular disease
12. LBBB — left bundle branch block
13. LVH — left ventricular hypertrophy
14. MAT — multifocal atrial tachycardia
15. MI — myocardial infarction
16. NSR — normal sinus rhythm
17. PAC — premature atrial contraction
18. PAT — paroxysmal atrial tachycardia
19. PST/PSVT — paroxysmal supraventricular tachycardia
20. PTCA — percutaneous transluminal coronary angioplasty
21. PVC — premature ventricular contraction
22. RBBB — right bundle branch block
23. RSR — regular sinus rhythm

UNIT I Anatomy, Terminology, and Pathophysiology

24.	RVH	right ventricular hypertrophy
25.	SVT	supraventricular tachycardia
26.	TEE	transesophageal echocardiography
27.	TST	treadmill stress test

MEDICAL TERMS

Acute Coronary Syndrome (ACS)	An umbrella term used to cover clinical symptoms compatible with acute myocardial ischemia
Anastomosis	Surgical connection of two tubular structures, such as two pieces of the intestine
Aneurysm	Abnormal dilation of vessels, usually an artery
Angina	Spasmotic, choking, or suffocative pain
Angiography	Radiography of blood vessels
Angioplasty	Procedure in a vessel to dilate vessel opening
Atherectomy	Removal of plaque from an artery (can be done by a percutaneous or open procedure)
Auscultation	Listening for sounds within body
Bundle of His	Muscular cardiac fibers that provide heart rhythm to ventricles
Bypass	To go around
Cardiopulmonary	Refers to heart and lungs
Cardiopulmonary bypass	Blood bypasses heart through a heart-lung machine
Cardioverter-defibrillator	Surgically placed or wearable device that directs an electric shock to the heart to restore rhythm
Circumflex	A coronary artery that circles heart
Cutdown	Incision into a vessel for placement of a catheter
Edema	Swelling due to abnormal fluid collection in tissue spaces
Electrode	Lead attached to a generator that carries electric current from the generator to atria or ventricles
Electrophysiology	Study of electrical system of heart, including study of arrhythmias
Embolectomy	Removal of blockage (embolism) from vessel
Endarterectomy	Incision into an artery to remove inner lining
Epicardial	Over heart
False aneurysm	Sac of clotted blood that has completely destroyed vessel and is being contained by tissue that surrounds vessel
Fistula	Abnormal opening from one area to another area or to outside of the body
Hematoma	Mass of blood that forms outside vessel
Hemolysis	Breakdown of red blood cells
Hypoxemia	Low level of oxygen in blood

Hypoxia	Low level of oxygen in tissue
Intracardiac	Inside heart
Invasive	Entering body, breaking skin
Noninvasive	Not entering body, not breaking skin
Nuclear cardiology	Diagnostic specialty that uses radiologic procedures to aid in diagnosis of cardiologic conditions
Order	Shows subordination of one thing to another; family or class
Pericardiocentesis	Procedure in which a surgeon withdraws fluid from pericardial space by means of a needle inserted percutaneously
Pericardium	Membranous sac enclosing heart and ends of great vessels
Swan Ganz catheter	A catheter that measures pressure in right side of heart and in pulmonary artery
Thoracostomy	Incision into chest wall and insertion of a chest tube
Thromboendarterectomy	Removal of thrombus and atherosclerotic lining from an artery (percutaneous or open procedure)
Transvenous	Through a vein

CARDIOVASCULAR SYSTEM ANATOMY AND TERMINOLOGY QUIZ

1. These carry blood to the heart:
   a. capillaries
   b. arteries
   c. arterioles
   d. veins

2. Relaxation phase of heartbeat:
   a. diastole
   b. systole

3. Nature's pacemaker is this node:
   a. atrioventricular
   b. Bundle of His
   c. sinoatrial
   d. mitral

4. Node located on interatrial septum:
   a. atrioventricular
   b. Bundle of His
   c. sinoatrial
   d. Purkinje

5. Which of following is NOT one of the three layers of chamber walls of the heart?
   a. endocardium
   b. myocardium
   c. epicardium
   d. parietal

6. Septum that divides upper two chambers of heart:
   a. intraventricular
   b. interatrial
   c. tricuspid
   d. myocardium

7. Valve between right atrium and right ventricle:
   a. pulmonary
   b. aortic
   c. bicuspid
   d. tricuspid

8. Outer two-layer covering of heart:
   a. pericardium
   b. mitral
   c. myocardium
   d. epicardium

UNIT I   Anatomy, Terminology, and Pathophysiology

9. These are chambers that receive blood:
   a. right and left ventricle
   b. left ventricle and right atrium
   c. right atrium and right ventricle
   d. right and left atria

10. This combining form means plaque:
    a. atri/o
    b. brachi/o
    c. cyan/o
    d. ather/o

CARDIOVASCULAR SYSTEM—PATHOPHYSIOLOGY

Vascular Disorders

Coronary Artery Disease (CAD)/Ischemic Heart Disease (IHD)
Thickening and hardening of arterial intima (innermost layer) with lipid and fibrous plaque (atherosclerosis)

- Produces narrowing and stiffening of vessel

Location of lesions leads to various vascular diseases

- Femoral and popliteal arteries = peripheral vascular disease
- Carotid arteries = stroke
- Aorta = aneurysms (dilation/weakening of vessel walls)
- Coronary arteries = ischemic heart disease or myocardial infarction

Resulting in decreased oxygen supply

Risk factors increased by:

- Age
- Family history of CAD
- Hyperlipidemia
- Low HDL-C (good cholesterol)
- Hypertension
- Cigarette smoking
- Diabetes mellitus
- Obesity, particularly abdominal

Ischemia
Deficiency of oxygenated blood

- Often due to constriction or obstruction of blood vessel

Localized myocardial ischemia—most common cause: atherosclerosis of vessels
Oxygen demand of tissues greater than supply

Presenting symptoms

- Chest pain (angina pectoris)
- Hypotension
- Changes in ECG

Transient ischemia
Heart muscle begins to perform at a low level due to lack of oxygen (reversible ischemia)

Irreversible ischemia—is cause of an MI (myocardial infarction)
Heart muscle dies—necrosis (myocardial infarction)

- Prolonged ischemia of 30 minutes or more
- Reestablishment of blood flow reduces residual necrosis
  - Thrombolytic agents to dissolve or split up thrombus
  - Primary percutaneous transluminal coronary angioplasty (PTCA)

Cardiac enzymes are released from damaged cells

- Blood test reveals elevation of enzymes, confirming myocardial infarction

Hypertension (HTN)
Normal is less than 120/80 for adults

- Fig. 1–20 illustrates new hypertension classifications

Leading cause of death in United States, due to damage to brain, heart, kidneys, eyes, and arteries of the lower extremities

Cause is unknown in 95% of cases

- Known as
  - Primary hypertension
  - Essential hypertension

5% of cases are secondary to underlying disease

Increased resistance damages heart and blood vessels

- Retinal vascular changes are monitored to assess therapy and disease progression

Chronic hypertension often leads to end-stage renal disease

- Result of progressive sclerosis of renal vessels

Treatment
Medications

- ACE (angiotensin-converting enzyme) inhibitor
- Alpha-adrenergic or beta-adrenergic receptor blocker
- Diuretic
- Calcium channel blocker

Lifestyle changes

Classification of blood pressure for adults aged 18 years or older[1]

Category	Systolic (mm Hg)	Diastolic (mm Hg)
Normal	<120	<80
Prehypertension (stays between)	120–139	80–89
Hypertension[2]		
Stage 1 (mild)	140–159	90–99
Stage 2 (moderate)	160–179	100–109
Stage 3 (severe)	≥180	≥110

[1] Not taking antihypertensive drugs and not acutely ill. When systolic and diastolic pressures fall into different categories, the higher category should be selected.

[2] Based on the average of two or more readings taken at each of two or more visits after an initial screening.

Figure **1-20** Classification of blood pressure.

Hypotension
Abnormally low blood pressure
Types
Orthostatic (postural) hypotension
- Fall in both systolic and diastolic arterial blood pressure on standing
- Associated with
  - Dizziness
  - Blurred vision
  - Fainting (syncope)
- Caused by insufficient oxygenated blood flow through brain
- Can be acute (temporary) or chronic

Chronic orthostatic hypotension—types
- Primary of unknown cause
- Secondary to certain disease processes
- Such as:
  - Endocrine
  - Metabolic
  - Central nervous system disorders
- Treatment for secondary hypotension is correction of underlying disease

Aneurysm
Dilation of an arterial blood vessel wall or cardiac chamber
- Danger is rupture of aneurysm

Atherosclerosis is common cause

Arteriosclerosis and hypertension also common in persons with aneurysms

True aneurysm
  Involves all three layers of arterial wall
  Causes weakening and ballooning of arterial wall

False or psuedoaneurysm
  Usually result of trauma
  Also known as saccular
  Separation of arterial wall layers (dissecting) in artery wall (crisis situation—a medical emergency)
  Bleeds into dissected space and is contained by arterial connective tissue wall

Thrombus
Blood clot that remains attached to vessel wall and occludes vessel

Dislodged thrombus is a thromboembolus

Causes
  Trauma

Interior wall lining irritation/roughening

Infection

Inflammation

Low blood pressure/blood stagnation

Obstruction

Atherosclerosis

Risks related to thrombus
Dislodge/moving to lungs, brain, heart

Grow to occlude blood flow

Treatment
Pharmacologic, anticoagulants

Heparin

Warfarin derivatives

Non-invasive intervention
Balloon-tipped catheter to remove or compress thrombus

Thrombophlebitis Caused by Inflammation (Phlebitis)
Causes
Trauma

Infection

Immobility

Commonly associated with
Endocarditis

Rheumatic heart disease

Embolism
Mass that is present and circulating in blood

Common types
Air bubble

Fat

Bacterial mass

Cancer cells

Foreign substances

Dislodged thrombus

Amniotic fluid

Obstructs vessel
Pulmonary emboli travel through venous side or right side of heart to the pulmonary artery

Systemic or arterial emboli originate in left side of the heart

Associated with
- Myocardial infarction
- Left-side heart failure

- Endocarditis
- Valvular conditions
- Dysrhythmias

Peripheral Arterial Disease

Thromboangiitis obliterans (Buerger's disease)
Occurs most often in young men who are heavy smokers

Inflammatory disease of peripheral arteries creating thombi and vasospasms

Involves small or medium arteries of feet and often hands

- May necessitate amputation

Raynaud's disease
Vasospasms and constriction of small arterioles of fingers and toes

Affects young women as a secodary condition

Triggered by cold temperatures, emotional stress, cigarette smoking

Fingertips thicken and nails become brittle

Raynaud's phenomenon is secondary to primary disease, such as

- Scleroderma
- Pulmonary hypertension

Treatment of underlying condition
No known origin or treatment

Varicose Veins
Blood pools in veins, distending them

Tends to be progressive/vein valve failure

Occurs most commonly in saphenous veins

Hemorrhoids are varicose veins of anus

Leads to
Swelling and discomfort

Fatigue when in legs

Possible ulcerations

Heart Disorders

Congestive Heart Failure (CHF)—heart cannot pump required amounts of blood
Can be left-sided or right-sided heart failure

Left-sided heart failure (systolic); cannot generate adequate output, causing pulmonary edema

Common causes:

Myocardial infarction

Myocarditis

Cardiomyopathies leading to ischemia

Symptoms of left-sided congestive heart failure include:

    Shortness of breath

    Fatigue

    Exercise intolerance

Right-sided heart failure (diastolic) results in right ventricle stasis, inadequate pulmonary circulation, and peripheral edema/hepatosplenomegaly

Abnormal Heart Rhythms (Conduction Irregularities)

Bradycardia and heart block (atrioventricular block)

    Inadequate conduction impulses from SA node though AV node to AV bundle

    Treatment

        Cardiac pacemaker to maintain proper heart rate

Flutter—rapid regular contractions (most commonly of atria)

    Symptoms—palpitations

    Treatment

        Cardioversion (electronic shock to heart)

    Ablation (radiofrequency catheter destroying tissue causing arrhythmia)

Fibrillation—rapid, erratic, inefficient contractions of atria and ventricles

    Atrial fibrillation—most common (electrical impulses move randomly in atria)

        Symptoms—palpitation, risk of stroke due to clot formations from poor atrial outputs

    Treatment

    Cardioversion

    Ablation

Ventricular fibrillation—life-threatening, random electrical impulses throughout ventricles

    Symptoms

        Cardiac death or arrest without immediate treatment

    Treatment

        Cardioversion

        Digoxin—drug used to slow heart rate

        Implantable cardioverter-defibrillator (ICD)

        Emergency treatment—automatic external defibrillators (AEDs)

        Radiofrequency catheter ablation (RFA) is a minimally invasive technique used to treat cardiac arrhythmias

Infective Endocarditis

Inflammation of interior most lining of heart

Leads to destruction and permanent damage to heart valves

Caused by
> Bacteria (most common streptococci and staphlococci)
>
> Virus
>
> Fungi
>
> Parasites

Patients with heart defects or damage usually take antibiotics prior to invasive procedures

Pericarditis
Inflammation of pericardium of heart

Common types
- Acute
- Pericardial effusion
- Constrictive

Rheumatic Fever/Rheumatic Heart Disease
Results in formation of scar tissue of the endocardium and heart valves

In 10% of cases leads to rheumatic heart disease

Family tendency to develop

Begins as carditis (inflammation of all layers of heart wall)

Long-term effect:

Mitral and/or aortic valve disease

> Stenosis
>
> Regurgitation
>
> Insuffiency

Tricuspid valve

> Affected in about 10% of cases

Pulmonary valve

> Rarely affected

Valvular Heart Disease

Valves are extensions of endocardial tissue

Endocardial damage can be congenital or acquired

Damage leads to stenosis and/or incompetent valve

Includes

- Valvular stenosis is narrowing, stiffness, thickening, fusion, or blockage of valve, creating resistance, resulting in increased pressure in cardiac chamber behind valve
- Valvular regurgitation is failure of valve leaflet to close tightly, allowing backflow of blood
  - Result of lesions causing valve leaflets to shrink
  - Functional valvular regurgitation results in increased chamber size (cardiomegaly)

Stenosis

Aortic valve stenosis

Caused by

Congenital malformation

Degeneration

Infection

Results in slowing blood circulatory rate

Symptoms

Bradycardia

Faint pulse

May lead to heart murmur and hypertrophy

Mitral valve stenosis

Impaired flow from left atrium to left ventricle

Caused by

Rheumatic fever

Bacterial infections

Symptom

Decreased cardiac output

May lead to

- Pulmonary hypertension
- Right ventricular heart failure
- And/or edema

Valvular Regurgitation

Flow in opposite direction from normal

Mitral regurgitation (MR)

Backflow of blood from left ventricle into left atrium

Aortic regurgitation (AR)

Backflow of blood from aorta into the left ventricle

Pulmonic regurgitation (PR)

Backflow of blood from pulmonary artery into right ventricle

Tricuspid regurgitation (TR)

Backflow of blood from right ventricle into the right atrium

Heart Wall Disorders

Acute Pericarditis

Roughening and inflammation of pericardium (sac around heart)

Treatment

Antiinflammatory drugs and pain medication

Constrictive Pericarditis (Restrictive Pericarditis)
Forms fibrous lesions that encase heart

Compresses heart—thickened pericardial sac prevents heart from expanding when blood enters it

> Tamponade occurs when fluid builds up in pericardial space
>
> Pressure stops heart from beating—pericardial effusion or bleeding after heart surgery

Reduces output

Pericardial Effusion
Accumulation of fluid in pericardial cavity

Results in pressure on heart

- Sudden development of pressure on heart is tamponade

Cardiomyopathies

Myocardium: muscular wall (middle layer) of heart musculature

Group of diseases that affect myocardium

Cause

> Idiopathic (most common)
>
> Underlying condition

Types of Cardiomyopathy
Dilated cardiomyopathy (congestive cardiomyopathy)

- Ventricular distention and impaired systolic function

Hypertrophic cardiomyopathy

- Cause is often hypertensive or valvular heart disease
- Results in thickened interventricular septum (septum between the ventricle chambers)

Restrictive cardiomyopathy

- Myocardium becomes stiffened
- Heart enlarges (cardiomegaly)
- Dysrhythmias common
- Caused by infiltrative diseases such as amyloidosis

Congenital Heart Defects

Coarctation of aorta (CoA)—narrowing of the aorta

- Treatment
  > Surgical removal of narrow segment/end to end anastomosis

Patent ductus arteriosus (PDA)—opening between aorta and pulmonary artery

- Treatment
  > Drugs to close/embolize or plug ductus or tying off surgically

Tetralogy of Fallot—malformation of heart including four defects

- Pulmonary artery stenosis—narrowing/obstruction

Ventricular septal defect

- Hole between two ventricles

Shift of aorta to right—aorta overrides the interventricular septum

- Hypertrophy of right ventricle

- Myocardium enlarges to pump blood through narrowed pulmonary artery

Septal defect—holes in the septa (wall) between the atria (atrial septal defect) or the ventricles (ventricular septal defect)

- Treatment

    Close hole using open heart technique and heart lung machine support or percutaneous transcatheter closure is used to close hole in septum

CARDIOVASCULAR SYSTEM PATHOPHYSIOLOGY QUIZ

1. Lesion of carotid artery may lead to:
   a. heart attack
   b. stroke
   c. peripheral vascular disease
   d. ischemic heart disease

2. This blood pressure is hypertension:
   a. 120/80
   b. 130/70
   c. 140/90
   d. 110/70

3. Tachyarrhythmia or fast heart rate is that in excess of _____ bpm.
   a. 60
   b. 80
   c. 90
   d. 100

4. Angina pectoris is:
   a. heart block
   b. heart murmur
   c. chest pain
   d. barrel chest

5. In this type of regurgitation there is a backflow of blood from left ventricle into left atrium:
   a. aortic
   b. pulmonic
   c. tricuspid
   d. mitral

6. In this type of heart wall disorder, fibrous lesions form and encase heart:
   a. constrictive pericarditis
   b. acute pericarditis
   c. pericardial effusion
   d. cardiomyopathy

7. Which of the following terms means "of unknown cause"?
   a. etiology
   b. manifestation
   c. idiopathic
   d. late effect

8. This condition is also known as congestive cardiomyopathy:
   a. hypertrophic
   b. valvular
   c. dilated
   d. restrictive

UNIT I Anatomy, Terminology, and Pathophysiology

9. This peripheral arterial disease most often occurs in young men who are heavy smokers:
   a. Buerger's
   b. Pick's
   c. Addison's
   d. Glasser's

10. This cardiomyopathy results in a thickened interventricular septum:
    a. restrictive
    b. congestive
    c. dilated
    d. hypertrophic

FEMALE GENITAL SYSTEM AND PREGNANCY

FEMALE GENITAL SYSTEM AND PREGNANCY—ANATOMY AND TERMINOLOGY

Terminology

Ovaries (Pair)
Produce ova (single female gamete) and hormones; ova: plural; ovum: singular (Fig. 1–21). Each ova/gamete contains 23 chromosomes.

Fallopian Tubes (Uterine Tubes or Oviducts)
Ducts from ovary to uterus

Uterus (Womb)
Muscular organ that holds embryo

Three layers
- Endometrium: inner mucosa
- Myometrium: middle layer/muscle
- Perimetrium/Uterine serosa: outer layer
  - Cervix: lower narrow portion of uterus
  - Fundus: the upper rounded part of the uterus

Vagina
Tube from uterus to outside of body

Vulva
External genitalia
- Clitoris: erectile tissue
- Labia majora: outer lips of vagina
- Labia minora: inner lips of vagina
- Urinary meatus: opening to urethra
- Bartholin's gland: glands on either side of vagina
- Hymen: membrane partially or wholly occludes entrance to vagina

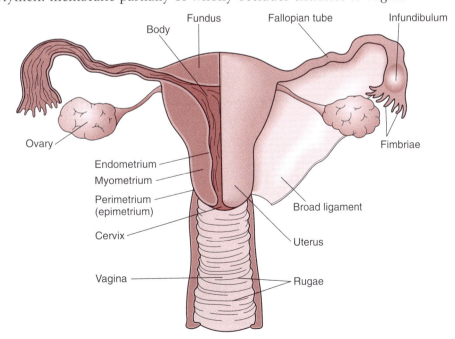

Figure **1-21** Female reproductive system.

Perineum
Area between anus and vaginal orifice

Accessory Organs (Fig. 1-22)
Breasts
Mammary glands

Composed of glandular tissue containing milk glands/lactiferous ducts

In response to hormones from pituitary gland, milk is produced in acini (also known as alveolua) (lactation)

Lactiferous ducts transfer milk to nipple

Nipple, surrounded by areola

Menstruation and Pregnancy
Proliferation Phase
Menstruation (Days 1-5): discharge of blood fluid containing endometrial cells, blood cells, and glandular secretions from endometrium

Endometrium repair (Days 6-12): maturing follicle in ovary produces estrogen (hormone) which causes endometrium to thicken and ovum (egg) to mature in graafian follicle

Secretory Phase
Ovulation (Days 13-14): occurs when graafian follicle ruptures and ovum travels down fallopian tube

Usually only one graffian follicle develops each month

Premenstruation (Days 15-28): a period of time in which graafian follicle converts to corpus luteum secreting progesterone to stimulate build-up of uterine lining. If after 5 days no fertilization occurs, cycle repeats.

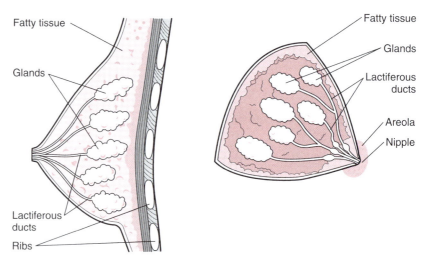

Figure **1-22** Breast structure.

Pregnancy

Prenatal stage of development from fertilization to birth (39 weeks)

Fertilized ovum or zygote develops in a double cavity: yolk sac (produces blood cells) and amniotic cavity (contains amniotic fluid)

Embryo, stage of development from 4th to 8th week

Fetus, unborn offspring, 9 weeks until birth

Placenta Forms Within Uterine Wall and Produces Hormone—Human Chorionic Gonadotropin (HCG)

HCG is horomone tested in urine pregnancy tests

HCG stimulates corpus luteum to produce estrogen and progesterone until the third month of pregnancy

Placenta then produces hormones

Expelled after delivery (afterbirth)

Gestation, Approximately 266 Days

280 days used when calculating Estimated Date of Delivery (EDD) or that time from last menstrual period (LMP)

Three trimesters

- First   LMP-12 weeks
- Second   13-27 weeks
- Third   28 weeks-EDD

COMBINING FORMS

1.	amni/o	amnion
2.	arche/o	first
3.	cephal/o	head
4.	cervic/o	cervix
5.	chori/o	chorion
6.	colp/o	vagina
7.	crypt/o	hidden
8.	culd/o	cul-de-sac
9.	episi/o	vulva
10.	fet/o	fetus
11.	galact/o	milk
12.	gynec/o	female
13.	gyn/o	female
14.	hymen/o	hymen
15.	hyster/o	uterus
16.	lact/o	milk

UNIT I Anatomy, Terminology, and Pathophysiology

17.	lapar/o	abdominal wall
18.	mamm/o	breast
19.	mast/o	breast
20.	men/o	menstruation, month
21.	metr/o	uterus, measure
22.	metr/i	uterus
23.	my/o, muscul/o	muscle
24.	nat/a	birth
25.	nat/i	birth
26.	obstetr/o	pregnancy/childbirth
27.	olig/o	few
28.	oo/o	egg
29.	oophor/o	ovary
30.	ov/o	egg
31.	ovari/o	ovary
32.	ovul/o	ovulation
33.	perine/o	perineum
34.	peritone/o	peritoneum
35.	phor/o	to bear
36.	salping/o	uterine tube, fallopian tube
37.	top/o	place
38.	uter/o	uterus
39.	vagin/o	vagina
40.	vulv/o	vulva

PREFIXES

1.	ante-	before
2.	dys-	painful
3.	ecto-	outside
4.	endo-	in
5.	extra-	outside
6.	in-	into
7.	intra-	within
8.	multi-	many
9.	neo-	new
10.	nulli-	none
11.	nulti-	none

12. post- — after
13. primi- — first
14. pseudo- — false
15. retro- — backwards
16. uni- — one

SUFFIXES

1. -arche — beginning
2. -cyesis — pregnancy
3. -gravida — pregnancy
4. -rrhexis — rupture
5. -para — woman who has given birth
6. -parous — to bear
7. -rrhea — discharge
8. -salpinx — uterine tube
9. -tocia — labor
10. -version — turning

MEDICAL ABBREVIATIONS

1. AFI — amniotic fluid index
2. AGA — appropriate for gestational age
3. ARM — artificial rupture of membrane
4. BPD — biparietal diameter
5. BPP — biophysical profile
6. BV — bacterial vaginosis
7. CHL — crown-to-heel length
8. CNM — certified nurse midwife
9. CPD — cephalopelvic disproportion
10. CPP — chronic pelvic pain
11. D&C — dilation and curettage
12. D&E — dilation and evacuation
13. DUB — dysfunctional uterine bleeding
14. ECC — endocervical curettage
15. EDC — estimated date of confinement
16. EDD — estimated date of delivery
17. EFM — electronic fetal monitoring
18. EFW — estimated fetal weight

UNIT I   Anatomy, Terminology, and Pathophysiology

19.	EGA	estimated gestational age
20.	EMC	endometrial curettage
21.	ERT	estrogen replacement therapy
22.	FAS	fetal alcohol syndrome
23.	FHR	fetal heart rate
24.	FSH	follicle-stimulating hormone
25.	HPV	human papillomavirus
26.	HSG	hysterosalpingogram
27.	HSV	herpes simplex virus
28.	IVF	in vitro fertilization
29.	LEEP	loop electrosurgical excision procedure
30.	LGA	large for gestational age
31.	PID	pelvic inflammatory disease
32.	PROM	premature rupture of membranes
33.	SHG	sonohysterogram
34.	SROM	spontaneous rupture of membrane
35.	SUI	stress urinary incontinence
36.	TAH	total abdominal hysterectomy
37.	VBAC	vaginal birth after cesarean

MEDICAL TERMS

Abortion	Termination of pregnancy
Amniocentesis	Percutaneous aspiration of amniotic fluid
Amniotic sac	Sac containing fetus and amniotic fluid
Antepartum	Before childbirth
Cesarean	Surgical opening through abdominal wall for delivery
Chorionic villus sampling	CVS, biopsy of outermost part of placenta
Cordocentesis	Procedure to obtain a fetal blood sample; also called a percutaneous umbilical blood sampling
Curettage	Scraping of a cavity using a spoon-shaped instrument
Cystocele	Herniation of bladder into vagina
Delivery	Childbirth
Dilation	Expansion (of cervix)
Ectopic	Pregnancy outside uterus (i.e., in fallopian tube)
Hysterectomy	Surgical removal of uterus
Hysterorrhaphy	Suturing of uterus
Hysteroscopy	Visualization of canal and cavity of uterus using a scope placed through vagina

Introitus	Opening or entrance to vagina
Ligation	Binding or tying off, as in constricting blood flow of a vessel or binding fallopian tubes for sterilization
Multipara	More than one pregnancy
Oophorectomy	Surgical removal of ovary(ies)
Perineum	Area between vulva and anus; also known as pelvic floor
Placenta	A structure that connects fetus and mother during pregnancy
Postpartum	After childbirth
Primigravida	First pregnancy
Primipara	First delivered infant/given birth to only one child
Salpingectomy	Surgical removal of uterine tube
Salpingostomy	Creation of a fistula into uterine tube
Tocolysis	Repression of uterine contractions
Vesicovaginal fistula	Abnormal opening/channel between vagina and bladder

FEMALE GENITAL SYSTEM AND PREGNANCY ANATOMY AND TERMINOLOGY QUIZ

1. This is NOT one of three layers of uterus:
   a. perimetrium
   b. endometrium
   c. myometrium
   d. barametrium

2. Located at the lower end of uterus is the:
   a. cervix
   b. vagina
   c. perineum
   d. labia majora

3. Approximate gestation of a human fetus is:
   a. 266 days
   b. 276 days
   c. 290 days
   d. 292 days

4. LMP is the:
   a. later maternity phase
   b. last menstrual period
   c. low metabolic pregnancy
   d. late menstruation phase

5. Name of stage that describes development of fetus from fertilization to birth is:
   a. postpartum
   b. antepartum
   c. prenatal
   d. natal

6. Which of the following correctly identifies three trimesters of gestation?
   a. LMP-12 weeks, 13-27 weeks, 28-EDD
   b. LMP-14 weeks, 15-27 weeks, 28-EDD
   c. LMP-14 weeks, 15-28 weeks, 29-EDD
   d. LMP-11 weeks, 12-26 weeks, 27-EDD

7. Combining form meaning few:
   a. oopho/o
   b. olig/o
   c. nati/i
   d. top/o

8. Combining form meaning hidden:
   a. amni/o
   b. crypt/o
   c. chori/o
   d. fet/o

UNIT I   Anatomy, Terminology, and Pathophysiology

9. Suffix meaning beginning:
   a. -cyesis
   b. -rrhea
   c. -arche
   d. -orrhexis

10. Prefix meaning within:
    a. ante-
    b. dys-
    c. ecto-
    d. endo-

FEMALE GENITAL SYSTEM AND PREGNANCY—PATHOPHYSIOLOGY

Menstrual and Hormonal Disorders

Dysmenorrhea

Painful menstruation

Common types
- Primary and secondary

Primary dysmenorrhea

No underlying condition but begins with commencement of ovulation

Cramping is caused by excess of prostaglandin

- Causes contractions and uterine ischemia
- Develops 24 to 48 hours prior to menstruation

Treatment
- Nonsteroidal antiinflammatory agents
- Progesterone

Secondary dysmenorrhea

Caused by an underlying disorder, such as

- Polyps
- Tumors
- Endometriosis
- Pelvic inflammatory disease

Treatment

Directed at underlying disorder

Amenorrhea

Amenorrhea is absence of menstruation

Common types
- Primary and secondary

Primary amenorrhea

Menstruation has never occurred

May be genetic disorder

- Turner's syndrome (ovaries do not function)

Secondary amenorrhea

Cessation of menstruation for 3 cycles or 6 months

- Individual has previously menstruated

Various causes of annovulation/amenorrhea

> *Examples:*
> - Tumors
> - Stress
> - Eating disorders
> - Competitive sports participation

Dysfunctional Uterine Bleeding (DUB)
Abnormal bleeding patterns

Occurs when no organic cause can be identified

Abnormal Menstruation Types
Oligomenorrhea: in excess of 6 weeks between periods

Polymenorrhea: less than 3 weeks between periods

Metrorrhagia: bleeding between cycles

Menorrhagia: increase in amount and duration of flow

Hypomenorrhea: light or spotty flow

Menometrorrhagia: irregular cycle with varying amounts and duration

Menorrhea: lengthy menstrual flow

Dysmenorrhea: painful menstruation

Premenstrual Syndrome (PMS)
Also known as premenstrual tension (PMT)

Occurs before onset of menses (luteal phase) and ends at onset of menses

Cluster of common symptoms
- Weight gain
- Breast tenderness
- Sleep disturbances
- Headache
- Irritability
- Cause is unknown

Treatment
- Vary depending on individual symptoms

Endometriosis
Endometrial tissue (uterine lining) develops outside the uterus (on ovaries, fallopian tubes, small intestine, etc.)

Responses to hormone cycle
Ectopic (out of place) endometrial tissue degenerates, sheds, and bleeds

Causes
- Irritation
- Inflammation
- Pain

Continued cycles produce fibrous tissue

- Adhesions and obstructions can then form
- Interferes with normal bodily function
- For example, fallopian tube endometriosis may lead to obstructed tubes

Primary symptom is dysmenorrhea

- May also cause painful intercourse (dyspareunia)

Risks
Increased risk for cancers
- Breast
- Ovaries
- Non-Hodgkin lymphoma

Treatment Includes
Hormonal suppression

Surgical removal of endometrial tissue
- May require hysterectomy and BSO (bilateral salpingo-oophorectomy)

Infection, Inflammation, and Sexually Transmitted Diseases

Pelvic Inflammatory Disease (PID)
Infection and inflammation of reproductive tract
- Primarily ovaries and fallopian tubes
- Usually originates in cervix or vagina
  - Migrates up through reproductive tract

Types
Acute

Chronic

Commonly forms adhesions and strictures
- May lead to infertility

Candidiasis
Yeast infection
- *Candida albicans (Monilia)*

Not sexually transmitted

Opportunistic infection may follow
- Infection treated with antibiotics
- Period of reduced resistance
- Increased glucose or glycogen levels (often associated with diabetes mellitus)

Affects mucous membranes

Produces a white, thick, curd-type discharge

Result may be dyspareunia and dysuria

Treatment
Antifungal substances such as nystatin

Identification and treatment of underlying condition

Chlamydia
Most common sexually transmitted disease (STD)

Cause
Bacteria, *Chlamydia trachomatis*

Symptoms
Asymptomatic or mild discharge and dysuria

Treatment
Antimicrobial

Genital Herpes
Cause
Virus, herpes simplex 2 (HSV-2)

Symptoms
Ulcers and vesicles

Treatment
Antiviral, manage outbreaks

There is no cure for genital herpes

Genital Warts
Cause
Virus, human papillomavirus

Symptoms
Polyps or grey lesions

Treatment
Excision

Prevention
Vaccine

There is no cure for genital warts

Gonorrhea
Cause
Bacteria, *Neisseria gonorrhoeae*

Some strains are drug-resistant

Symptoms
Dysuria

Discharge

Treatment
Antibacterial drugs

Syphilis
Cause
Bacteria, *Treponema pallidum*

Symptoms
Primary syphilis

- Ulcer or chancre at site of entry

Secondary syphilis
- Headache
- Fever
- Rash
- Tertiary
  - Affects cardiovascular and nervous systems

Treatment
Penicillin

Trichomoniasis
Cause
Protozoa, *Trichomonas vaginalis*

Symptoms
Usually asymptomatic

Treatment
Antimicrobial drugs

Benign Lesions

Leiomyomas—Uterine Fibroids
Well-defined, solid uterine tumor

Also known as
- Uterine fibroids
- Fibromyoma
- Fibroma
- Myoma
- Fibroid

Classification is based on location of tumor within uterine wall

Submucous: beneath endometrium

Subserous: beneath serosa

Intramural: in muscle wall

Symptoms
May be asymptomatic

Abnormal uterine bleeding

Pressure on nearby structures, such as bladder and rectum

Constipation

Pain

Sensation of heaviness

Treatment
Surgical excision of lesions

Hysterectomy may be necessary

Adenomyosis
Within uterine myometrium

Symptoms
- Usually asymptomatic
- Abnormal menstrual bleeding
- Enlarged uterus

Commonly develops in late reproductive years

Common in those taking Tamoxifen

Treatment
- Symptomatic in mild cases
- Surgical in severe cases
  - Excision of adenomyosis or hysterectomy

Malignant Lesions

Carcinoma of Breast
Accessory of reproductive system

Most often develops in upper outer quadrant
- Due to location, often spreads to lymph nodes
- May metastasize to lungs, brain, bone, liver, etc.

Majority arise from epithelial cells of ducts and lobules

Second most common cancer of women

Most are adenocarcinoma
- Invasive ductal carcinoma most common type
- Invasive lobular carcinoma second most common type
- Lymph node spread is determined by biopsying sentinel node (SNB)
- Small primary tumors are excised in a lumpectomy (tumor and immediate surrounding tissue only)
- Mastectomy is alternative surgical procedure removing entire breast
- Chemotherapy and radiation may be indicated to prevent reoccurrence

If neoplasm is responsive to hormone, hormone-blocking agents are administered

Increased risks
- Heredity
  - Especially history of mother or sister who developed breast cancer
  - Mutated breast cancer gene (BRCA-1)
  - Familial breast cancer syndrome associated with BRCA-2
- Lower socioeconomic status
- Radiation exposure

Carcinoma of Uterus (Endometrial Cancer)

Most frequent pelvic cancer

Usually postmenopausal

Associated with higher levels of estrogen

Increases risk
- Obesity (estrogen produced by fat tissue)
- Early menarche
- Delayed menopause
- Hypertension
- Diabetes mellitus
- Nulliparity (no viable births)
- Some types of colorectal cancer
- Oral contraceptives (estrogen)
- Estrogen-producing tumors

Symptoms
- Abnormal, excessive uterine bleeding
- Postmenopausal bleeding

No simple screening test available
- Uterine cells may be aspirated for evaluation

Staging of endometrial, cervical, and ovarian malignancies
- I—Confined to corpus
- II—Involves corpus and cervix
- III—Extends outside uterus but not outside true pelvis
- IV—Extends outside true pelvis or involves rectum or bladder

Treatment
- Pharmaceutical
- Surgical
- Irradiation
- Chemotherapy
- Combination of above

Carcinoma of Cervix

Routinely found on Papanicolaou smear

Dysplasia is an early change in cervical epithelium

Increases risks
- Herpes simplex virus type 2 (HSV-2)
- Human papillomavirus (HPV)
- Young age of sexual activity

Smoking

Lower socioeconomic status

Stages of cervical cancer

Stage 1 Carcinoma of cervix

Stage 2 Carcinoma spread from cervix to upper vagina

Stage 3 Carcinoma spread to lower portion of vagina/pelvic wall

Stage 4 Most invasive stage spreading to other body parts

Symptoms
Early stages asymptomatic

Later stages

- Bleeding
- Discharge

Biopsy is used to confirm

Treatment
Pharmaceutical

Surgical

Irradiation

Chemotherapy

Combination of above

Carcinoma of Ovary
Cause is unknown—considered silent killer

Increased risks
Genetic factors (BRCA-1)

Endocrine

- Nulliparous
- Early menarche
- Late menopause
- Non-breast feeding
- Late first pregnancy
- Postmenopausal estrogen replacement therapy (ERT)

Tumor categories
Germ cell tumors
Arise from primitive germ cells, usually the testis and ovum

Types
- Germinoma
- Yolk sac

- Endodermal sinus tumor
- Teratoma
- Embryonal carcinoma
- Polyembryoma
- Gonadoblastoma
- Some types of choriocarcinoma

Categories
- Dermoid cysts (benign)
- Malignant tumors
- Primitive malignant
  - Embryonic
  - Extraembryonic cells

Epithelial tumors
Most common gynecologic cancer

Gonadal stromal tumors
Symptoms
    Pelvic heaviness

    Dysuria

    Increased urinary frequency

    Sometimes vaginal bleeding

Treatment
    Excision

        Hysterectomy, including bilateral salpingo-oophorectomy with omentectomy (fold of peritoneum)

    Chemotherapy

    Radiation therapy

    Combination of above

Carcinoma of Fallopian Tubes
Primary fallopian tube tumors
Rare

Must be located within tube to be considered primary

- Adenocarcinoma most common primary tumor

Most tumors are secondary

Symptoms
    Often asymptomatic

    Bleeding or discharge

    Irregular menstruation

    Pain

Treatment
Hysterectomy, including bilateral salpingo-oophorectomy with any necessary omentectomy (fold of peritoneum)

Chemotherapy

Radiation therapy

Combination of above

Carcinoma of Vulva
Usually squamous cell carcinoma (90%)

Increased risk with STDs

Symptoms
Can be asymptomatic

Pruritic vulvular lesion

Treatment
Radical vulvectomy with node dissection

Wide local excision

Carcinoma of Vagina
Usually squamous cell carcinoma

Increased risk
Human papillomavirus (HPV)

Postmenopausal hysterectomy

History of abnormal Pap

History of other carcinomas

Symptoms
Often asymptomatic

Vaginal pain, discharge, or bleeding

Treatment
Squamous cell—radiation

Early tumors may be excised

Vaginectomy

Hysterectomy

Lymph node dissection

Pregnancy

Placenta Previa
Opening of cervix is obstructed by displaced placenta

Types (Fig. 1-23)
Marginal

Partial

Total

Female Genital System and Pregnancy—Pathophysiology

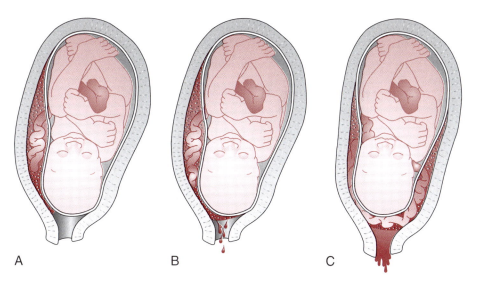

Figure **1-23** **A,** Marginal placenta previa. **B,** Partial placenta previa. **C,** Total placenta previa.

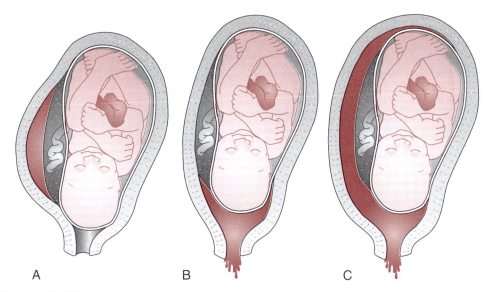

Figure **1-24** Abruptio placentae is classified according to the grade of separation of the placenta from uterine wall. **A,** Mild separation in which hemorrhage is internal. **B,** Moderate separation in which there is external hemorrhage. **C,** Severe separation in which there is external hemorrhage and extreme separation.

Abruptio Placentae (Fig. 1-24)
Premature separation of placenta from uterine wall

Eclampsia
Serious condition of pregnancy characterized by

- Hypertension
- Edema
- Proteinuria

Ectopic Pregnancy (Extrauterine) (Fig. 1-25)
Implantation of fertilized ovum outside uterus

- Often fallopian tubes (tubal pregnancy)

Hydatidiform Mole
Benign tumor of placenta

Secretes hormone (chorionic gonadotropic hormone, CGH)

Indicates positive pregnancy test

Malpositions and Malpresentations (Fig. 1-26)
Vaginal Delivery
Breech

Vertex

Face

Brow

Shoulder

Abortion
Types

    Spontaneous

- Miscarriage
- Happens naturally
- Uterus completely empties

    Incomplete

- Uterus does not completely empty
- Requires intervention to remove remaining fetal material

    Missed

- Fetus dies naturally
- Requires intervention to remove fetal material

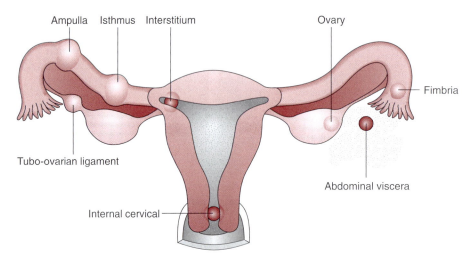

Figure **1-25** Ectopic pregnancy most often occurs in fallopian tube. Pregnancy outside the uterus may end in life-threatening rupture.

Female Genital System and Pregnancy—Pathophysiology

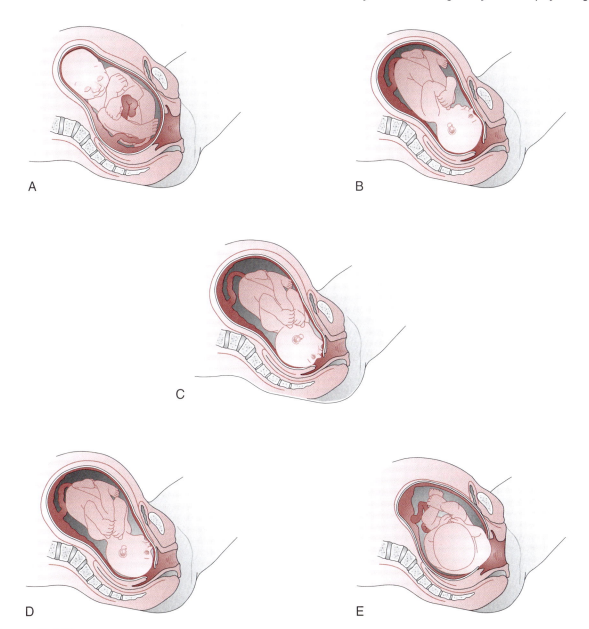

Figure **1-26** Five types of malposition and malpresentation of fetus: **A,** Breech. **B,** Vertex. **C,** Face. **D,** Brow. **E,** Shoulder.

Septic

- Similar to missed
- Has added complication of infection
- Requires intervention to remove fetal material
- Vigorous treatment of infection

Methods
  D&C

- Dilation and curettage (scraping)

Evacuation (suction)

Intra-amniotic injections
- Saline (salt) solution

Vaginal suppositories
- Such as prostaglandin

FEMALE GENITAL SYSTEM AND PREGNANCY PATHOPHYSIOLOGY QUIZ

1. Most common solution used for intra-amniotic injections is:
   a. prostaglandin
   b. saline
   c. estrogen
   d. chorionic gonadotropic hormone

2. This type of dysmenorrhea is treated with nonsteroidal antiinflammatory agents and progesterone:
   a. secondary
   b. constrictive
   c. periodic
   d. primary

3. In this type of amenorrhea there is a cessation of menstruation:
   a. secondary
   b. constrictive
   c. periodic
   d. primary

Match the abnormal menstruation type with correct definition.

4. oligomenorrhea _____   a. increased amount and duration of flow

5. metrorrhagia _____   b. bleeding between cycles

6. menorrhagia _____   c. in excess of 6 weeks

7. Increased risks of breast cancer, ovarian cancer, and non-Hodgkin lymphoma exist with this condition:
   a. endometriosis
   b. pelvic inflammatory disease
   c. sexually transmitted disease
   d. dysfunctional uterine bleeding

8. This benign lesion is also known as uterine fibroids:
   a. adenomyosis
   b. squamous cell
   c. leiomyoma
   d. extraembryonic cell primitive

9. Marginal, partial, and total are types of this condition:
   a. abruptio placentae
   b. placenta previa
   c. ectopic pregnancy
   d. hydatidiform mole

10. Which of the following is NOT a malposition of fetus?
    a. breech
    b. shoulder
    c. back
    d. brow

MALE GENITAL SYSTEM

MALE GENITAL SYSTEM—ANATOMY AND TERMINOLOGY

Function, reproduction

Structure, essential organs, and accessory organs (Fig. 1–27)

Essential Organs

Testes (Gonads)

Produce sperm (male gamete with 23 chromosomes) in seminiferous tubules

Covered by tunica albuginea, located in scrotum

Produce testosterone in Leydig cells

Vas Deferens

Is a tube

End of epididymis

Accessory Organs

Ducts (carry sperm from testes to exterior), sex glands (produce solutions that mix with sperm), and external genitalia

Seminal vesicles produce most seminal fluid

Prostate gland produces some seminal fluid and activates sperm

Bulbourethral gland (Cowper's glands) secretes a very small amount of seminal fluid

External genitalia: penis and scrotum

- Penis contains three columns of erectile tissue: two corpora cavernosa and one spongiosum
- Urethra passes through corpora spongiosum
- Scrotum encloses testes

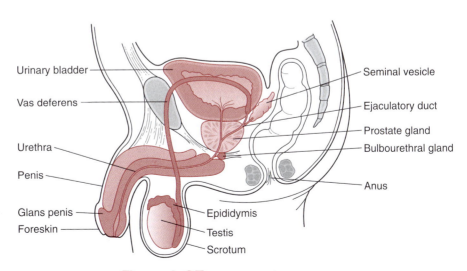

Figure **1-27** Male reproductive system.

UNIT I Anatomy, Terminology, and Pathophysiology

Passage of sperm from production to exterior

Sperm are produced in seminiferous tubules (testes) and pass into

Epididymis then to vas deferens (within seminal vesicles) to

Ejaculatory duct then through urethra (prostate gland and Cowper's [bulbourethral] gland)

Passes though penis to outside of body

COMBINING FORMS

1.	andr/o	male
2.	balan/o	glans penis
3.	cry/o	cold
4.	crypt/o	hidden
5.	epididym/o	epididymis
6.	gon/o	seed
7.	hydr/o	water, fluid
8.	orch/i	testicle
9.	orch/o	testicle
10.	orchi/o	testicle
11.	orchid/o	testicle
12.	prostat/o	prostate gland
13.	semin/i	semen
14.	sperm/o	sperm
15.	spermat/o	sperm
16.	test/o	testicle
17.	varic/o	varicose veins
18.	vas/o	vessel, vas deferens
19.	vesicul/o	seminal vesicles

SUFFIXES

1.	-one	hormone
2.	-pexy	fixation
3.	-ectomy	removal
4.	-stomy	new opening

MEDICAL ABBREVIATIONS

1.	BPH	benign prostatic hypertrophy
2.	PSA	prostate-specific antigen
3.	TURBT	transurethral resection of bladder tumor
4.	TURP	transurethral resection of prostate

MEDICAL TERMS

Cavernosa	Connection between cavity of penis and a vein
Cavernosography	Radiographic recording of a cavity, e.g., pulmonary cavity or main part of penis
Cavernosometry	Measurement of pressure in a cavity, e.g., penis
Chordee	Condition resulting in penis being bent downward
Corpora cavernosa	The two cavities of penis
Epididymectomy	Surgical removal of epididymis
Epididymis	Tube located at the top of testes that stores sperm
Epididymovasostomy	Creation of a new connection between vas deferens and epididymis
Meatotomy	Surgical enlargement of opening of urinary meatus
Orchiectomy	Castration, removal of testes
Orchiopexy	Surgical procedure to release undescended testis and fixate within scrotum
Penoscrotal	Referring to penis and scrotum
Plethysmography	Determining changes in volume of an organ part or body
Priapism	Painful condition in which penis is constantly erect
Prostatotomy	Incision into prostate
Transurethral resection, prostate	Procedure performed through urethra by means of a cystoscopy to remove part or all of prostate
Tumescence	State of being swollen
Tunica vaginalis	Covering of testes
Varicocele	Swelling of a scrotal vein
Vas deferens	Tube that carries sperm from epididymis to ejaculatory duct and seminal vesicles
Vasectomy	Removal of segment of vas deferens
Vasogram	Recording of the flow in vas deferens
Vasotomy	Incision in vas deferens
Vasorrhaphy	Suturing of vas deferens
Vasovasostomy	Reversal of a vasectomy
Vesiculectomy	Excision of seminal vesicle
Vesiculotomy	Incision into seminal vesicle

MALE GENITAL SYSTEM ANATOMY AND TERMINOLOGY QUIZ

1. This gland activates sperm and produces some seminal fluid:
   a. seminal vesicle
   b. bulbourethral gland
   c. prostate gland
   d. scrotum

2. Carries sperm from testes to ejaculatory duct:
   a. vans deferens
   b. sex gland
   c. tunica
   d. seminal

3. Penis contains these erectile tissues:
   a. one corpora cavernosa and two spongiosa
   b. two corpora cavernosa and two spongiosa
   c. one corpora cavernosa and one spongiosum
   d. two corpora cavernosa and one spongiosum

4. Also known as Cowper's gland:
   a. seminal vesicles
   b. bulbourethral gland
   c. prostate gland
   d. scrotum

5. Which of the following is NOT an accessory organ?
   a. gonads
   b. seminal vesicles
   c. prostate
   d. penis

6. Combining form meaning male:
   a. andr/o
   b. balan/o
   c. orchi/o
   d. test/o

7. Combining form meaning glans penis:
   a. balan/o
   b. vas/o
   c. vesicul/o
   d. orch/o

8. Testes are covered by the:
   a. seminal vesicles
   b. androgen
   c. chancre
   d. tunica albuginea

UNIT I Anatomy, Terminology, and Pathophysiology

9. This abbreviation describes a surgical resection of prostate that is accomplished by means of an endoscope inserted into urethra:
   a. TURBT
   b. BPH
   c. UPJ
   d. TURP

10. This abbreviation describes a condition of prostate in which there is an enlargement that is benign:
    a. TURBT
    b. BPH
    c. UPJ
    d. TURP

MALE GENITAL SYSTEM—PATHOPHYSIOLOGY

Male Genital System Disorders

Disorders of Scrotum, Testes, and Epididymis

Cryptorchidism

Undescended testes—condition at birth

- Unilateral or bilateral
- Primarily result from obstruction
- Risk neoplastic processes

Treatment

- May descend spontaneously
- Administration of hormone to stimulate testosterone production
- Surgical intervention (orchiopexy) near age 1 to avoid risk of infertility

Orchitis

Inflammation of testes

Most common cause is virus

- Such as mumps orchitis
- Atrophy with irreversible loss of sperm production at risk

May be associated with

- Mumps or epidemic parotitis
- Gonorrhea
- Syphilis
- Tuberculosis

Symptoms

- Mild to severe pain in testes
- Mild to severe edema
- Feeling of weight in testicular area

Treatment

- Depends upon presence of underlying condition

Epididymitis

Inflammation of epididymis

Inflammatory response to trauma or infection

Abscess may form

Types

Sexually transmitted epididymitis

- Gonorrhea
- *T. pallidum*
- *T. vaginalis*

Nonspecific bacterial epididymitis

- *E. coli*
- *Streptococci*
- *Staphylococci*
- Associated with underlying urological disorder

Symptoms
Scrotal pain

Swelling

Erythema

Perhaps hydrocele formation

Treatment
Antibiotic

Bed rest

Ice packs

Scrotal support

Analgesics

Hydrocele (Fig. 1–28)
Collection of fluid in membranes of tunica vaginalis

May be congenital or acquired (response to infection or tumors)

Congenital hydrocele may reabsorb due to a communication between the scrotal sac and peritoneal cavity and require no intervention

Symptoms
Scrotal enlargement

Usually painless
- Unless infection is present

Varicocele
Abnormal dilation of plexus of veins

Decreases sperm production and motility

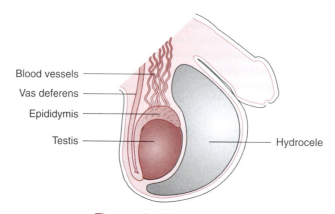

Figure **1-28** Hydrocele.

Symptoms
Usually painless

In elderly, may signal renal tumor

Treatment
Surgical intervention

Torsion of testes (Fig. 1-29)
Twisting of testes

Congenital abnormal development of tunica vaginalis and spermatic cord

Trauma may precipitate

Symptoms
Sudden onset of severe pain

Nausea

Vomiting

Scrotal edema and tenderness

Fever

Treatment
Immediate surgical intervention

Cancer of testes
Rare form of cancer

Cure rate high (95%)

Cause unknown

Usually occurs in younger men

Two main groups
- Germ cell tumors (GCT)—90% testicular tumors
- Sex cord-stromal tumors

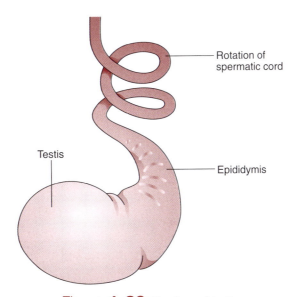

Figure **1-29** Torsion of testis.

Cancer of scrotum
Rare form of cancer

- Squamous cell carcinoma

Symptoms
Asymptomatic in early stages

Ulcerations in later stages

Treatment
Wide local excision

Mohs micrographic surgery

- Precise removal of tumor
- Layers are removed until no further microscopic evidence of abnormal cells is seen

Laser therapy

Lymph nodes are examined for metastasis

Disorders of Urethra
Epispadias
Congenital anomaly

Urethral meatus is located on dorsal side of penis

Usually occurs in conjunction with other abnormalities

Treatment
Surgical reconstruction

Hypospadias
Most common abnormality of penis

Urethral opening on ventral side of penis

Results in curvature of penis

- Due to chordee

Treatment
Surgical reconstruction

Urethritis
Inflammation of urethra

Infectious urethritis can be gonococcal or nongonococcal

Nongonococcal organisms

- *C. trachomatis*
- *U. urealyticum*

Symptoms
Discharge

Inflammation of meatus

Burning

Itching

Urgent and frequent urination

In nongonococcal, symptoms are less

Treatment
Antibiotics based on organism

Disorders of Penis
Balanitis
Inflammation of glans

Causes
Syphilis

Trichomoniasis

Gonorrhea

Candida albicans

Tinea

Underlying disease diabetes mellitus and candidiasis

No circumcision

Symptoms
Irritation

Tenderness

Discharge

Edema

Ulceration

Swelling of lymph nodes

Treatment
Culture of discharge

Saline irrigation

Antibiotics

Phimosis and paraphimosis
Phimosis
Condition in which prepuce (foreskin) is constricted

- Prepuce cannot be retracted over glans penis

Can occur at any age

Associated with poor hygiene and chronic infection in uncircumcised males

Symptoms
Erythema

Edema

Tenderness

Purulent discharge

Treatment
Surgical circumcision

Paraphimosis
Condition in which prepuce (foreskin) is constricted

Prepuce is retracted over glans penis and cannot be moved forward

Symptom
Edema

Treatment
Surgical

Peyronie's disease
Also known as bent nail syndrome

Fibrotic condition

- Results in lateral curvature of penis during erection

Occurs most often in middle-aged men

Cause is unknown but associated with

- Diabetes
- Keloid development
- Dupuytren's contracture (flexion deformity of toes and fingers)

Treatment
Sometimes spontaneous remission

Pharmacologic oxygenation increasing therapies

Surgical resection of fibrous bands

Cancer of penis
Rare form of cancer

Occurs most often in men over 60

Squamous cell carcinoma

Increased risks

- More common in uncircumcised men
- Sexual partner with cervical carcinoma
- Human papillomavirus

Usually begins with small lesion beneath prepuce

Intraepithelial neoplasia is also known as

- Bowen's disease
- Erythroplasia of Queyrat
- Begins as noninvasive

Progresses to invasive if untreated

Metastasis to lymph nodes

Treatment
Excision

Mohs micrographic surgery

Radiation therapy

Laser therapy

Cryosurgery

Advanced tumors are treated with partial or total penectomy and chemotherapy

Disorders of Prostate Gland
Benign prostatic hyperplasia/hypertrophy (BPH)
Multiple fibroadenomatous nodules; usually located on outside of gland so easily palpable on digital exam

- Related to aging; common in men over 60 years of age
- Enlarging prostate obstructs bladder neck and urethra
- Decreases urine flow

It is thought that increased levels of estrogen/androgen cause BPH

Symptoms
Increased frequency and urgency of urination

Nocturia

Incontinence

Hesitancy

Diminished force

Postvoiding dribble

Screening
Prostate-specific antigen (PSA)

Digital rectal examination (DRE)

Treatment
Partial prostatectomy

Transurethral resection of prostate (TURP)

Excision of nodules

Hormone therapy

Placement of urethral stents

Pharmaceuticals—those that inhibit production of testosterone and those that relax smooth muscle of gland and neck of bladder

Prostatitis
Inflammation of prostate

- Acute or chronic bacterial prostatitis

Causes
Escherichia coli

Enterococci

Staphylococci

Streptococci

Chlamydia trachomatis

Ureaplasma urealyticum

Neisseria gonorrhea

Nonbacterial
Spontaneous

Prostatodynia

Symptoms
Acute prostatitis
Fever and chills

Lower back pain

Perineal pain

Dysuria

Tenderness, suprapubic

Urinary tract infection

Chronic prostatitis
Recurring

Same as acute only with no infection in urinary tract

Treatment
Acute
Antibiotic based on culture

Chronic
No treatment available

Cancer of prostate
Most common diagnosed malignancy in men, occuring in men over age 60

Indications are cause is related to androgens

Predominately adenocarcinoma (95%)

No relationship between BPH and cancer of prostate

Symptoms
Asymptomatic in early stages

Later symptoms include

- Dysuria
- Back pain
- Hematuria
- Frequent urination

- Urinary retention
- Increased incidence of uremia

Stages
Two systems used to stage prostate cancer

- Whitmore-Jewett stages as indicated in Fig. 1–30
- Tumor node metastasis (TNM) as indicated in Fig. 1–31

Treatment
Dependent upon stage

WHITMORE-JEWETT STAGES:
Stage A is clinically undetectable tumor confined to the gland and is an incidental finding at prostate surgery.
A1: well-differentiated with focal involvement
A2: moderately or poorly differentiated or involves multiple foci in the gland
Stage B is tumor confined to the prostate gland.
B0: nonpalpable, PSA-detected
B1: single nodule in one lobe of the prostate
B2: more extensive involvement of one lobe or involvement of both lobes
Stage C is a tumor clinically localized to the periprostatic area but extending through the prostatic capsule; seminal vesicles may be involved.
C1: clinical extracapsular extension
C2: extracapsular tumor producing bladder outlet or ureteral obstruction
Stage D is metastatic disease.
D0: clinically localized disease (prostate only) but persistently elevated enzymatic serum acid phosphatase
D1: regional lymph nodes only
D2: distant lymph nodes, metastases to bone or visceral organs
D3: D2 prostate cancer patients who relapse after adequate endocrine therapy

Figure **1-30** Whitmore-Jewett stages.

TNM STAGES:

Primary Tumor (T)
TX: Primary tumor cannot be assessed
T0: No evidence of primary tumor
T1: Clinically inapparent tumor not palpable or visible by imaging
    T1a: Tumor incidental histologic finding in 5% or less of tissue resected
    T1b: Tumor incidental histologic finding in more than 5% of tissue resected
    T1c: Tumor identified by needle biopsy (e.g., because of elevated PSA)
T2: Tumor confined within the prostate
    T2a: Tumor involves half a lobe or less
    T2b: Tumor involves more than half of a lobe, but not both lobes
    T2c: Tumor involves both lobes; extends through the prostatic capsule
T3a: Unilateral extracapsular extension
T3b: Bilateral extracapsular extension
T3c: Tumor invades the seminal vesicle(s)
T4: Tumor is fixed or invades adjacent structures other than the seminal vesicle(s)
    T4a: Tumor invades any of bladder neck, external sphincter, or rectum
    T4b: Tumor invades levator muscles and/or is fixed to the pelvic wall

Regional lymph nodes (N)
NX: Regional lymph nodes cannot be assessed
N0: No regional lymph node metastasis
N1: Metastasis in a single lymph node, 2 cm or less in greatest dimension
N2: Metastasis in a single lymph node, more than 2 cm but not more than 5 cm in greatest dimension; or multiple lymph node metastases, none more than 5 cm in greatest dimension
N3: Metastasis in a single lymph node more than 5 cm in greatest dimension

Distant metastases (M)
MX: Presence of distant metastasis cannot be assessed
M0: No distant metastasis
M1: Distant metastasis
    M1a: Nonregional lymph node(s)
    M1b: Bone(s)
    M1c: Other site(s)

Figure **1-31** TNM stages.

MALE GENITAL SYSTEM PATHOPHYSIOLOGY QUIZ

1. What is the condition in which testes do not descend?
   a. cryptorchidism
   b. Bowen's disease
   c. torsion
   d. hypospadias

2. Orchitis is most often caused by a:
   a. bacteria
   b. virus
   c. parasite
   d. fungus

3. A condition that can be either congenital or acquired through trauma and that involves twisting of testes is:
   a. hydrocele
   b. hypospadias
   c. cryptorchidism
   d. torsion

4. Cancer of _____ is divided into two main groups of germ cell tumors and sex stromal cord tumors.
   a. testes
   b. penis
   c. scrotum
   d. prostate

5. This type of surgical technique involves excision of a lesion in layers until no further evidence of abnormality is seen:
   a. Bowen's
   b. Addison's
   c. Mohs
   d. laser

6. Epispadias is a disorder of urethra in which urethral meatus is located on _____ side of penis:
   a. ventral
   b. dorsal
   c. lateral
   d. medial

7. Inflammation of glans is:
   a. phimosis
   b. paraphimosis
   c. urethritis
   d. balanitis

8. This disease is also known as bent nail syndrome:
   a. Bowen's
   b. Peyronie's
   c. Addison's
   d. Whitmore-Jewett

UNIT I Anatomy, Terminology, and Pathophysiology

9. Condition in which multiple fibroadenomatous nodules form and lead to decreased urine flow. Condition is thought to be related to increased levels of estrogen/androgen.
   a. BPH
   b. DRE
   c. GCT
   d. TNM

10. Cancer of prostate is predominately this type of cancer:
    a. sex cord
    b. adenocarcinoma
    c. squamous cell
    d. seminoma

URINARY SYSTEM

URINARY SYSTEM—ANATOMY AND TERMINOLOGY

Removes metabolic waste materials (nitrogenous waste: urea, creatinine, and uric acid)

Conserves nutrients and water

Balances: electrolytes (acids/bases balance)

    Electrolytes are electronically charged molecules required for nerve and muscle function

Assists liver in detoxification

Organs (Fig. 1-32)

Kidneys
Ureters
Urinary bladder
Urethra

Kidneys (Fig. 1-33)

Electrolytes and fluid balance
Controls pH balance (acid/base)

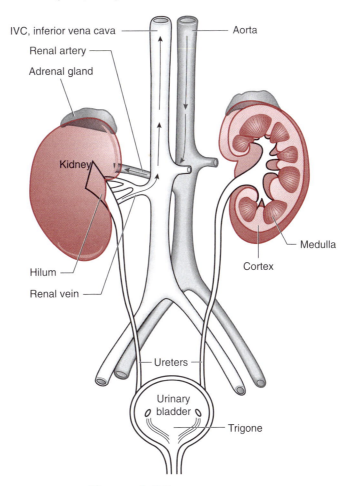

Figure **1-32** Urinary system.

UNIT I   Anatomy, Terminology, and Pathophysiology

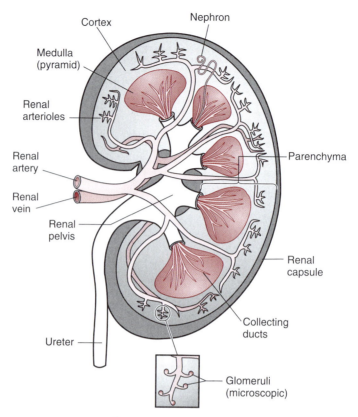

Figure **1-33** Kidney.

Secrete berenin which affects blood pressure and erythropoietin which stimulates red blood cell production in bone marrow

Secrete active vitamin D required for calcium absorption from intestines

Two organs located behind peritoneum (retroperitoneal space)

Kidney Structure

Cortex (outer layer)

Medulla (inner portion)

Hilum (depression on medial border through which blood ressels and nerves pass)

Pyramids (divisions of medulla)

Papilla (inner part of pyramids)

Pelvis (receptacle for urine within kidney)

Calyces surround top of renal pelvis

Nephrons (3 types) are operational units of kidney

Ureters
Narrow tubes transporting urine from kidneys to bladder

Urinary Bladder
Reservoir for urine

Shaped like an upside down pear with three surfaces

- Posterior (base)
- Anterior (neck)
- Superior (peritoneum)

Trigone

- Smooth triangular area inside bladder—size never changes
- Formed by openings of ureters and urethra

Urethra
Canal from bladder to exterior of body
Urinary meatus, outside opening of urethra

COMBINING FORMS

1. albumin/o — albumin
2. azot/o — urea
3. bacteri/o — bacteria
4. cali/o — calyx
5. cyst/o — urinary
6. dips/o — thirst
7. glomerul/o — glomerulus
8. glyc/o — sugar
9. glycos/o — sugar
10. hydr/o — water
11. ket/o — ketone bodies/ketoacidosis
12. lith/o — stone
13. meat/o — meatus
14. nephr/o — kidney
15. noct/i — night
16. olig/o — scant, few
17. pyel/o — renal pelvis
18. ren/o — kidney
19. son/o — sound
20. tripsy — to crush
21. tryg/o — trigone region/kidney
22. ur/o — urine
23. ureter/o — ureter
24. urethr/o — urethra
25. uria — urination/urinary condition
26. urin/o — urine
27. vesic/o — bladder

UNIT I   Anatomy, Terminology, and Pathophysiology

PREFIXES

1.	dys-	painful
2.	peri-	surrounding
3.	poly-	many
4.	retro-	behind

SUFFIXES

1.	-eal	pertaining to
2.	-lithiasis	condition of stones
3.	-lysis	separation
4.	-plasty	repair
5.	-rrhaphy	suture
6.	-tripsy	crush

MEDICAL ABBREVIATIONS

1.	ARF	acute renal failure
2.	BUN	blood urea nitrogen
3.	ESRD	end-stage renal disease
4.	HD	hemodialysis
5.	IVP	intravenous pyelogram
6.	KUB	kidney, ureter, bladder
7.	pH	symbol for acid/base level
8.	PKU	phenylketonuria
9.	sp gr	specific gravity
10.	UA	urinalysis
11.	UPJ	ureteropelvic junction
12.	UTI	urinary tract infection

MEDICAL TERMS

Bulbocavernosus	Muscle that constricts vagina in a female and urethra in a male
Bulbourethral	Gland with duct leading to urethra
Calculus	Concretion of mineral salts, also called a stone
Calycoplasty	Surgical reconstruction of recess of renal pelvis
Calyx	Recess of renal pelvis
Cystolithectomy	Removal of a calculus (stone) from urinary bladder
Cystometrogram	CMG, measurement of pressures and capacity of urinary bladder
Cystoplasty	Surgical reconstruction of bladder
Cystorrhaphy	Suture of bladder

Urinary System—Anatomy and Terminology

Cystoscopy	Use of a scope to view bladder
Cystostomy	Surgical creation of an opening into bladder
Cystotomy	Incision into bladder
Cystourethroplasty	Surgical reconstruction of bladder and urethra
Cystourethroscopy	Use of a scope to view bladder and urethra
Dilation	Stretching or expansion
Dysuria	Painful urination
Endopyelotomy	Procedure involving bladder and ureters, including insertion of a stent into renal pelvis
Extracorporeal	Occurring outside of body
Fundoplasty	Repair of the bottom of bladder
Hydrocele	Sac of fluid
Kock pouch	Surgical creation of a urinary bladder from a segment of the ileum
Nephrocutaneous fistula	An abnormal channel from kidney to skin
Nephrolithotomy	Removal of a kidney stone through an incision made into the kidney
Nephrorrhaphy	Suturing of kidney
Nephrostomy	Creation of a channel into renal pelvis of kidney
Transureteroureterostomy	Surgical connection of one ureter to other ureter
Transvesical ureterolithotomy	Removal of a ureter stone (calculus) through bladder
Ureterectomy	Surgical removal of a ureter, either totally or partially
Ureterocutaneous fistula	Channel from ureter to exterior skin
Ureteroenterostomy	Creation of a connection between intestine and ureter
Ureterolithotomy	Removal of a stone from ureter
Ureterolysis	Freeing of adhesions of ureter
Ureteroneocystostomy	Surgical connection of ureter to a new site on bladder
Ureteropyelography	Ureter and renal pelvis radiography
Ureterotomy	Incision into ureter
Urethrocystography	Radiography of bladder and urethra
Urethromeatoplasty	Surgical repair of urethra and meatus
Urethropexy	Fixation of urethra by means of surgery
Urethroplasty	Surgical repair of urethra
Urethrorrhaphy	Suturing of urethra
Urethroscopy	Use of a scope to view urethra
Vesicostomy	Surgical creation of a connection of viscera of bladder to skin

URINARY SYSTEM ANATOMY AND TERMINOLOGY QUIZ

1. The outer covering of kidney:
   a. medulla
   b. pyramids
   c. cortex
   d. papilla

2. Which is not a division of kidneys?
   a. pelvis
   b. pyramids
   c. cortex
   d. trigone

3. The inner portion of kidneys:
   a. medulla
   b. pyramids
   c. cortex
   d. papilla

4. The smooth area inside bladder:
   a. pyramids
   b. calyces
   c. trigone
   d. cystocele

5. The narrow tube connecting kidney and bladder:
   a. urethra
   b. ureter
   c. meatus
   d. trigone

6. Which of the following is NOT a surface of urinary bladder?
   a. posterior
   b. anterior
   c. superior
   d. inferior

7. Combining form that means stone:
   a. azot/o
   b. cyst/o
   c. lith/o
   d. olig/o

8. Term meaning painful urination:
   a. pyuria
   b. dysuria
   c. diuresis
   d. hyperemia

UNIT I Anatomy, Terminology, and Pathophysiology

9. Combining form meaning scant:
   a. glyc/o
   b. hydr/o
   c. meat/o
   d. olig/o

10. Term that describes renal failure that is acute:
    a. ARF
    b. ESRD
    c. HD
    d. BPH

URINARY SYSTEM—PATHOPHYSIOLOGY

Renal Failure

Acute Renal Failure
Sudden onset of renal failure

Cause
- Extreme hypotension
- Trauma
- Infection
- Inflammation
- Toxicity
- Obstructed vascular supply

Symptoms
- Uremia
- Oliguria (decreased output) or anuria (no output)
- Hyperkalemia (high potassium in blood)
- Pulmonary edema

Types
- Prerenal
  - Associated with poor systemic perfusion
  - Decreased renal blood flow
    - Such as with congestive heart failure
- Intrarenal
  - Associated with renal parenchyma disease (functional tissue of kidney)
    - Such as acute interstitial nephritis, glomerulopathies, and malignant hypertension
- Postrenal
  - Resulting from urine flow obstruction outside kidney (ureters or bladder neck)

Treatment
- Underlying condition
- Dialysis
- Monitoring of fluid and electrolyte balance

Chronic Renal Failure
Gradual loss of function
- Progressively more severe renal insufficiency until end stage of
  - Renal disease
  - Irreversible kidney failure

Stages—based on level of creatinine clearance
- Stage I: Blood flow through kidney increases, kidney enlarges
- Stage II: (mild) Small amounts of blood protein (albumin) leak into urine (microalbuminuria)

Stage III: (moderate) Albumin and other protein losses increase; patient may develop high blood pressure and kidney loses ability to filter waste

Stage IV: (severe) Large amounts of urine pass through kidney; blood pressure increases

Stage V: End-stage renal failure. Ability to filter waste nearly stops; dialysis or transplant only option

Cause
Long-term exposure to nephrotoxins

Diabetes

Hypertension

Symptoms
No symptoms until well advanced

Polyuria

Nausea or anorexia

Dehydration

Neurologic manifestations

Stages of nephron loss
Decreased reserve
- 60% loss

Renal insufficiency
- 75% loss

End-stage renal failure
- 90% loss

Treatment
No cure

Dialysis

Kidney transplant

Urinary Tract Infections (UTI)

Cystitis—Bacterial
Cause
Bacteria, usually *E. coli*

Symptoms
Lower abdominal pain

Dysuria

Lower back pain

Urinary frequency and urgency

Cloudy, foul-smelling urine

Systemic signs
Fever

Malaise

Nausea

Treatment
Antibiotics

Increased fluid intake

Cystitis—Nonbacterial
Cause
Unknown

May later produce bacterial infection

Symptoms
Urinary frequency and urgency

Dysuria

Negative urine culture

Treatment
No known treatment

Acute Pyelonephritis (Fig. 1-34)
Bacterial infection with multiple abcesses of renal pelvis and medullary tissue

- May involve one or both kidneys

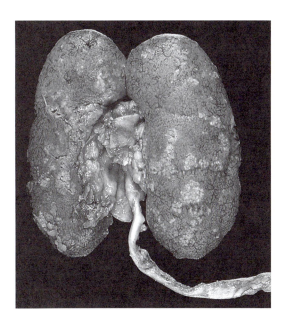

Figure **1-34** Acute pyelonephritis. Cortical surface exhibits grayish white areas of inflammation and abscess formation. (From Kumar V, Abbas AK, Fausto N: *Robbins and Cotran Pathologic Basis of Disease*, ed 7, Philadelphia, 2005, Saunders.)

Cause
    E. coli

    Proteus

    Pseudomonas

    Obstruction and reflux of urine from bladder

Symptoms
    Fever

    Chills

    Groin or flank pain

    Dysuria

    Pyuria

    Nocturia

Treatment
    Antibiotics

    Surgical correction of obstruction

Chronic Pyelonephritis

Recurrent infection that causes scarring of kidney

Cause is difficult to determine

- Repeated infections
- Obstructive conditions

Symptoms
    Hypertension

    Dysuria

    Flank pain

    Increased frequency of urination

Treatment
    Antibiotics for extended periods when reoccurring

    Surgical reduction of obstruction

Glomerular Disorders

May be acute or chronic

Function of glomerulus is blood filtration

Glomerulonephritis

Inflammation of glomerulus

Cause
    Drugs or toxins

    Systemic disorder affecting many organs or idiopathic

    May follow acute infections—most commonly streptococcal infections

    Vascular pathology

    Immune disorders

Treatment
Follows cause

Nephrotic Syndrome (Nephrosis)
Disease of kidneys that includes damage to membrane of the glomerulus causing excessive protein loss to urine

Accompanied by
- Hypoalbuminemia
- Hypercholesterolemia
- Hypercoagulability (excessive clotting)
- Prone to infections
- Edema
- Protein loss of >3.5 g

Damage to glomerulus results from
- Infection
- Immune response
  - Most predominant cause of dysfunction is exposure to toxins

May be a manifestation of an underlying condition, such as diabetes

Symptoms
Edema
Weight gain
Pallor
Proteinuria
Lipiduria

Treatment
Glucocorticoids, such as prednisone
- Reduces inflammation

Sodium and fat reduced diet
Protein supplements
Careful monitoring for continued inflammation

Acute Poststreptococcal Glomerulonephritis (APSGN)
Cause
Streptococcus infection
- With certain types of group A beta-hemolytic *Streptococcus*

Creates an antigen-antibody complex
- Infiltrates glomerular capillaries
- Results in inflammation in kidneys
- Inflammation interferes with normal kidney function
- Fluid and waste build-up
- Can lead to acute renal failure and scarring

Usually occurs in children 3 to 7 years of age
- Most often in boys

Symptoms
    Back and flank pain

    Cloudy, dark urine

    Oliguria (decreased output)

    Edema

    Elevated blood pressure

    Fatigue

    Malaise

    Headache

    Nausea

Treatment
    Sodium reduction

    Antibiotics

    Careful monitoring for continued inflammation

Urinary Tract Obstructions

Interference with urine flow

Causes urine backup behind obstruction of urinary system

Damage occurs to structures behind blockages

Increased urinary tract infection

Obstruction can be

- Functional
- Anatomic
  - Also known as obstructive uropathy

Kidney Stones (nephrolithiasis—renal calculi)
Formed of mineral salts (uric and calcuim)

Develop anywhere in urinary tract

Tend to form in presence of excess salt and decreased fluid intake

- Most stones are formed of calcium salts
- Staghorn calculus forms in renal pelvis

Symptoms
    Asymptomatic until obstruction occurs

    Obstruction results in renal colic

- Extremely intense pain in flank
- Nausea
- Vomiting
- Cold, clammy skin
- Increased pulse rate

Urinary System—Pathophysiology

Treatment
Stone usually passes spontaneously

May use extracorporeal ultrasound or laser lithotripsy to break up stone (also known as extracorporeal shock wave lithotripsy or ESWL)

Drugs may be used to dissolve stone

Preventative treatment to adjust pH level

- Increased fluid intake

Bladder Carcinoma
Malignant tumor
Most common site of malignancy in urinary system

Tumors originate in transitional epithelial lining

Tends to recur

Often metastatic to liver and bone

Tumor staging for renal cancer
Stage I tumor of kidney capsule only

Stage II tumor invading renal capsule/vein but within fascia

Stage III tumor extending to regional lymph/vena cava

Stage IV other organ metatasis

Symptoms
Often asymptomatic in early stage

Hematuria

Dysuria

Frequent urination

Infections common

Increased Risks
Cigarette smoking

Males age 50+

Working with industrial chemicals

Analgesics used in large amounts

Recurrent bladder infections

Treatment
Immunotherapy (bacillus Calmette-Guérin vaccine, BCG)

Excision

Chemotherapy

Radiation therapy

Hydronephrosis
Distention of kidney with urine

- Due to an obstruction
- Usually as a result of a kidney stone

- May also be due to scarring, tumor, edema from infection, or other obstruction

Symptoms
Usually asymptomatic

Mild flank pain

Infection may develop

May lead to chronic renal failure

Treatment
Treat underlying condition, such as removal of stone or antibiotics for infection

Dilation of stricture

Vascular Disorders

Nephrosclerosis
Excessive hardening and thickening of vascular structure of kidney

- Reduces blood supply
  - Increases blood pressure
  - Results in atrophy and ischemia of structures
  - May lead to chronic renal failure

Symptoms
Asymptomatic in early stages

Treatment
Diuretics

ACE (angiotensin-converting enzyme) inhibitors

Beta blockers that block release of resin

Antihypertensive drugs

Sodium intake reduction

Congenital Disorders

Polycystic Kidney (PKD)
Numerous kidney cysts

Genetic disease

Symptoms
Asymptomatic until 40s

Cysts progressive in development (both kidneys)

Nephromegaly, hematuria, URT, hypertension, uremia

Develops chronic renal failure

Cysts may spread to other organs, such as liver

Treatment
As for chronic renal failure

Urinary System—Pathophysiology

Wilms' Tumor—Nephroblastoma

Usually unilateral kidney tumors

Most common tumor in children

Usually advanced at time of diagnosis

- Metastasis to lungs at time of diagnosis is common

Symptoms

Asymptomatic until abdominal mass becomes apparent at age 1 to 5

Treatment

Excision

Radiation therapy

Chemotherapy

Usually a combination of above

URINARY SYSTEM PATHOPHYSIOLOGY QUIZ

1. Which of the following is NOT a type of acute renal failure?
   a. prerenal
   b. intrarenal
   c. interrenal
   d. postrenal

2. The loss of nephron function in end-stage renal disease is:
   a. 60%
   b. 70%
   c. 80%
   d. 90%

3. The cause of bacterial cystitis is usually:
   a. Proteus
   b. *Pseudomonas*
   c. *Staphylococci*
   d. *E. coli*

4. The primary treatment for acute pyelonephritis would be:
   a. prednisone
   b. sodium reduction
   c. antibiotics
   d. BCG

5. APSGN stands for:
   a. advanced poststaphylococcal glomerulonephritis
   b. acute poststreptococcal glomerulonephritis
   c. acute poststaphylococcal glomerulonephritis
   d. advanced poststreptococcal glomerulonephritis

6. Obstructive uropathy is also known as:
   a. pyelonephritis
   b. renal failure
   c. urinary tract obstruction
   d. nephrotic syndrome

7. A treatment for kidney stone may be:
   a. ESWL
   b. prednisone
   c. open surgical procedure
   d. diuretics

8. The treatment for hydronephrosis involves:
   a. an open surgical procedure
   b. use of diuretics
   c. treatment of the underlying condition
   d. BCG

UNIT I Anatomy, Terminology, and Pathophysiology

9. This is a congential condition in which numerous cysts form in the kidney:
   a. Wilms' tumor
   b. polycystic kidney
   c. nephrosclerosis
   d. nephrotic syndrome

10. The treatment of Wilms' tumor would NOT include which of the following?
    a. excision
    b. chemotherapy
    c. diuretic
    d. radiation therapy

DIGESTIVE SYSTEM

DIGESTIVE SYSTEM—ANATOMY AND TERMINOLOGY

Function: digestion, absorption, and elimination

Includes gastrointestinal tract (alimentary canal) and accessory organs

Mouth (Fig. 1–35)

Roof: hard palate, soft palate, uvula (projection at back of mouth)

Floor: contains tongue (Fig. 1–36), muscles, taste buds, and lingual frenulum, which anchors tongue to floor of mouth

Teeth

Thirty-two teeth (permanent)

Names of teeth: incisor, cuspid, bicuspid, and tricuspid

Tooth has crown (outer portion), neck (narrow part below gum line), root (end section), and pulp cavity (core)

Salivary Glands (Fig. 1–37)

Surround mouth and produce saliva—1.5 liters daily

Parotid

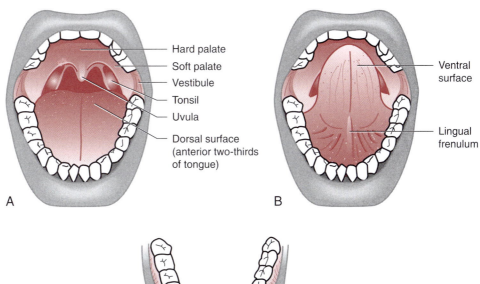

Figure **1-35** Anatomic structures of the mouth.

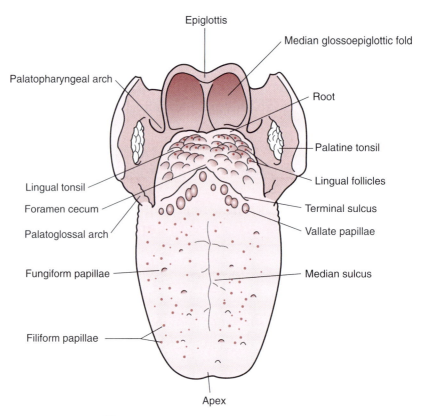

Figure **1-36** Dorsum of the tongue.

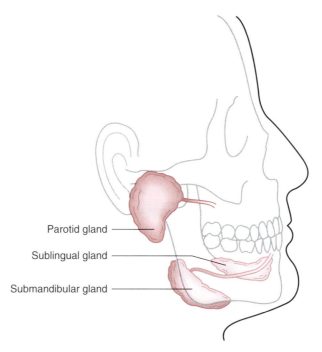

Figure **1-37** Major salivary glands.

Submandibular

Sublingual

Pharynx or Throat (Fig. 1–38)

Muscular tube (5 inches long) lined with mucus membrane through which air and food/water travel

Epiglottis covers larynx/esophagus when swallowing

Esophagus

Muscular tube (9-10 inches long) that carries food from pharynx to stomach by means of peristalsis (rhythmic contractions)

Stomach

Sphincter (ring of muscles) at entry into stomach (gastroesophageal or cardiac)

Three parts of stomach:

   Fundus (upper part)

   Body (middle part)

   Antrum/pylorus (lower part)

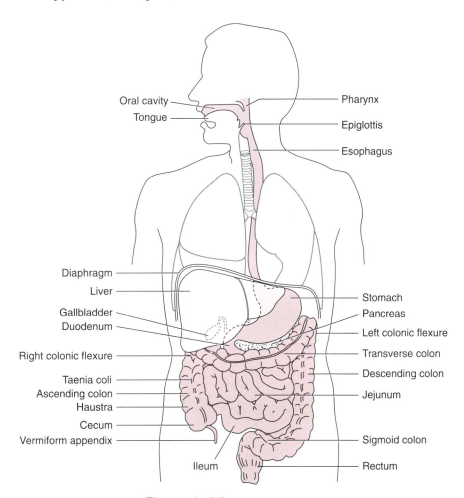

Figure **1-38** Digestive system.

Lined with rugae (folds of mucosal membrane)

Pyloric sphincter opens to allow chyme (thick liquid) to leave stomach and enter small intestine

Small Intestine

Duodenum (2 inches long): first portion beyond stomach—bile and pancreatic juice delivered here

Jejunum (96 inches long): connects duodenum to ileum

Ileum (132 inches long): attaches to large intestine

Large Intestine

Extends from ileum to anus

Cecum, from which appendix extends, connects ileum and colon

Colon (60 inches long), divided into:

 Ascending

 Transverse

 Descending

 Sigmoid

Sigmoid colon, connected to rectum, which terminates at anus

Accessory Organs

Liver produces bile, sent to gallbladder via hepatic duct and cystic duct

Gallbladder stores bile, sent to duodenum from cystic duct into common bile duct

Bile emulsifies fat (breaks up large globules)

Pancreas produces enzymes sent through pancreatic duct to hepatopancreatic ampulla (ampulla of Vater) then to duodenum

Pancreatic cells—Islets of Langerhans produce insulin and glucagon

Peritoneum

Serous membrane lines abdominal cavity and maintains organs in correct anatomic position

Food passes through digestive tract via:

 Mouth—including salivary glands

 Pharynx

 Esophagus

 Stomach

 Duodenum—pancreatic enzymes and bile produced in liver and stored in gallbladder enter

 Jejunum

Ileum

Cecum

Ascending colon

Transverse colon

Descending colon

Sigmoid colon

Rectum

Anus

COMBINING FORMS

1.	abdomin/o	abdomen
2.	an/o	anus
3.	appendic/o	appendix
4.	bil/i	bile
5.	bilirubin/o	bile pigment
6.	bucc/o	cheek
7.	cec/o	cecum
8.	celi/o	abdomen
9.	cheil/o	lip
10.	chol/e	gall/bile
11.	cholangio/o	bile duct
12.	cholecyst/o	gallbladder
13.	choledoch/o	common bile duct
14.	col/o	colon
15.	dent/i	tooth
16.	diverticul/o	diverticulum
17.	duoden/o	duodenum
18.	enter/o	small intestine
19.	esophag/o	esophagus
20.	faci/o	face
21.	gastr/o	stomach
22.	gingiv/o	gum
23.	gloss/o	tongue
24.	hepat/o	liver
25.	herni/o	hernia
26.	ile/o	ileum
27.	jejun/o	jejunum

UNIT I Anatomy, Terminology, and Pathophysiology

28.	labi/o	lip
29.	lapar/o	abdomen
30.	lingu/o	tongue
31.	lip/o	fat
32.	lith/o	stone
33.	or/o	mouth
34.	ordont/o	tooth
35.	palat/o	palate
36.	pancreat/o	pancreas
37.	peritone/o	peritoneum
38.	pharng/o	throat
39.	polyp/o	polyp
40.	proct/o	rectum
41.	pylor/o	pylorus
42.	rect/o	rectum
43.	sial/o	saliva
44.	sialaden/o	salivary gland
45.	sigmoid/o	sigmoid colon
46.	steat/o	fat
47.	stomat/o	mouth
48.	uvul/o	uvula

SUFFIXES

1.	-ase	enzyme
2.	-cele	hernia
3.	-chezia	defecation
4.	-iasis	abnormal condition
5.	-phagia	eating
6.	-prandial	meal

MEDICAL ABBREVIATIONS

1.	EGD	esophagogastroduodenoscopy
2.	EGJ	esophagogastric junction
3.	ERCP	endoscopic retrograde cholangiopancreatography
4.	GERD	gastroesophageal reflux disease
5.	GI	gastrointestinal
6.	HJR	hepatojugular reflux

7. LLQ   left lower quadrant
8. LUQ   left upper quadrant
9. PEG   percutaneous endoscopic gastrostomy
10. RLQ   right lower quadrant
11. RUQ   right upper quadrant

MEDICAL TERMS

Anastomosis	Surgical connection of two tubular structures, such as two pieces of intestine
Biliary	Refers to gallbladder, bile, or bile duct
Cholangiography	Radiographic recording of bile ducts
Cholecystectomy	Surgical removal of gallbladder
Cholecystoenterostomy	Creation of a connection between gallbladder and intestine
Colonoscopy	Fiberscopic examination of entire colon that may include part of terminal ileum
Colostomy	Artificial opening between colon and abdominal wall
Diverticulum	Protrusion in wall of an organ
Dysphagia	Difficulty swallowing
Enterolysis	Releasing of adhesions of intestine
Eventration	Protrusion of bowel through an opening in abdomen
Evisceration	Pulling viscera outside of the body through an incision
Exstrophy	Condition in which an organ is turned inside out
Fulguration	Use of electric current to destroy tissue
Gastrointestinal	Pertaining to stomach and intestine
Gastroplasty	Operation on stomach for repair or reconfiguration
Gastrostomy	Artificial opening between stomach and abdominal wall
Hernia	Organ or tissue protruding through wall or cavity that usually contains it
Ileostomy	Artificial opening between ileum and abdominal wall
Imbrication	Overlapping
Incarcerated	Regarding hernias, a constricted, irreducible hernia that may cause obstruction of an intestine
Intussusception	Slipping of one part of intestine into another part
Jejunostomy	Artificial opening between jejunum and abdominal wall
Laparoscopy	Exploration of the abdomen and pelvic cavities using a scope placed through a small incision in abdominal wall
Lithotomy	Incision into an organ or a duct for the purpose of removing a stone
Lithotripsy	Crushing of a stone by sound wave or force

UNIT I   Anatomy, Terminology, and Pathophysiology

Paraesophageal or hiatal hernia	Protrusion of any structure through esophageal hiatus of diaphragm
Proctosigmoidoscopy	Fiberscopic examination of sigmoid colon and rectum
Sialolithotomy	Surgical removal of a stone of salivary gland or duct
Varices	Varicose veins
Volvulus	Twisted section of intestine

DIGESTIVE SYSTEM ANATOMY AND TERMINOLOGY QUIZ

1. This is NOT a part of the small intestine:
   a. ileum
   b. cecum
   c. duodenum
   d. jejunum

2. Term meaning a ring of muscles:
   a. pyloric
   b. parotid
   c. epiglottis
   d. sphincter

3. The throat is also known as the:
   a. larynx
   b. epiglottis
   c. esophagus
   d. pharynx

4. The three parts of the stomach:
   a. pyloric, rugae, fundus
   b. fundus, body, antrum
   c. antrum, pyloric, rugae
   d. ilium, fundus, pyloric

5. The projection at the back of the mouth:
   a. palate
   b. sublingual
   c. uvula
   d. parotid

6. Mucosal membrane that lines the stomach:
   a. cecum
   b. rugae
   c. frenulum
   d. fundus

7. The parts of the colon are:
   a. ascending, transverse, descending, sigmoid
   b. ascending, descending, sigmoid
   c. transverse, descending, sigmoid
   d. descending, sigmoid

8. Combining form meaning abdomen:
   a. an/o
   b. cec/o
   c. celi/o
   d. col/o

UNIT I Anatomy, Terminology, and Pathophysiology

9. Term that means connecting two ends of a tube:
   a. anastomosis
   b. amylase
   c. aphthous stomatitis
   d. atresia

10. Abbreviation that means a scope placed through the esophagus, into the stomach, and to the duodenum:
    a. ERCP
    b. EGD
    c. GERD
    d. PEG

DIGESTIVE SYSTEM—PATHOPHYSIOLOGY

Disorders of Oral Cavity

Cleft Lip and Cleft Palate (Orofacial Cleft) (Fig. 1-39)
Congenital defect

Cleft lip and palate

    Lip and palate do not properly join together

Causes feeding problems

- Infants cannot create sufficient suction for feeding
- Danger of aspirating food
- Results in speech defects

Treatment
    Surgical repair of defects

Ulceration
Canker sore—caused by herpes simplex virus

- Ulceration of oral mucosa

Also known as

- Aphthous ulcer (aphtha: small ulcer)
- Aphthous stomatitis

Heals spontaneously

Infections
Candidiasis
Candida albicans is naturally found in mouth

Thrush (oral candidiasis) is overarching infection

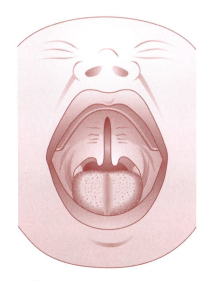

Figure **1-39** Cleft palate.

Causes

Antibiotic regimen

Chemotherapy

Glucocorticoids

Common in diabetics and AIDS patients

Treatment

Nystatin (topical fungal agent)

Herpes simplex type 1

Herpetic stomatitis

- Viral cold sores and blisters
- Associated with herpes simplex virus type 1 (HSV-1)

Treatment

No cure

May be alleviated somewhat by antiviral medications

Cancer of Oral Cavity

Most common type is squamous cell carcinoma

- Kaposi's sarcoma is type seen in AIDS patients

Increased in smokers

    Lip cancer also increased in smokers, particularly pipe

Poor prognosis

Usually asymptomatic until later stages

Metastasis through lymph nodes

Esophageal Disorders

Scleroderma

Also known as progressive systemic sclerosis

Atrophy of smooth muscles of lower esophagus

Lower esophageal sphincter (LES) does not close properly

- Leads to esophageal reflux
- Strictures form

Symptom

Predominantly dysphagia

Esophagitis

Inflammation of esophagus

Types

Acute

Most common type is that caused by hiatal hernia

Infectious esophagitis is common in patients with AIDS

Ingestion of strong alkaline or acid substances

- Such as those in household cleaners

Inflammation leads to scarring

Chronic
Most common type is that caused by LES reflux

Cancer of Esophagus
Most common type is squamous cell or secondary adenocarcinoma

Usually caused by continued irritation

- Smoking
- Alcohol
- Hiatal hernia
- Chronic esophagitis/GERD

Poor prognosis

Hiatal Hernia (Diaphragmatic hernia)
Diaphragm goes over stomach

- Esophagus passes through diaphragm at natural opening (hiatus)
- Part of the stomach protrudes (herniates) through opening in diaphragm into thorax

Types (Fig. 1–40)
Sliding

- Stomach and gastroesophageal junction protrude through the hiatus

Paraesophageal/rolling hiatal

- Part of fundus protrudes

Symptoms
   Heartburn

   Reflux

   Belching

   Lying down causes discomfort

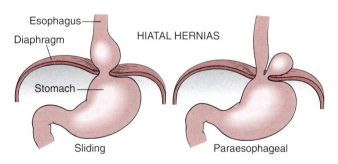

Figure **1-40** Sliding and paraesophageal hernias (hiatal hernias).

Dysphagia

Substernal pain after eating

Gastroesophageal Reflux Disease (GERD)
Associated with hiatal hernias

- Reflux of gastric contents

Lower esophageal sphincter does not constrict properly

Treatment
Reduce irritants, such as

- Smoking
- Spicy foods
- Alcohol

Antacids

Elevate head of bed

Avoid tight clothing

Stomach and Duodenum Disorders

Gastritis
Inflammation of stomach mucosa

Acute superficial gastritis
Mild, transient irritation

Causes
Excessive alcohol

Infection

Food allergies

Spicy foods

Aspirin

H. pylori (Helicobacter pylori)

Symptoms
Nausea

Vomiting

Anorexia

Bleeding in more severe cases

Epigastric pain

Treatment
Usually spontaneous remission in 2 to 3 days

Removal of underlying irritation

Antibiotics for infection

Chronic atrophic gastritis
Progressive atrophy of epithelium

Types

Type A, atrophic or fundal

- Involves fundus of stomach
- Autoimmune disease
  - Decreases acid secretion
  - Results in high gastrin levels

Type B, antral

- Involves antrum region of stomach
- Often associated with elderly
  - May be associated with pernicious anemia
- Low gastrin levels
- Usually caused by infection
- Irritated by alcohol, drugs, and tobacco

Symptom abatement

- Bland diet
- Alcohol avoidance
- ASA avoidance
- Antibiotics for *H. pylori*

Peptic Ulcers

Erosive area on mucosa

- Extends below epithelium
- Chronic ulcers have scar tissue at base of erosive area

Ulcers can occur anyplace on gastrointestinal tract but typically are found on the

- Lower esophagus
- Stomach
- Proximal duodenum

Some causes

Alcohol

Smoking

Aspirin

Severe stress

Bacterial infection caused by *Helicobacter pylori (H. pylori)*, 90% of the time

Genetic factor

Constant use of anti-inflammatory drugs

Symptoms

Epigastric pain when stomach is empty

- Relieved by food or antacid

Burning

May include
- Vomiting blood
- Nausea
- Weight loss
- Anorexia

Severe cases may include
- Obstruction
- Hemorrhage
- Perforation

Treatment
Surgical intervention

Antacids

Dietary restrictions

Rest

Antibiotics

Gastric Cancer (malignant tumor of stomach)
Most often occurs in men over 40

Cause is unknown, but often associated with *Helicobacter pylori* (bacterial infection)

Predisposing Factors
Atrophic gastritis

Pernicious anemia

History of nonhealing gastric ulcer

Blood type A

Geographic factors

Environmental factors

Carcinogenic foods
- Smoked meats
- Nitrates
- Pickled foods

Symptoms
Usually asymptomatic in early stages

Treatment
Excision

Chemotherapy

Radiation (not good response)

Prognosis is poor

Pyloric Stenosis
Narrowing of the pyloric sphincter

Signs appear soon after birth
- Failure to thrive
- Projectile vomiting

Treatment
Surgery to relieve stenosis (pyloromyotomy)

Intestinal Disorders

■ Small Intestine

Malabsorption Conditions

Celiac disease
Most important malabsorption condition

Villi atrophy in response to food containing gluten and lose ability to absorb

- Gluten is a protein found in wheat, rye, oats, and barley

Symptoms
Malnutrition

Muscle wasting

Distended abdomen

Diarrhea

Fatigue

Weakness

Steatorrhea (excess fat in feces)

Treatment
Gluten-free diet

Steroids when necessary

Lactase deficiency
Enzyme deficiency

- Secondary to gastrointestinal damage, such as
  - Regional enteritis
  - Infection
- Common in blacks, occurring in adulthood

Symptoms
Intolerance to milk

Intestinal cramping

Diarrhea

Flatulence

Treatment
Elimination of milk products

Crohn's disease (regional enteritis)
Inflammatory bowel disease (IBD)—affects terminal ileum and colon

Cause
Unknown

Symptoms
Vary greatly/inflammatory disease of GI tract

Diarrhea

Gas

Fever

Abdominal pain

Malaise

Anorexia

Weight loss

Treatment
No specific treatment

Palliative medications to control symptoms

Resection of affected section of intestine with anastomosis

Diet modifications

Duodenal Ulcers
Most common ulcer

Develop in younger population

Common in type O blood types

Appendicitis
Inflammation of vermiform appendix that projects from cecum

Obstruction of lumen leads to infection

- Appendix becomes hypoxic (decreased oxygen levels)
- May cause gangrene
- May rupture, causing peritonitis

Symptoms
Periumbilical (around umbilicus) pain, initially

Right lower quadrant (RLQ) pain as inflammation progresses

Nausea

Vomiting

Possible diarrhea

Treatment
Appendectomy

Management of any perforation or abscess

Meckel's Diverticulum—an appendage of ileum near cecum derived from an unobliterated yolk stalk in fetal development. Symptoms can mimic appendicitis.

Peritonitis
Inflammation of peritoneum (membrane that lines abdominal cavity)

Usually a result of

- Spread of infection from abdominal organ
- Puncture wound to abdomen
- Rupture of gastrointestinal tract—appendicitis or Meckel's diverticulum

Abscesses form, resulting in adhesions

- May result in obstruction

Types
Acute

Chronic

Symptoms
Abdominal pain

Vomiting

Rigid abdomen

Fever

Leukocytosis (increased white cells in blood)

Treatment
Antibiotics

Suction of stomach and intestines

If possible, surgical removal of origin of infection, such as appendix

Fluid replacement

Bed rest

Obstruction
Any interference with passage of intestinal contents

May be

- Acute
- Chronic
- Partial
- Total

Types
Nonmechanical
- Paralytic ileus
- Result of trauma or toxin

Mechanical
- Result of tumors, adhesions, hernias
- Simple mechanical obstruction
  - One point of obstruction
- Closed-loop obstruction
  - At least two points of obstruction

Diverticulosis

  Twisted bowel (volvulus)

  Telescoping bowel (intussception)

Symptoms
Abdominal distention

Pain

Vomiting

Total constipation

Treatment
Surgical intervention

Symptomatic treatment

Large Intestine

Diverticulosis

Herniation of intestinal mucosa

- Forms sacs in lining, called diverticula

Diverticulitis

Sacs fill and become inflamed

- Common in aged

Symptoms
- Diarrhea or constipation
- Gas
- Abdominal discomfort

Complications
- Perforation
- Bleeding
- Peritonitis
- Abscess
- Obstruction

Treatment
- Antimicrobials as necessary
- High-fiber diet (greater than 20 g daily)
- Stool softeners
- Dietary restrictions of solid foods
- Surgical intervention if necessary

Ulcerative Colitis (Fig. 1-41)

Inflammation of rectum that progresses to sigmoid colon

Intermittent exacerbations and remissions

May develop into toxic megacolon

- Leads to obstruction and dilation of colon

Increased risk of colorectal cancer

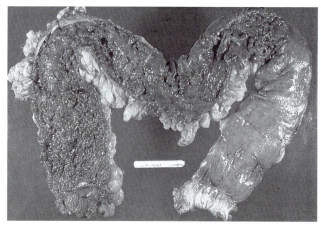

Figure **1-41** Ulcerative colitis. (From Damjanov I: *Pathology for the Health Professions,* ed 3, St. Louis, 2006, Saunders.)

Symptoms
Diarrhea
- Blood and mucus may be present

Cramping

Fever

Weight loss

Treatment
Remove physical or emotional stressors

Anti-inflammatory medications

Antimotility agents

Nutritional supplementation

Surgical intervention, if necessary

Colorectal Cancer
Usually develop from polyp
- In those 55 and older

Increased risks
Genetic factors

40 years of age and older

Diets high in
- Fat
- Sugar
- Red meat

Low-fiber diets

Symptoms
Asymptomatic until advanced

Some may experience
- Cramping
- Ribbon stools
- Feeling of incomplete evacuation
- Fatigue
- Weight loss
- Change in bowel habits
- Blood in stool

Treatment
Surgical excision

Radiation

Chemotherapy

Combination of above

Disorders of Liver, Gallbladder, and Pancreas

Disorders of Liver

Jaundice (Hyperbilirubinemia)
A symptom of biliary disease, not a disease itself

- Results in yellow eyes (sclera) and skin

Types
Prehepatic

- Excess destruction of red blood cells
- Result of hemolytic anemia or reaction to transfusion

Intrahepatic

- Impaired uptake of bilirubin and decreased blending of bilirubin by hepatic cells
- Result of liver disease, such as cirrhosis or hepatitis

Posthepatic

- Excess bile flows into blood
- Result of obstruction
  - Due to conditions such as inflammation of liver, tumors, cholelithiasis

Treatment
Removal of cause

Cancer of Liver
Most commonly a metastasis/primary CA rare

Risk for primary liver CA

- Hepatitis B, C, and D
- Cirrhosis
- Myotoxins
- Heavy smoking/alcohol use

Treatment
Surgical resection if localized

Survival typically 3 or 4 months

Viral Hepatitis
Liver cells are damaged

Results in inflammation and necrosis

Damage can be mild or severe

Scar tissue forms in liver

- Leads to ischemia

Hepatitis A (HAV)
Infectious hepatitis—caused by hepatitis A virus

Transmission

- Most commonly oral-fecal route—contaminated food or water

Does not have a chronic state

Slow onset—complete recovery characteristic

Vaccine available for those who are traveling

Gamma globulin may be administered to those just exposed

Hepatitis B (HBV)
Serum hepatitis

Carrier state is common

Caused by hepatitis B virus

- Asymptomatic but contagious

Long incubation period

Transmission

- Intravenous drug users
- Transfusion
- Exposure to blood and bodily fluids
- Sexual transmission
- Mother-to-fetus transmission
- Immune globulin is temporary prophylactic
- Vaccine is now routine for children and is given to those at risk

Severe forms cause liver cell destruction, cirrhosis, death

Hepatitis C (HCV)
Transmission of virus

- Most commonly by transfusion
- IV drug users

Half of cases develop into chronic hepatitis

Increases risk of hepatocellular cancer

Carrier state may develop

Hepatitis D (HDV)
Transmission of hepatitis D virus

- Blood
- Intravenous drug users

Hepatitis B is present for this type to develop

Hepatitis E (HEV)
Transmission of hepatitis E virus

- Oral-fecal route

Does not develop into chronic or carrier

Hepatitis G
Transmission of hepatitis G virus

- IV drug use
- Sexual transmission

Symptoms of hepatitis
Stages
Preicteric
- Anorexia
- Nausea and vomiting

Liver enzymes may be elevated—indication of liver cell damage
- Fatigue
- Malaise
- Generalized pain with low grade fever
- Cough

Icteric
- Jaundice
- Hepatomegaly (enlarged liver)
- Biliary obstruction
- Light-colored stools and dark urine
- Pruritus
- Abdominal pain

Posticteric (recovery)
- Reduction of symptoms

Treatment
None

In early stages gamma globulins may be used

Interferon may be used for cases of chronic hepatitis B and C

Nonviral hepatitis
Hepatitis that results from hepatotoxins

Symptoms
- Similar to viral hepatitis

Treatment
- Removal of hepatotoxin

Cirrhosis
Profuse liver damage
- Extensive fibrosis
  - Results in inflammation

Progressive disorder

Leads to liver failure

Types
Alcoholic liver
- Known as Laënnec's cirrhosis or portal
- Largest group

Biliary
- Associated with immune disorders

- Obstructions (intrahepatic or extrahepatic blood vessels) occur and disrupt normal function

Postnecrotic

- Associated with chronic hepatitis (A or C) and exposure to toxins

Symptoms
Asymptomatic in early stages

Nausea

Vomiting

Fatigue

Weight loss

Pruritus

Jaundice

Edema

Treatment
Symptomatic

Dietary restrictions

- Reduced protein and sodium
- Increased vitamins and carbohydrates

Diuretics

Antibiotics

Liver transplant

■ Disorders of Gallbladder

Cholecystitis
Inflammation of gallbladder and cystic duct

Cholangitis
Inflammation of bile duct

Cholelithiasis
Formation of gallstones (Fig. 1–42)

- Consists of cholesterol or bilirubin

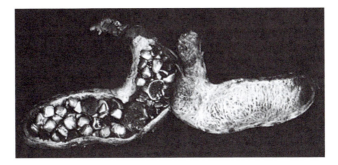

Figure **1-42** Resected gallbladder containing mixed gallstones. (From Kissane JM, editor: *Anderson's pathology*, ed 9, St Louis, 1990, Mosby.)

- Occurs most often in those with high levels of cholesterol, calcium, or bile salts

Stones cause irritation and inflammation
- May lead to infection
- Obstruction
  - May result in pancreatitis
  - Rupture is possible

Symptoms
Often asymptomatic

Dietary intolerance particularly to fat

Right upper quadrant (RUQ) pain

Pain in back and/or shoulder

Epigastric discomfort

Bloating heartburn, flatulence

Treatment
Surgical intervention (laparoscopic cholecystectomy)

Lithotripsy

Medical management by use of drugs that break down stone

■ Disorders of Pancreas

Pancreatitis
Inflammation of pancreas resulting from digestive enzyme attack to pancreas

Acute and chronic forms

Commonly associated with alcoholism/biliary tract obstruction, drug toxicity, gallstone obstruction of common bile duct and viral infections

Symptoms
Severe pain

Fever

Acute form is a medical emergency

Neurogenic shock

Septicemia

General sepsis

Complications
Adult respiratory distress syndrome (ARDS)

Renal failure

Treatment
No oral intake
- IV fluids given and carefully monitored

Analgesics

Stop process of autodigestion

Prevent systemic shutdown

Pancreatic Cancer
Increased risk
Cigarette smoking

Diet high in fat and protein

Symptoms
Weight loss

Jaundice

Anorexia

Most types of pancreatic cancer are asymptomatic until well advanced

Treatment
Palliative

Pain management

DIGESTIVE SYSTEM PATHOPHYSIOLOGY QUIZ

1. This type of hyperbilirubinemia is hallmarked by excess bile flow into the blood:
   a. intrahepatic
   b. prehepatic
   c. posthepatic
   d. jaundice

2. This type of hepatitis is transmitted by the oral-fecal route:
   a. A
   b. B
   c. C
   d. D

3. Which of the following is the recovery stage of hepatitis?
   a. prehepatic
   b. posthepatic
   c. preicteric
   d. posticteric

4. This type of cirrhosis is also known as portal cirrhosis:
   a. biliary
   b. alcoholic liver
   c. postnecrotic
   d. traumatic

5. This condition is the inflammation of the bile ducts:
   a. cholangitis
   b. cholecystitis
   c. cholelithiasis
   d. cholangioma

6. Formation of gallstones most often occurs with high levels of the following:
   a. bile salts and toxins
   b. cholesterol and toxins
   c. cholesterol and bile salts
   d. toxins

7. The primary factor that increases the risk of pancreatic cancer is:
   a. smoking
   b. alcohol
   c. intravenous drug use
   d. hepatitis

8. A potential complication of this condition is ARDS:
   a. hyperbilirubinemia
   b. hepatitis
   c. pancreatitis
   d. pancreatic cancer

UNIT I Anatomy, Terminology, and Pathophysiology

9. The primary treatment for jaundice is:
   a. removal of cause
   b. antibiotics
   c. dialysis
   d. vaccine

10. This condition has as the largest group those that abuse alcohol:
    a. cirrhosis
    b. hepatitis
    c. pancreatitis
    d. pancreatic cancer

MEDIASTINUM AND DIAPHRAGM
MEDIASTINUM AND DIAPHRAGM—ANATOMY AND TERMINOLOGY

Not an organ system

Mediastinum

That area between lungs that a median (partition) divides (Fig. 1–43) into

- Superior
- Anterior
- Posterior
- Middle

Space that houses heart, thymus gland, trachea, esophagus, nerves, lymph and blood vessels and major blood vessels

- Aorta
- Inferior vena cava

Diaphragm

A dome-shaped muscular partition that separates abdominal cavity from thoracic cavity

- Assists in breathing
  - Expands to assist lungs in exhalation/relaxation of diaphragm
  - Flattens out during inspiration/contraction of diaphragm
- Diaphragmatic hernia: esophageal hernia

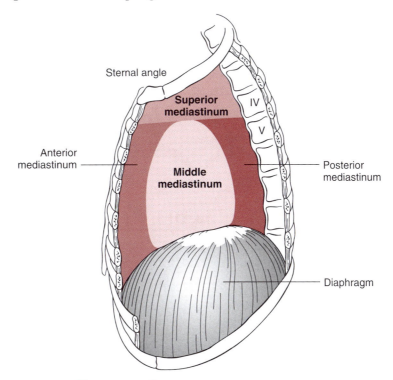

Figure **1-43** Mediastinum and diaphragm.

MEDIASTINUM AND DIAPHRAGM ANATOMY AND TERMINOLOGY QUIZ

1. The mediastinum is NOT an organ system.
   a. true
   b. false

2. The mediastinum is divided into:
   a. superior, anterior, posterior
   b. superior, anterior, posterior, middle
   c. anterior, posterior, middle
   d. middle, anterior, superior

3. During inspiration, the diaphragm:
   a. expands
   b. moves upward
   c. collapses
   d. flattens out

4. Term meaning partition:
   a. middle
   b. aspect
   c. median
   d. diaphragm

5. The diaphragm is said to be this shape:
   a. square
   b. flat
   c. dome
   d. round

6. This separates the abdominal cavity from the thoracic cavity:
   a. mediastinum
   b. diaphragm
   c. superior
   d. inferior

7. This is the area between the lungs:
   a. mediastinum
   b. diaphragm
   c. superior
   d. inferior

8. This is an esophageal hernia:
   a. mediastinal
   b. diaphragmatic
   c. paraesophageal
   d. hiatal

UNIT I Anatomy, Terminology, and Pathophysiology

9. A diaphragmatic hernia is also known as:
   a. esophageal
   b. epiglottis
   c. partitional
   d. medial

10. The diaphragm assists in:
    a. percussion
    b. auscultation
    c. contraction
    d. breathing

■ HEMIC AND LYMPHATIC SYSTEM
HEMIC AND LYMPHATIC SYSTEM—ANATOMY AND TERMINOLOGY

Hemic refers to blood

Lymphatic system removes excess tissue fluid

- Lymph tissue is scattered throughout body
- Composed of lymph nodes, vessels, and organs

Lymph

Colorless fluid containing lymphocytes and monocytes

Originates from blood and after filtering, returns to blood

Transports interstitial fluids and proteins that have leaked from blood system into venous system

Absorbs and transports fats from villi of small intestine to venous system

Assists in immune function

Lymph Vessels

Similar to veins

Organized circulatory system throughout body

Lymph Organs

Lymph nodes, spleen, bone marrow, thymus, tonsils, and Peyer's patches (lymphoid tissue on mucosa of small intestine)

Lymph nodes, areas of concentrated tissue (Fig. 1–44)

Spleen, located in left upper quadrant (LUQ) of abdomen

- Composed of lymph tissue
  - Function is to filter blood; activates lymphocytes and B-cells to filter antigens
  - Stores blood

Thymus secretes thymosin causing T-cells to mature

- Larger in infants and shrinks with age

Tonsils

- Palatine tonsils
- Pharyngeal tonsils/adenoids

Hematopoietic Organ

Bone marrow, contains tissue that produces RBCs, WBCs, and platelets

- Produces stem cells

COMBINING FORMS

1. aden/o   gland
2. adenoid/o   adenoids

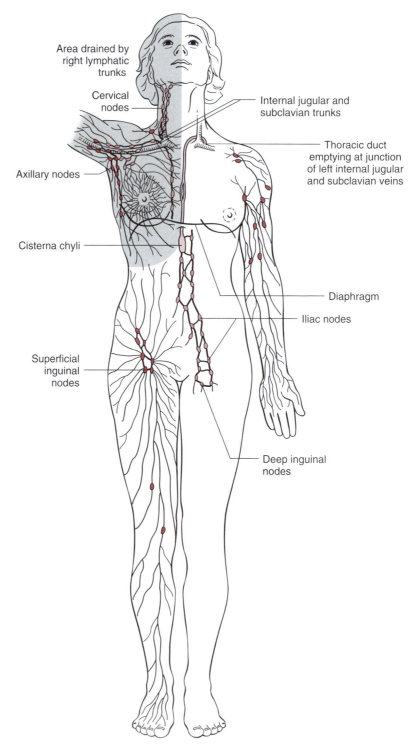

Figure **1-44** Lymphatic system.

Hemic and Lymphatic System—Anatomy and Terminology

3.	axill/o	armpit
4.	cervic/o	neck/cervix
5.	immun/o	immune
6.	inguin/o	groin
7.	lymph/o	lymph
8.	lymphaden/o	lymph gland
9.	splen/o	spleen
10.	thym/o	thymus gland
11.	tonsill/o	tonsil
12.	tox/o	poison

PREFIXES

1.	hyper-	excess
2.	inter-	between
3.	retro-	behind

SUFFIXES

1.	-ectomy	removal
2.	-edema	swelling
3.	-itis	inflammation
4.	-megaly	enlargement
5.	-oid	resembling
6.	-oma	tumor
7.	-penia	deficient
8.	-pexy	fixation
9.	-phylaxis	protection
10.	-poiesis	production

MEDICAL TERMS

Axillary nodes	Lymph nodes located in armpit
Cloquet's node	Also called a gland; it is highest of deep groin lymph nodes
Inguinofemoral	Referring to groin and thigh
Jugular nodes	Lymph nodes located next to large vein in neck
Lymph node	Station along lymphatic system
Lymphadenectomy	Excision of a lymph node or nodes
Lymphadenitis	Inflammation of a lymph node
Lymphangiography	Radiographic recording of lymphatic vessels and nodes

Lymphangiotomy	Incision into a lymphatic vessel
Lymphangitis	Inflammation of lymphatic vessel or vessels
Parathyroid	Produces a hormone to mobilize calcium from bones to blood
Splenectomy	Excision of spleen
Splenography	Radiographic recording of spleen
Splenoportography	Radiographic procedure to allow visualization of splenic and portal veins of spleen
Stem cell	Immature blood cell
Thoracic duct	Largest lymph vessel which collects lymph from portions of body below diaphragm and from left side of body above diaphragm
Transplantation	Grafting of tissue from one source to another

HEMIC AND LYMPHATIC SYSTEM ANATOMY AND TERMINOLOGY QUIZ

1. The spleen is located in this quadrant of the abdomen:
   a. RUQ
   b. LUQ
   c. LLQ
   d. LRQ

2. Produces RBCs and platelets:
   a. thymus
   b. tonsils
   c. lymph node
   d. bone marrow

3. Which of the following is NOT a lymph organ?
   a. adrenal
   b. spleen
   c. thymus
   d. tonsil

4. Lymph transports fluids and _____ that have leaked from the blood system back to veins.
   a. stem cells
   b. lymphocytes
   c. B-cells
   d. proteins

5. This is largest in infants and shrinks with age:
   a. tonsils
   b. spleen
   c. thymus
   d. bone marrow

6. Combining form meaning gland:
   a. axill/o
   b. thym/o
   c. aden/o
   d. tox/o

7. Prefix meaning excess:
   a. hyper-
   b. hypo-
   c. inter-
   d. retro-

8. Suffix meaning enlargement:
   a. -edema
   b. -poiesis
   c. -penia
   d. -megaly

UNIT I Anatomy, Terminology, and Pathophysiology

9. Lymph node located on neck:
   a. thoracic
   b. jugular
   c. Cloquet's
   d. axillary

10. These cells originate in the bone marrow:
    a. B-cells
    b. antigens
    c. erythrocytes
    d. stem cells

HEMIC AND LYMPHATIC SYSTEM—PATHOPHYSIOLOGY

Anemia

Reduction in number of erythrocytes or decrease in quality of hemoglobin

- Less oxygen is transported in the blood

Aplastic Anemia
Diverse group of anemias

Characterized by bone marrow failure with reduced numbers of red and white cells and platelets

Causes
Genetic or acquired (primary or secondary)

Toxins/chemical agents
    Benzene and antibiotics such as chloramphenicol

Irradiation

Immunologic

Idiopathic (unknown)

Treatment
Blood transfusion

Bone marrow transplant

Iron Deficiency Anemia
Characterized by small erythrocytes and a reduced amount of hemoglobin

Caused by low or absent iron stores or serum iron concentrations

- Blood loss
- Decreased intake of iron
- Malabsorption of iron

Symptoms
Pallor

Headache

Stomatitis

Oral lesions

Gastrointestinal complaints

Retinal hemorrhages

Thinning, brittle nails and hair

Treatment
Iron supplement

Pernicious Anemia
Megaloblastic anemia (large stem cells)

Inability to absorb vitamin B_{12} due to a lack of intrinsic factor (found in gastric juices)

Usually in older adults

Caused by impaired intestinal absorption of vitamin B_{12}

Symptoms
Pallor

Weakness

Neurologic manifestations

Gastric discomfort

Treatment
Injections of vitamin B_{12}

Transfusions

Hemolytic Anemia
May be acute or chronic

Shortened survival of mature erythrocytes—excessive destruction of RBC

- Inability of bone marrow to compensate for decreased survival of erythrocytes

Treatment
Treat cause

Sickle Cell Anemia
Occurs primarily in those of West African descent

Abnormal sickle-shaped erythrocytes (sickle cell) caused by an abnormal type of hemoglobin (hemoglobin S)

Symptoms
Abdominal pain

Arthralgia

Ulceration of lower extremities

Fatigue

Dyspnea

Increased heart rate

Treatment
Symptomatic

Granulocytosis

Increase in granulocytes

- Neutrophils
- Eosinophils
- Basophils

Eosinophilia

Increase in number of eosinophilic granulocytes

Cause
Allergic disorders

Dermatologic disorders

Parasitic invasion

Drugs

Malignancies

Basophilia
Increase in basophilic granulocytes seen in leukemia

Monocytosis
Increased number of monocytes

Cause
Infection

Hematologic factors

Leukocytosis
Increased number of leukocytes

Cause
Acute viral infections, such as hepatitis

Chronic infections, such as syphilis

Leukocytopenia
Decreased number of leukocytes

Cause
Neoplasias

Immune deficiencies

Drugs

Virus

Radiation

Infectious Mononucleosis
Acute Infection of B Cells
Epstein-Barr virus most common cause

Symptoms
Fatigue

Fever

Weakness (asthenia)

Pharyngitis

Atypical lymphocytes in blood

Lymph node enlargement

Splenomegaly

Hepatomegaly

Transmission
Saliva

- Known as kissing disease

Treatment
Rest

Treatment of symptoms

Leukemia

Malignant disorder of blood and blood-forming organs

Leads to dysfunction of cells

- Primarily leads to proliferation of abnormal leukocytes—filling bone marrow and bloodstream

Acute Myelogenous Leukemia (AML)
Rapid onset

Short survival time

Symptoms
Abrupt onset

Fatigue

Lymphadenopathy

Bone pain and tenderness

Anemia

Bleeding

Fever

Infection

Anorexia

Splenomegaly

Hepatomegaly

Headache, vomiting, paralysis

Treatment
Chemotherapy

Bone marrow transplant following high-dose chemotherapy eradicating leukemic cells

Acute Lymphocytic Leukemia (ALL)
Immature lymphocytes (lymphoblasts)

Most cases occur in children and adolescents

Sudden onset

Treatment
    Chemotherapy with drugs that suppress cell division/destroy rapid dividing cells

    Remission

    Relapse—leukemia cells in bone marrow and blood requiring treatment

Chronic Myelogenous Leukemia (CML)
Mature and immature granulocytes in bone marrow and blood

Slow progressive disease (those over 55 years live many years without life threat)

Cells are more differentiated

Gradual onset with milder symptoms

- Majority of cases are in adults

Symptoms
Extreme fatigue

Weight loss

Splenomegaly

Night sweats

Fever

Infections

Treatment
    Chemotherapy—target abnormal proteins

      Bone marrow transplant—following high-dose chemotherapy

Chronic Lymphocytic Leukemia (CLL)
Increased numbers of mature lymphocytes in marrow, lymph nodes, spleen

Most common form seen in elderly

Slowly progressive

Treatment
    Chemotherapy

Lymphadenopathy

Lymphadenopathy
Any abnormality of lymph node

Enlargement of lymph node

Lymphangitis
Inflammation of lymphatic vessel

Lymphadenitis
Inflammation of lymph node

Localized inflammation associated with inflamed lesion

Generalized inflammation associated with disease

Inflammation can occur as result of
- Trauma
- Infection
- Drug reaction
- Autoimmune disease
- Immunologic disease

Malignant Lymphoma

Hodgkin's Disease
Initial sign is a painless mass commonly located on neck

Giant Reed-Sternberg cells are present in lymphatic tissue

Presentation
Enlarged spleen (splenomegaly)

Abdominal mass

Mediastinal mass

Localized node involvement
- Orderly spreading of node involvement
- Cervical, axillary, inguinal, and retroperitoneal lymph node involvement

Symptoms
Night sweats

Fever

Weight loss

Itching (pruritus)

Anorexia

Weakness

Treatment
If localized: radiation therapy and chemotherapy

If systemic: chemotherapy alone

High probability of cure with new treatments

Non-Hodgkin's Lymphoma
No giant Reed-Sternberg cells present

Involves multiple nodes scattered throughout body (follicular lymphoma)

Large cell lymphoma (large lymphocytes in diffuse nodes and lymph tissue)
- Noncontiguous spread of node involvement
- Not localized

Usually begins as a painless enlargement of node

Symptoms
Presents similar to Hodgkin's disease

Treatment
Chemotherapy cures or stops disease progression

Burkitt's Lymphoma
Type of non-Hodgkin's lymphoma

Usually found in Africa and New Guinea

Characterized by lesions in jaw and face

Epstein-Barr (herpes virus) has been found in Burkitt's lymphoma

Treatment
Radiation and chemotherapy for African type

Myeloma

Multiple Myeloma
B-cell cancer—lymphocytes that produce antibodies destroying bone tissue

- Also known as plasma cell myeloma

Increased plasma cells replace bone marrow

Overproduction of immunoglobulins—Bence Jones protein (found in urine)

Multiple tumor sites cause bone destruction

Results in weakened bone

Hypercalcemia

Anemia

Renal damage

Increased susceptibility to infections

Cause
Unknown

Treatment
Chemotherapy

Radiotherapy

Autologous bone marrow transplant (ABMT)—prolongs remission—may be a cure

Palliative treatments

HEMIC AND LYMPHATIC SYSTEM PATHOPHYSIOLOGY QUIZ

1. This condition involves a reduced number of erythrocytes and decreased quality of hemoglobin:
   a. monocytosis
   b. eosinophilia
   c. anemia
   d. leukocytosis

2. This condition is hallmarked by a shortened survival of mature erythrocytes and inability of bone marrow to compensate for decreased survival:
   a. hemolytic anemia
   b. granulocytosis
   c. eosinophilia
   d. monocytosis

3. The most common cause of this disease is Epstein-Barr virus:
   a. leukocytopenia
   b. infectious mononucleosis
   c. leukocytosis
   d. hemolytic anemia

4. Inflammation of the lymphatic vessels is:
   a. lymphadenitis
   b. lymphoma
   c. lymphadenopathy
   d. lymphangitis

5. What giant cell is present in Hodgkin's disease?
   a. B cell
   b. Reed-Sternberg
   c. T cell
   d. C cell

6. The average number of years of survival for multiple myeloma is:
   a. 5
   b. 10
   c. 3
   d. 20

7. Injection of vitamin B may be prescribed for this type of anemia:
   a. pernicious
   b. aplastic
   c. sideroblastic
   d. sickle cell

8. These are large stem cells:
   a. megaloblasts
   b. leukocytes
   c. erythrocytes
   d. granulocytes

UNIT I   Anatomy, Terminology, and Pathophysiology

9. This is known as the kissing disease:
   a. monocytosis
   b. leukocytopenia
   c. infectious mononucleosis
   d. granulocytosis

10. This lymphoma is usually found in Africa:
    a. multiple
    b. Burkitt's
    c. B-cell
    d. T-cell

ENDOCRINE SYSTEM

ENDOCRINE SYSTEM—ANATOMY AND TERMINOLOGY

Regulates body through hormones (chemical messengers)

Ductless endocrine glands secrete hormones directly to bloodstream

Affects growth, development, and metabolism

Endocrine Glands (Fig. 1-45)

Pituitary (Hypophysis): Master Gland
Located at base of brain in a depression in skull (sella turcica)

Anterior pituitary (adenohypophysis)

- Adrenocorticotropic hormone (ACTH)—stimulates adrenal cortex and increases production of cortisol

- Follicle-stimulating hormone (FSH)—males, stimulates sperm and testosterone production; females, with luteinizing hormone (LH) stimulates secretion of estrogen and follicle development and ovulation

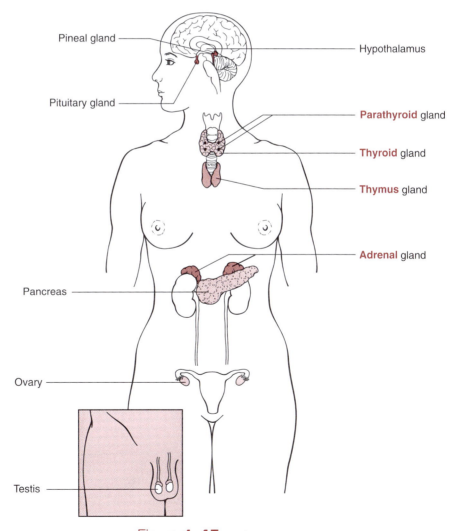

Figure **1-45** Endocrine system.

- Growth hormone (GH or somatotropin STH)—stimulates protein processing resulting in growth of bones, muscle, and fat metabolism, and maintains blood glucose levels
- Luteinizing hormone (LH)—males, stimulates testosterone production; females, stimulates secretion of progesterone and estrogen
- Melanocyte-stimulating hormone (MSH)—increases skin pigmentation
- Prolactin (PRL)—secreted by anterior pituitary, stimulates milk production and breast development
- Thyroid-stimulating hormone (TSH or thyrotropin)—stimulates thyroid gland

Posterior pituitary (neurohypophysis)—stores and releases hormones

- Antidiuretic hormone (ADH) or vasopressin—stimulates reabsorption of water by kidney tubules and increases blood pressure by constricting arterioles
- Oxytocin (OT)—stimulates contractions during childbirth, production and release of milk

Thyroid
Two lobes overlying trachea

Secretes two hormones that increase cell metabolism—thyroxine (T_4) and triiodothyronine (T_3)—synthesized from iodine

Secretes one hormone that decreases blood calcium—thyrocalcitonin (nasal spray used to treat osteoporosis)

Parathyroid Glands (4)
Located on posterior side of thyroid

Secretes PTH (parathyroid hormone) or parathoromone

Promotes calcium homeostasis in bloodstream

Adrenal Gland (Pair)
Located on top of each kidney

Adrenal cortex—outer region that secretes corticosteroids

- Cortisol—increases blood glucose
- Aldosterone—increases reabsorption of sodium (salt)
- Androgen, estrogen, progestin—sexual characteristics

Adrenal medulla—inner region that secretes catecholamines (epinephrine to dilate blood vessels to lower blood pressure, increase heart rate, dilate bronchial tubes, and release glycogen for energy and norepinephrine to constrict blood vessels to raise blood pressure)

Pancreas
Located behind stomach

Contains specialized cells (islets of Langerhans) that produce insulin and glycogen hormones

Insulin (decreases blood glucose), glucagon (converts glycogen to glucose, raising blood sugar), and somatostatin (regulates other cells of pancreas)

Thymus
Located behind sternum

Atrophies during adolescence

Produces thymosin—stimulates T-lymphocytes, effecting a positive immune response

Hypothalamus (Part of Brain)
Located below thalamus and above pituitary gland

Stimulates anterior pituitary to release hormones and posterior hypothalamus to store and release horomones

Pineal
Located between two cerebral hemispheres and above third ventricle

Secretes melatonin—more so at night, which affects sleep cycle

Also responsible for delaying sexual maturation in children

Also has neurotransmitters such as somatostatin, norepinephrine, seratonin, and histamine

Ovaries (Pair, Females)
Estrogen production stimulates ova production and secondary female sex characteristics

Progesterone—prepares the uterus for and maintains pregnancy

Placenta
Produces HCG (human chorionic gonadotropin) to sustain a pregnancy

Testes (Pair, Males)
Testosterone—male sex characteristics

COMBINING FORMS

1.	aden/o	in relationship to a gland
2.	adren/o	adrenal gland
3.	adrenal/o	adrenal gland
4.	andr/o	male
5.	calc/o, calc/i	calcium
6.	cortic/o	cortex
7.	crin/o	secrete
8.	dips/o	thirst
9.	estr/o	female
10.	gluc/o	sugar
11.	glyc/o	sugar
12.	gonad/o	ovaries and testes
13.	home/o	same
14.	hormon/o	hormone

UNIT I Anatomy, Terminology, and Pathophysiology

15.	kal/i	potassium
16.	lact/o	milk
17.	myx/o	mucus
18.	natr/o	sodium
19.	pancreat/o	pancreas
20.	parathyroid/o	parathyroid gland
21.	phys/o	growing
22.	pituitar/o	pituitary gland
23.	somat/o	body
24.	ster/o, stere/o	solid, having three dimensions
25.	thry/o	thyroid gland
26.	thyroid/o	thyroid gland
27.	toc/o	child birth
28.	toxic/o	poison
29.	ur/o	urine

PREFIXES

1.	eu-	good/normal
2.	oxy-	sharp, oxygen
3.	pan-	all
4.	tetra-	four
5.	tri-	three
6.	tropin-	act upon

SUFFIXES

1.	-agon	assemble
2.	-drome	run, relationship to conducting, to speed
3.	-emia	blood condition
4.	-in	a substance
5.	-ine	a substance
6.	-tropin	act upon
7.	-uria	urine

MEDICAL TERMS

Adrenals	Glands, located at top of kidneys, that produce steroid hormones (cortex) and catecholamines (medulla)
Contralateral	Opposite side
Hormone	Chemical substance produced by body's endocrine glands

Endocrine System—Anatomy and Terminology

Isthmus	Connection of two regions or structures
Isthmus, thyroid	Tissue connection between right and left thyroid lobes
Isthmusectomy	Surgical removal of isthmus
Lobectomy	Removal of a lobe
Thymectomy	Surgical removal of thymus
Thymus	Gland that produces hormones important to immune response
Thyroglossal duct	A duct in embryo between thyroid and posterior tongue which occasionally persists into adult life and causes cysts, fistulas, or sinuses
Thyroid	Part of endocrine system that produces hormones that regulate metabolism
Thyroidectomy	Surgical removal of thyroid

ENDOCRINE SYSTEM ANATOMY AND TERMINOLOGY QUIZ

1. Which of the following is NOT affected by the endocrine system?
   a. digestion
   b. development
   c. progesterone
   d. metabolism

2. Gland that overlies the trachea:
   a. parathyroid
   b. adrenal
   c. pancreas
   d. thyroid

3. Gland that is located on the top of each kidney:
   a. parathyroid
   b. adrenal
   c. pancreas
   d. thyroid

4. The outer region of the adrenal gland that secretes corticosteroids:
   a. cortex
   b. medulla
   c. sternum
   d. medullary

5. Located on the thyroid:
   a. hypophysis
   b. thymus
   c. pineal
   d. parathyroid

6. Located at the base of the brain in a depression in the skull:
   a. pituitary
   b. thymus
   c. adrenal
   d. pineal

7. Stimulates contractions during childbirth:
   a. cortisol
   b. PTH
   c. ADH
   d. oxytocin

8. Produced only during pregnancy by the placenta:
   a. estrogen and progesterone
   b. melatonin
   c. thymosin
   d. adrenocorticotropic hormone

UNIT I Anatomy, Terminology, and Pathophysiology

9. Combining form meaning secrete:
   a. dips/o
   b. crin/o
   c. gluc/o
   d. kal/i

10. Prefix meaning good:
    a. tri-
    b. tropin-
    c. pan-
    d. eu-

ENDOCRINE SYSTEM—PATHOPHYSIOLOGY

Diabetes Mellitus

Caused by a deficiency in insulin production or poor use of insulin by body cells

Islets of Langerhans (pancreatic cells) secrete glucagon and insulin to regulate fat, carbohydrate, and protein metabolism

Types of Diabetes Mellitus

Type 1, IDDM (insulin-dependent diabetes mellitus), immune mediated
Onset before age 30—peak onset age 12

Includes beta islet cell destruction, insulin deficiency

Acute onset

Positive family history

Requires insulin

Ketoacidosis (fats improperly burned leads to ketones and acids circulating)

Type 2, NIDDM (non–insulin-dependent diabetes mellitus)
Adult onset, after age 30, but it is now occurring earlier

Insidious onset/asymptomatic

Positive in immediate family

Dietary management and/or oral hypoglycemics and/or insulin

Most common type—85% are obese at onset

Insulin is present

Ketoacidosis does not occur

Symptoms
Polyuria

Polydipsia

Glycosuria

Hyperglycemia

Polyphagia

Unexplained weight loss

Acute complications
Hypoglycemia

Diabetic ketoacidosis

Chronic complications
Diabetic neuropathy (Fig. 1–46)

Retinopathy

Coronary artery disease (atherosclerosis)

Stroke

Peripheral vascular disease

Infection

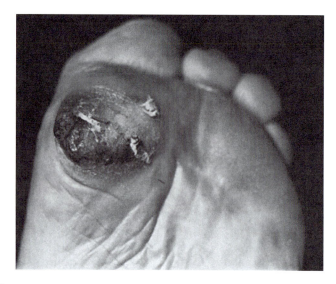

Figure **1-46** Patient with diabetes mellitus and neuropathy had severe claw toes, and shear forces across plantar surface of first metatarsal head caused recurrent ulceration. (From Canale ST, Beaty JH, *Campbell's Operative Orthopaedics*, ed 11, Philadelphia, 2008, Mosby.)

Gestational diabetes mellitus—predisposition to diabetes
Most often recognized in third trimester

Glucose intolerance may be temporary occurring only during pregnancy

Majority will develop diabetes mellitus within 15 years

Pituitary Disorders

Tumors

    Most common cause of pituitary disorders

    May secrete hormone

        Such as prolactin and ACTH

Anterior Pituitary
Dwarfism (hypopituitarism)
Can be caused by deficiency of somatotrophin (growth hormone)

Gigantism (Fig. 1-47) (hyperpituitarism)
Can be caused by excess of somatotrophin (growth hormone) in childhood

Treatment
Resection of tumor or irradiation of pituitary

Acromegaly (hyperpituitarism)
Increased GH in adulthood

Enlargement of facial bones, feet, and hands

Treatment
Pituitary adenoma is irradiated or removed

Endocrine System—Pathophysiology

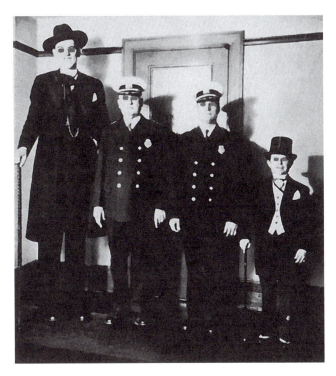

Figure **1-47** Gigantism. A pituitary giant and dwarf contrasted with normal-size men. (From Thibodeau GA, Patton KT: *Anatomy & physiology,* ed 5, St Louis, 2003, Mosby.)

Posterior Pituitary
Diabetes insipidus
Insufficient antidiuretic hormone—kidney tubules fail to retain needed water and salts

Causes polyuria, polydipsia, and dehydration

ADH or SIADH—syndrome of inadequate antidiuretic hormone

Excessive secretion of antidiuretic hormone

Causes excessive water retention

Treatment
Some types have no treatment

Others can be controlled with vasopressin (drugs)

Thyroid Disorders

Goiter (Fig. 1–48)
Enlargement of thyroid gland in the neck

Cause
Hypothyroid disorders

Hyperthyroid disorders

Hyperthyroidism—Thyrotoxicosis
Excessive thyroid hormone production

Most common form: Graves' disease (familial)—results of autoimmune process

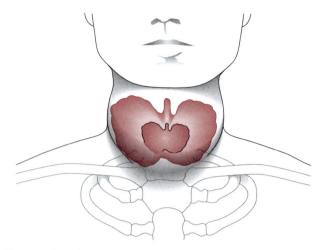

Figure **1-48** Goiter is an enlargement of thyroid gland.

Characterized by
Goiter

Tachycardia

Atrial fibrillation

Dyspnea

Palpitations

Fatigue

Tremor

Nervousness

Weight loss

Exophthalmos (protruding eyes)

- Decreased blinking

Treatment
Medication (antithyroid drugs)

Radioactive iodine

Surgical excision

Thyrotoxicosis storm/crisis

Thyroid storm/crisis is an acute life-threatening hypermetabolic state induced by excessive release of thyroid horomones

Most extreme state of thyrotoxicosis

Hypothyroidism
Primary: inadequate thyroid hormone production

Resulting in increasing levels of thyroid-stimulating hormone (TSH) production

Secondary: inadequate amounts of thyroid-stimulating hormone synthesized

Types
Cretinism

Endocrine System—Pathophysiology

- Congenital
- Occurs in children
- If not treated, it will cause a severe delay in physical/mental development

Treatment
Thyroid hormone

Myxedema

- Severe form
- Occurs in adults
  - Atherosclerosis
- Symptoms
  - Cold intolerance
  - Weight gain
  - Mental sluggishness
  - Fatigue

Treatment
Thyroid hormone

Hashimoto's thyroiditis

- Autoimmune disorder

Treatment
Medication (levothyroxine synthetic hormone replacement)

Parathyroid Disorders

Hyperparathyroidism—Excessive Parathyroid Hormone (PTH)
Leads to hypercalcemia

- Affects heart and bones and damages kidneys

Symptoms
Brittle bones

Kidney stones

Cardiac disturbances

Treatment
Surgical excision

Hypoparathyroidism—Abnormally Low PTH
Leads to hypocalcemia

Symptoms
Nerve irritability—twitching or spasms

Muscle cramps

Tingling and burning (parathesias) fingertips, toes, and lips

Anxiety, nervousness

Tetany (constant muscle contraction)

Treatment
Calcium and vitamin D

Adrenal Gland Disorders

Cushing Syndrome—Hypercortisolism
Excess levels of adrenocorticotropic hormone (ACTH)

Cause
Hyperfunction of adrenal cortex

Long-term use of steroid medications

Symptoms
Weight gain

- Fat deposits on face (moonface) and trunk (buffalo hump)

Glucose intolerance

Hypernaturemia

Hypokalemia

Virilization

Hypertension

- Diabetes may develop (20%)

Muscle wasting

Osteoporosis

Change in mental status

Delayed healing

Treatment
Medication

Radiation therapy

Surgical intervention

Addison's Disease—Primary Adrenal Insufficiency
Deficiency of adrenocortical hormones resulting from destruction of adrenal glands
- Glucocorticoids
- Mineralocorticoids

Cause
Tumors

Autoimmune disorders

Viral

Tuberculosis

Infection

Symptoms
Decreased blood glucose levels

Elevated serum ACTH

Fatigue

Lack of ability to handle stress

Weight loss

Infections

Hypotension

Decreased body hair

Hyperpigmentation

Treatment
Hormone (glucocorticoid) replacement

Hyperaldosteronism
Excess aldosterone secreted by adrenal cortex

Types
Primary hyperaldosteronism (Conn's syndrome)
- Caused by an abnormality of adrenal cortex
  - Usually an adrenal adenoma

Secondary hyperaldosteronism
- Caused by other than adrenal stimuli

Symptoms
Hypertension

Hypokalemia

Neuromuscular disorders

Treatment
Treat the underlying condition that caused hyperaldosteronism
- Such as adrenal adenoma

Adrenal Medulla
Hypersecretion
  Pheochromocytoma—benign tumor of medulla
  Excessive production of epinephrine and norepinephrine

Symptoms
  Severe headaches
  Sweating
  Flushing
  Hypertension
  Muscle spasms

Treatment
  Antihypertensive drugs
  Remove tumor

Androgen and Estrogen Hypersecretion
Androgen, male characteristic hormone

- Virilization, development of male characteristics

Feminization, hypersecretion of estrogen, female characteristic hormone

Cause
Underlying condition

- Adrenal tumor
- Cushing syndrome
- Adenomas or carcinomas
- Defects in steroid metabolism

Treatment
Surgical intervention for tumor

Underlying condition

ENDOCRINE SYSTEM PATHOPHYSIOLOGY QUIZ

1. This type of diabetes typically occurs before age 30:
   a. type 1
   b. type 2

2. The acronym that indicates that insulin is not required is:
   a. IDDM
   b. NIDDM
   c. PIDDM
   d. NDDMI

3. The most common cause of pituitary disorders is:
   a. hypersecretion
   b. hyposecretion
   c. tumor
   d. infection

4. In excess, this hormone can cause gigantism:
   a. somatotrophin
   b. thyroid
   c. mineralocorticoids
   d. adrenocortical

5. Goiter can be caused by which of the following:
   a. hypothyroidism
   b. parathyroidism
   c. hyperthyroidism
   d. both a and c

6. This type of hypothyroidism is an autoimmune disorder:
   a. myxedema
   b. Hashimoto's
   c. cretinism
   d. hypokalemia

7. Tetany can be caused by:
   a. hypoparathyroidism
   b. hyperthyroidism
   c. hyperparathyroidism
   d. hyperaldosteronism

8. Conn's syndrome is also known as:
   a. primary hypoparathyroidism
   b. primary hyperthyroidism
   c. primary hyperparathyroidism
   d. primary hyperaldosteronism

UNIT I   Anatomy, Terminology, and Pathophysiology

9. Development of male characteristics is known as:
   a. virilization
   b. feminization
   c. hypertrophy
   d. hyperaldosteronism

10. The treatment for Addison's disease is often:
    a. chemotherapy
    b. radiation
    c. hormone replacement
    d. all of the above

NERVOUS SYSTEM

NERVOUS SYSTEM—ANATOMY AND TERMINOLOGY

Controlling, regulating, and communicating system

Organization

- Central nervous system (CNS), brain and spinal cord
- Peripheral nervous system (PNS), cranial and spinal nerves
  - Autonomic nervous system—motor and sensory nerves of viscera (involuntary)
  - Somatic nervous system—motor and sensory nerves of skeletal muscles

Cells of the Nervous System (Fig. 1-49)

Neurons—Primary Cells of Nervous System

Classified according to function (afferent [sensory], efferent [motor], interneurons [associational])

- Dendrites (receive signals)
- Cell body (nucleus, within cell body)
- Axon (carries signals from cell body)
- Myelin sheath (insulation around axon)

Glia

Astrocytes

   Star shaped—transport water and salts between capillaries and neurons

Microglia

   Multiple branching processes—protect neurons from inflammation

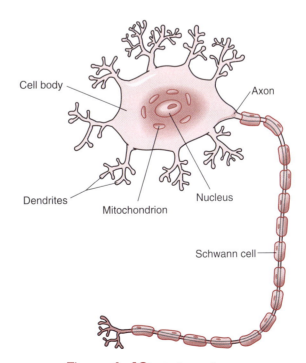

Figure **1-49** Myelinated axon.

UNIT I   Anatomy, Terminology, and Pathophysiology

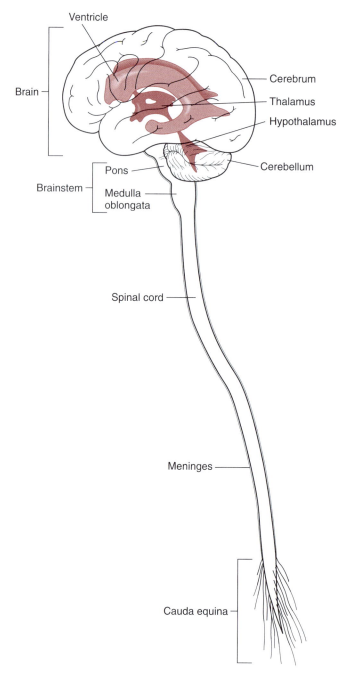

Figure **1-50** Brain and spinal cord.

Oligodendrocytes
   Form myelin sheath
Ependymal
   Lining membrane of brain and spinal cord where central spinal fluid circulates

Divisions of Central Nervous System (CNS) (Fig. 1-50)

Brain—Housed in Cranium (Box Comprised of 8 Bones)—Functioning to Enclose and Protect
Listing from inferior to superior

Nervous System—Anatomy and Terminology

Brainstem

Medulla oblongata—cross over area left to right and center of respiratory and cardiovascular systems

Pons—connection of nerves (face and eyes)

Midbrain

Diencephalon

Hypothalamus controls autonomic nervous system, body temperature, sleep, apetite, and control of pituitary

Thalamus relays impulses to cerebral cortex for sensory system (pain)

Cerebellum

Controls voluntary movement and balance

Cerebrum

Largest part of brain

Functions

Mental processes, personality, sensory interpretation, movements, and memory

Two hemispheres

Right controls left side of body

Left controls right side of body

Divided into five lobes
- Frontal
- Parietal
- Temporal
- Occipital
- Insula

Vertebral Column—33 Vertebrae

7 cervical

12 thoracic

5 lumbar

5 sacrum (fused)

4 coccygeal (fused)—tailbone

Spinal Cord—housed within vertebrae from medulla oblongata to second lumbar

Spinal and brain meninges (coverings—dura mater [external], archnoid, pia mater [internal])

Spine and brain spaces bathed by cerebrospinal fluid (CSF) (subarachnoid space)

Cavities within brain contain cerebrospinal fluid (ventricles)

Peripheral Nervous System (PNS)

Cranial nerves, 12 pair

Spinal nerves, 31 pair

Autonomic Nervous System (ANS)—Housed within Both PNS and CNS

Two divisions

- Sympathetic system—functions in fight and flight (stress)
- Parasympathetic system—functions to restore and conserve energy

COMBINING FORMS

1.	cephal/o	head
2.	cerebell/o	cerebellum
3.	cerebr/o	cerebrum
4.	crani/o	cranium
5.	dur/o	dura mater
6.	encephal/o	brain
7.	gangli/o	ganglion
8.	ganglion/o	ganglion
9.	gli/o	glial cells
10.	lept/o	slender
11.	mening/o	meninges
12.	meningi/o	meninges
13.	ment/o	mind
14.	mon/o	one
15.	myel/o	bone marrow, spinal cord
16.	neur/o	nerve
17.	phas/o	speech
18.	phren/o	mind
19.	poli/o	gray matter
20.	pont/o	pons
21.	psych/o	mind
22.	quadr/i	four
23.	radic/o	nerve root
24.	radicul/o	nerve root
25.	rhiz/o	nerve root
26.	vag/o	vagus nerve

PREFIXES

1.	hemi-	half
2.	per-	through

Nervous System—Anatomy and Terminology

    3. quadri-   four
    4. tetra-   four

SUFFIXES

1. -algesia — pain sensation
2. -algia — pain
3. -cele — hernia
4. -esthesia — feeling
5. -iatry — medical treatment
6. -ictal — pertaining to
7. -kines/o — movement
8. -paresis — incomplete paralysis
9. -plegia — paralysis

MEDICAL ABBREVIATIONS

1. ANS — autonomic nervous system
2. CNS — central nervous system
3. CSF — cerebrospinal fluid
4. CVA — stroke/cerebrovascular accident
5. EEG — electroencephalogram
6. LP — lumbar puncture
7. PNS — peripheral nervous system
8. TENS — transcutaneous electrical nerve stimulation
9. TIA — transient ischemic attack

MEDICAL TERMS

Burr	Drill used to create an entry into the cranium
Central nervous system	Brain and spinal cord
Craniectomy	Permanent, partial removal of skull
Craniotomy	Opening of the skull
Cranium	That part of the skeleton that encloses the brain
Diskectomy	Removal of a vertebral disk
Electroencephalography	Recording of the electric currents of the brain by means of electrodes attached to the scalp
Laminectomy	Surgical excision of posterior arch of vertebra—includes spinal process
Peripheral nerves	12 pairs of cranial nerves, 31 pairs of spinal nerves, and autonomic nervous system; connects peripheral receptors to the brain and spinal cord

UNIT I Anatomy, Terminology, and Pathophysiology

Shunt	An artificial passage
Skull	Entire skeletal framework of the head
Somatic nerve	Sensory or motor nerve
Stereotaxis	Method of identifying a specific area or point in the brain
Sympathetic nerve	Part of the peripheral nervous system that controls automatic body function and sympathetic nerves activated under stress
Trephination	Surgical removal of a disk of bone
Vertebrectomy	Removal of vertebra

NERVOUS SYSTEM ANATOMY AND TERMINOLOGY QUIZ

1. Portion of nervous system that contains cranial and spinal nerves:
   a. central
   b. peripheral
   c. autonomic
   d. parasympathetic

2. Part of neuron that receives signals:
   a. dendrites
   b. cell body
   c. axon
   d. myelin sheath

3. NOT associated with glia:
   a. monocytes
   b. astrocytes
   c. microglia
   d. oligodendrocytes

4. Largest part of brain:
   a. cerebellum
   b. cerebrum
   c. cortex
   d. pons

5. Divided into two hemispheres:
   a. cerebellum
   b. cerebrum
   c. cortex
   d. pons

6. Number of pairs of cranial nerves:
   a. 10
   b. 11
   c. 12
   d. 13

7. Controls right side of body:
   a. left cerebrum
   b. right cerebrum
   c. right cortex
   d. left cortex

8. Combining form that means brain:
   a. mening/o
   b. mon/o
   c. esthesi/o
   d. encephal/o

UNIT I   Anatomy, Terminology, and Pathophysiology

9. Prefix that means four:
   a. per-
   b. tetra-
   c. para-
   d. bi-

10. Combining form that means speech:
    a. phas/o
    b. rhiz/o
    c. poli/o
    d. myel/o

NERVOUS SYSTEM—PATHOPHYSIOLOGY

Dementias—Classified by Causative Factor

Cognitive deficiencies

Causes
Alzheimer's disease

Vascular disease

Head trauma

Tumors

Infection

Toxins

Substance abuse

AIDS

Alzheimer's Disease
Most common type of dementia

Progressive intellectual impairment

- Results in damage to neurons (neurofibrillary tangles)
- Fatal within 3 to 20 years

Causes
Mostly unknown

Perhaps genetic defect, autoimmune reaction, or virus

Symptoms
Behavior change

Memory loss

Confusion

Disorientation

Restlessness

Speech disturbances

Personality change—anxiety, depression

Irritability

Inability to complete activities of daily living

Treatment
- No cure
- Aricept (drug has modest effect in early stages)
- Symptomatic treatment
- Support for family

Vascular Dementia
Result of brain infarctions (vascular occlusion resulting in loss of brain function)

Nutritional Degenerative Disease
Deficiency

- B vitamins
- Niacin
- Pantothenic acid

Associated with alcoholism

Amyotrophic Lateral Sclerosis (ALS)
Motor neuron disease (MND)

Also known as Lou Gehrig's disease

- Baseball player who died of ALS

Deterioration of neurons of spinal cord and brain

Results in atrophy of muscles and loss of fine motor skills

Difficulty walking, talking, and breathing

Mental functioning remains normal

Survival is 2 to 5 years after diagnosis

Genetic cause/familial chromosome 21 aberration

- Death usually results from respiratory failure

Treatment
Symptomatic only

Emotional support

No cure

Huntington's Disease—Chorea
Inherited progressive atrophy of cerebrum

Symptoms
Restlessness

Rapid, jerky movements in arms and face (uncontrollable jerking and facial grimacing)

Rigidity

Intellectual impairment/bradyphrenia/apathy

Treatment
Genetic defect of chromosome 4

No cure

Symptomatic

Parkinson's Disease (Parkinsonism)
Decreased secretion of dopamine

Typically occurs after age 40

Cause

Unknown

Symptoms
Muscle rigidity and weakness

Bradykinesia—slow voluntary movements

Postural instability, stooped

Shuffling gait

Tremors at rest

Masklike facial appearance

Depression

Treatment
Medications to reduce symptoms

Dopamine replacement

Multiple Sclerosis (MS)
Common neurologic condition

- Demyelination of central nervous system—replaced by sclerotic tissue

Affects young adults 20–40 years old

Results in myelin destruction and gliosis of white matter of central nervous system

Speculation that it is an autoimmune condition or result of a virus

Exacerbations and remission patterns

Symptoms
Precipitated by "an event," i.e., infection, pregnancy, stress

Loss of feeling (paresthesias)

Vision problems

Bladder disorder

Mood disorders

Weakness of limbs—unsteady gait and paralysis

Treatment
Symptomatic

Management of relapses

Reducing relapses and disease progression—disease-modifying drugs (DMDs)

Myasthenia Gravis (MG)
Means grave muscle weakness

Autoimmune neuromuscular condition—antibodies block neurotransmission to muscle cells

Most have pathologic changes of thymus

Symptoms
Insidious

Muscle weakness and fatigability

May be localized or generalized

Often affects
- Swallowing
- Breathing
- Compromised swallowing and breathing may lead to crisis

Treatment

Anticholinesterase drugs
- Restores normal muscle strength and recoverability after fatigue

Corticosteroids (prednisone) and immunosuppressive drugs

Thymectomy

Tourette syndrome

Symptoms

Spasmodic, twitching movements, uncontrollable vocal sounds, inappropriate words

Begins with twitching eyelids and facial muscles (tics)

Verbal outbursts

Cause

Unknown

Excess dopamine or hypersensitivity to dopamine

Treatment

Antipsychotic drugs

Antidepressant drugs

Mood-elevating drugs

Poliomyelitis

Contagious viral disease

Affects motor neurons

Causes paralysis and respiratory failure

Prevent with vaccination

Postpolio Syndrome (PPS)

Also known as postpoliomyelitis neuromuscular atrophy

Progressive muscle weakness
- Past history of paralytic polio

Symptoms

Muscle weakness and fatigability
- May include atrophy and muscle twitching

Treatment

Symptomatic

Maintenance of respiratory function

Guillain-Barré Syndrome
Also known as

- Idiopathic polyneuritis
- Acute inflammatory polyneuropathy
- Landry's ascending paralysis

Demyelination of peripheral nerves—acquired disease

Symptoms
Primary ascending motor paralysis

Variable sensory disturbances

Treatment
Supportive

Congenital Neurologic Disorders

Hydrocephalus
Excessive amounts circulating of cerebrospinal fluid in ventricles of brain

Circulation is impaired in brain or spinal cord

Compresses brain

Treatment
Surgical placement of a shunt

Spina Bifida (Fig. 1-51)
Developmental birth defect which causes incomplete development of spinal cord and its coverings.

Vertebrae overlying open portions of spinal cord do not fully form and remain unfused and open.

- Spina bifida occulta—may not be noticed, no protrusion through defect
- Spina bifida manifesta which includes:
  - Myelomeningocele (spina bifida cystical)
    - Meninges and spinal cord protrude through defect
  - Meningocele
    - Meninges herniated through defect

Results in neurologic deficiencies

Treatment
Surgical repair

Mental Disorders

Schizophrenia
Variety of syndromes

Results in changes in brain

Hereditary factors are considered a cause

- Also, fetal brain damage is caused by viral infections, complications of pregnancy, nutritional deficiencies

Stress usually precipitates onset

UNIT I Anatomy, Terminology, and Pathophysiology

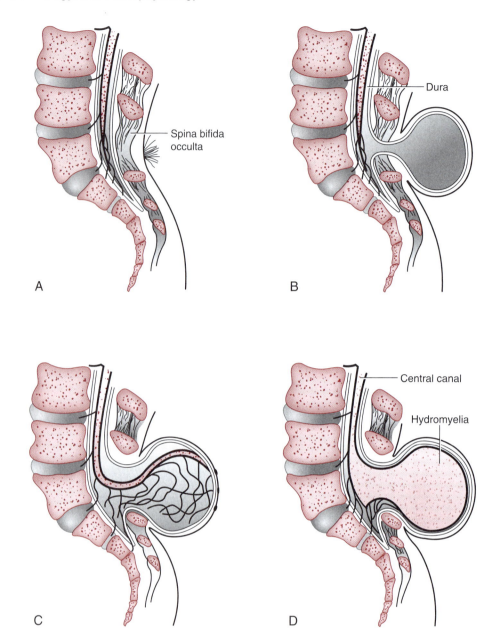

Figure 1-51 **A,** Spina bifida occulta. **B,** Meningocele. **C,** Myelomeningocele. **D,** Myelocystocele or hydromyelia.

Symptoms

Delusions of persecution and/or grandeur

Disorganized thought

Repetitive behaviors

Behavior issues

Decreased speech

Decreased ability to solve problems

Loss of emotions/flat affect

Hallucinations

Types are based on characteristics

Treatment
Antipsychotic drugs

Drugs have very unpleasant side effects such as tardive dyskinesia, with symptoms as follows:

- Excessive movement
- Grimacing
- Jerking
- Tremors
- Shuffling gait
- Dry mouth
- Blurred vision

Depression
Mood (sustained emotional state) disorder

Exact cause is unknown

Symptoms
Sadness

Hopelessness

Lethargy

Insomnia

Anorexia

Treatment
Antidepressant drugs

Electroconvulsive therapy

Central Nervous System (CNS) Disorders
■ Vascular Disorder
Transient Ischemic Attack (TIA)
Temporary reduction of blood flow to brain which produces strokelike symptoms but no lasting damage

Often a warning sign of cerebrovascular accident

Symptoms
Depend on location of ischemia

- Usual recovery in 24 hours

No loss of consciousness

Slurred, indiscernible speech

May display muscle weakness in legs/arms

Paresthesia (numbness) of face

Mental confusion may be present

Repeated attacks common in the presence of atherosclerotic disease

Cerebrovascular Accident (CVA) or Stroke

Infarction of brain due to lack of blood/oxygen flow

Necrosis of tissue with total occlusion of vessel

Causes

Atherosclerotic disease—thrombus formation

Embolus

Hemorrhage—arterial aneurysm

Symptoms

Depend on location of obstruction

- Thrombus
  - Gradual onset
  - Often occurs at rest
  - Intracranial pressure (ICP) minimal
  - Localized damage
- Embolus
  - Sudden onset
  - Occurs anytime
  - ICP minimal
  - Localized damage unless multiple emboli
- Hemorrhage
  - Sudden onset
  - Occurs most often with activity
  - ICP high
  - Widespread damage
  - May be fatal

Treatment

Anticoagulant drugs (clot dissolving) if caused by thrombus or embolus—tissue plasminogen activator (tPA)

Carotid endarterectomy (removes artherosclerotic plaque)

Oxygen treatment

Underlying condition treated, such as

- Hypertension
- Atherosclerosis
- Thrombus

Aneurysm—Cerebral

Dilation of artery

- May be localized or multiple

Rupture possible, often on exertion

- Fatal if rupture is massive

Symptoms
May display visual effects, such as

- Loss of visual fields

- Photophobia

- Diplopia

Headache

Confusion

Slurred speech

Weakness

Stiff neck (nuchal rigidity)

Treatment
Dependent on diagnosis prior to rupture

Surgical intervention

Encephalitis
Infection of parenchymal tissue of brain or spinal cord

- Often viral

Accompanying inflammation

Usually results in some permanent damage

Symptoms
Stiff neck

Headaches

Vomiting

Fever

May have seizure

Lethargy

Some types of encephalitis
Herpes simplex

Lyme disease

West Nile fever

Western equine

Treatment
Symptomatic

Supportive

Reye's Syndrome
Associated with viral infection

- Especially when aspirin has been administered

Changes occur in brain and liver

- Leads to increased intracranial pressure

Symptoms
Headaches

Vomiting

Lethargy

Seizures

Treatment
Symptomatic treatment

Brain Abscess
Localized infection

Necrosis of tissue

Usually spread from infection elsewhere, such as ears or sinus

Symptoms
Neurologic deficiencies

Increased intracranial pressure

Treatment
Antibiotics for bacterial infections

Surgical drainage

■ Epilepsies
Chronic seizure disorder

Types
Partial seizures (focal)
State of altered focus but conscious—simple

Impaired consciousness—complex

Specialized epileptic seizures

Aura

- Auditory or visual sign that precedes a seizure

Generalized seizures
Absence seizures—petit mal

- Brief loss of awareness
- Most common in children (febrile causation)

Tonic-clonic—grand mal or ictal event

- Loss of consciousness
- Alternate contraction and relaxation
- Incontinence
- No memory of seizure

Causes
Tumor

Hemorrhage

Trauma

Edema

Infection

Excessive cerebrospinal fluid

High fever

Treatment

Correct cause

Anticonvulsant drugs

Neurosurgery

Postictal event—after seizure—neurologic symptoms (weakness, etc.)

▪ Trauma

Head Injury—Traumatic Brain Injury (TBI)
Concussion
Mild blow to head

Temporary axonal disturbances

Grade 1: temporary confusion and amnesia (brief)

Grade 2: memory loss for very recent events and confusion

Grade 3: amnesia for recent events and disorientation (longer duration)

Results in reversible interference with brain function

- Recover in 24 hours with no residual damage

Contusion
Bruising of brain

Force of blow determines outcome

Hematomas—blood accumulation (clot)
Compresses surrounding structures

Classified based on location

- Epidural
  - Develops between dura and skull
- Subdural
  - Develops between dura and arachnoid
    - Development within 24 hours is acute
    - Development within a week is subacute
  - ICP increases with enlargement of hematoma
- Subarachnoid
  - Develops between pia and arachnoid
  - Blood mixes with cerebrospinal fluid
    - No localized hematoma forms

- Intracerebral
  - As a result of a contusion

Symptoms
Increased ICP

Others dependent on location and severity of injury

Treatment
Identification of the location of hematoma

Medications to decrease edema

Antibiotics

Surgical intervention—Burr hole if necessary to decrease the ICP

Spinal Cord Injury
Result of trauma to vertebra, cord, ligaments, intervertebral disc

Vertebra injuries classified as
- Simple—affects spinous or transverse process
- Compression—anterior fracture of vertebrae
- Comminuted—vertebral body is shattered
- Dislocation—vertebrae are out of alignment
- Flexion injury in which hyperflexion compresses vertebra

Dislocation

Rotation

Symptoms
Depend on vertebral level and severity

Paralysis

Loss of sensation

Drop in blood pressure

Loss of bladder and rectal control

Decreased venous circulation

Treatment
Identification of area of injury

Immobilization

Corticosteroids to decrease edema

Bladder and bowel management

Rehabilitation

■ Tumors of Brain and Spinal Cord

Increases ICP

Life threatening

Rarely metastasize outside of central nervous system

Secondary brain tumors are common

Metastasis from lung or breast

Gliomas Common Type

Primary malignant tumor—encapsulated and invasive

Types based on cell from which tumor arises and location of tumor

Glioblastoma
Located in cerebral hemispheres (deep in white matter)

Highly aggressive

Oligodendrocytoma
Usually located in frontal lobes

Oligodendroblastoma, more aggressive form

Ependymoma
Located in ventricles

Most often occurs in children

Ependymoblastoma, more aggressive form

Astrocytoma
Located anywhere in brain and spinal cord

Invasive but slow growing

Pineal Region
Germ cell tumors
Usually in adolescents

Rare

Variable growth rate

Several other pineal tumors
Pineocytoma

Teratoma

Germinoma

Blood Vessel
Angioma
Usually located in posterior cerebral hemispheres

Slow growing

Hemangioblastoma
Located in cerebellum

Slow growing

Medulloblastoma
Aggressive tumor

Located in posterior cerebellar vermis (fourth ventricle roof)

Meningioma
Originates in arachnoid

Slow growing

Pituitary Tumor
Related to aging

Slow growing

- Such as macroadenomas

Cranial Nerve Tumors
Neurilemmomas most common location: cranial nerve VIII

Slow growing

Metastatic

Spinal Cord Tumors
Symptoms are based on location of spinal compression

Intramedullary

- Originates in neural tissue

Extramedullary

- Originates outside the spinal cord

Metastatic tumors of spinal cord are more common

- Myeloma—marrow
- Lymphoma—lymph
- Carcinomas—lung, breast, prostate

Most common type of primary extramedullary tumor

- Meningiomas—anyplace in spine
- Neurofibromas—common in thoracic and lumbar

NERVOUS SYSTEM PATHOPHYSIOLOGY QUIZ

1. Most common dementia is:
   a. Alzheimer's disease
   b. secondary
   c. nutritional degenerative disease
   d. Lou Gehrig's disease

2. MND stands for:
   a. maximal neuron disorder
   b. migrating niacin disorder
   c. motor neuron disease
   d. motor neuropathic disorder

3. Dopamine replacement is useful in treating:
   a. multiple sclerosis
   b. Parkinson's disease
   c. Huntington's disease
   d. CVA

4. Condition in which primary symptoms are muscle weakness and fatigability:
   a. amyotrophic lateral sclerosis
   b. multiple sclerosis
   c. dyskinesis
   d. myasthenia gravis

5. Another name for idiopathic polyneuritis is:
   a. Guillain-Barré syndrome
   b. multiple sclerosis
   c. amyotrophic lateral sclerosis
   d. postpolio syndrome

6. This condition is thought to be caused by genetic factors and possibly fetal brain damage:
   a. Parkinson's
   b. schizophrenia
   c. spina bifida
   d. Guillain-Barré syndrome

7. This condition is associated with viral infection, especially when aspirin has been administered:
   a. Reye's syndrome
   b. Guillain-Barré syndrome
   c. Lou Gehrig's disease
   d. Conn's syndrome

8. Concussion is a mild blow to the head in which recovery is expected within _____ hours.
   a. 12
   b. 24
   c. 48
   d. 1 week

UNIT I Anatomy, Terminology, and Pathophysiology

9. ICP means:
   a. intercranial pressure
   b. intracranial pressure
   c. interior cranial pressure
   d. intensive cranial pressure

10. In this type of hematoma, blood mixes with cerebrospinal fluid:
    a. epidural
    b. subdural
    c. subarachnoid
    d. intracerebral

SENSES

SENSES—ANATOMY AND TERMINOLOGY

Sight	Eyes
Hearing	Ears
Smell	Nose
Taste	Tongue
Touch	Skin

Sight: Three Layers of Eye (Fig. 1-52)

Cornea (Outer Layer)
Fibrous, transparent layer that extends over dome of eye

Refracts (bends) light to focus on receptor cells (posterior eye)

Avascular (nourished by sclera)

Sclera (Extension of Outer Layer)
White of eye

Extends from cornea (anterior or surface) to optic nerve (posterior surface)

- Lies over iris

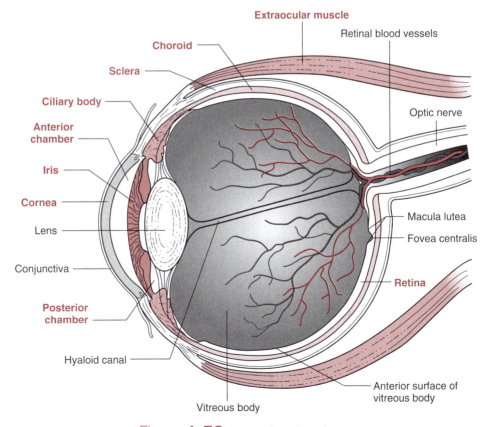

Figure **1-52** Eye and ocular adnexa.

Choroid (Middle Layer)
Pigment layer

Ciliary muscle and iris on front portion of layer

- Contracts

Retina (Inner Layer)
Contains rods and cones

- Rods provide night and peripheral vision
- Cones provide day and color vision and are stimulated by primary colors of red, green, and blue

Conjunctiva
Covers front of sclera and lines eyelid (contiguous layer)

Lens
Behind pupil

Lens is connected by zonules to ciliary body

Ciliary body muscles cause lens to change shape to refract light rays (accommodation)

Fluids
Aqueous humor (front of lens)—watery substance secreted by ciliary body

    Maintains shape of front portion of eye

    Refracts light

Vitreous humor (behind lens)—gel-like substance (not readily reformed) filling large space behind lens

    Maintains shape of eyeball

    Refracts light

Optic Nerve
Light rays from rods and cones travel from eye to brain via optic nerve

Optic nerve meets retina in optic disc (no light receptors)—blind spot

Pathway of light ray

    Cornea—refraction site

    Anterior chamber (aqueous humor)—refraction site

    Pupil

    Lens—refraction site

    Posterior chamber (vitreous humor)—refraction site

    Retina (rods and cones)

    Optic nerve fibers—first portion of brain that light is transmitted

    Optic chiasm

    Thalamus

    Cerebral cortex (occipital lobe)—light is interpreted

Hearing, Three Divisions of Ear

External Ear
Auricle (pinna)—sound waves enter ear

External auditory canal—tunnel from auricle to middle ear

Middle Ear
Begins with tympanic membrane (eardrum)

Ossicles—small bones conducting sound waves from middle to inner ear

- Malleus
- Incus
- Stapes

Eustachian tube—leads to pharynx

Inner Ear (Labyrinth)
Vestibule

Semicircular canals/vestibular apparatus

Cochlea contains perilymph and endolymph (liquids through which sound waves are conducted)

    Organ of Corti—auditory receptor area

Auditory nerve—electrical impulse is conducted to cerebral cortex for interpretation (hearing)

Pathway of sound vibration (exterior to brain)

    Pinna

    External auditory canal

    Tympanic membrane

    Malleus

    Incus

    Stapes

    Oval window

    Cochlea

    Auditory fluid/receptors in organ of Corti

    Auditory nerve

    Cerebral cortex

Smell

Olfactory Sense Receptors
Located in nasal cavity

Closely related to sense of taste

Cranial nerve I

Taste

Gustatory sense—sweet, salt, and sour differentiated

Taste buds located on anterior portion of tongue

Cranial nerves VII and IX

Touch

Mechanoreceptors
Widely distributed throughout body

Reacts to touch and pressure

- Meissner corpuscles (touch)
- Pacinian corpuscles (pressure)

Proprioceptors
Position and orientation

Dysfunctions

- Vestibular nystagmus—involuntary movement of eyes
- Vertigo—sense of spinning/dizziness

Thermoreceptors
Under skin

Sense temperature changes

Nociceptors
Pain sensors

In skin and internal organs

COMBINING FORMS

1.	ambly/o	dim, dullness
2.	aque/o	water
3.	audi/o	hearing
4.	blephar/o	eyelid
5.	conjunctiv/o	conjunctiva
6.	cor/o, core/o	pupil
7.	corne/o	cornea
8.	cycl/o	ciliary body
9.	dacry/o	tear
10.	essi/o, esthesi/o	sensation
11.	glauc/o	gray
12.	ir/o	iris
13.	irid/o	iris

Senses—Anatomy and Terminology

14.	kerat/o	cornea
15.	lacrim/o	tear
16.	mi/o	smaller
17.	myring/o	eardrum
18.	ocul/o	eye
19.	ophthalm/o	eye
20.	opt/o	eye, vision
21.	optic/o	eye
22.	ot/o	ear
23.	palpebr/o	eyelid
24.	papill/o	optic nerve
25.	phac/o	eye lens
26.	phak/o	eye lens
27.	phot/o	light
28.	presby/o	old age
29.	pupill/o	pupil
30.	retin/o	retina
31.	scler/o	sclera
32.	scot/o	darkness
33.	staped/o	stapes
34.	tympan/o	eardrum
35.	uve/o	uvea
36.	vitre/o	glassy
37.	xer/o	dry

PREFIXES

1.	audi-	hearing
2.	eso-	inward
3.	exo-	outward

SUFFIXES

1.	-opia	vision
2.	-omia	smell
3.	-tropia	to turn

MEDICAL ABBREVIATIONS

1.	AD	right ear
2.	AS	left ear
3.	AU	both ears

UNIT I   Anatomy, Terminology, and Pathophysiology

4.	H or E	hemorrhage or exudate
5.	IO	intraocular
6.	IOL	intraocular lens
7.	OD	right eye
8.	OS	left eye
9.	OU	each eye
10.	PERL	pupils equal and reactive to light
11.	PERRL	pupils equal, round, and reactive to light
12.	PERRLA	pupils equal, round, and reactive to light and accommodation
13.	REM	rapid eye movement
14.	TM	tympanic membrane

MEDICAL TERMS

Anterior segment	Those parts of eye in the front of and including lens, orbit, extraocular muscles, and eyelid
Apicectomy	Excision of a portion of temporal bone
Astigmatism	Condition in which refractive surfaces of eye are unequal
Aural atresia	Congenital absence of external auditory canal
Blepharitis	Inflammation of eyelid
Cataract	Opaque covering on or in lens
Chalazion	Granuloma around sebaceous gland
Cholesteatoma	Tumor that forms in middle ear
Conjunctiva	The lining of eyelids and covering of sclera
Dacryocystitis	Blocked, inflamed infection of nasolacrimal duct
Dacryostenosis	Narrowing of lacrimal duct
Ectropion	Eversion (outward sagging) of eyelid
Entropion	Inversion of eyelid (lashes rubbing cornea)
Enucleation	Removal of an organ or organs from a body cavity
Episclera	Connective covering of sclera
Exenteration	Removal of an organ all in one piece, commonly used to describe radical excision
Exophthalmos	Protrusion of eyeball
Exostosis	Bony growth
Fenestration	Creation of a new opening in inner wall of middle ear
Glaucoma	Eye diseases that are characterized by an increase of intraocular pressure
Hordeolum	Stye—infection of sebaceous gland (nodule on lid margin)
Hyperopia	Farsightedness, eyeball is too short from front to back
Keratomalacia	Softening of cornea associated with a deficiency of vitamin A

Senses—Anatomy and Terminology

Keratoplasty	Surgical repair of the cornea
Labyrinth	Inner connecting cavities, such as internal ear
Labyrinthitis	Inner ear inflammation
Lacrimal	Related to tears
Mastoidectomy	Removal of mastoid bone
Ménière's disease	Condition that causes dizziness, ringing in ears, and deafness
Myopia	Nearsightedness, eyeball too long from front to back
Myringotomy	Incision into tympanic membrane
Ocular adnexa	Orbit, extraocular muscles, and eyelid
Ophthalmoscopy	Examination of the interior of eye by means of a scope, also known as funduscopy
Otitis media	Noninfectious inflammation of middle ear; serous otitis media produces liquid drainage (not purulent), and suppurative otitis media produces purulent (pus) matter
Otoscope	Instrument used to examine ear
Papilledema	Swelling of optic disk (papilla)
Posterior segment	Those parts of eye behind lens
Ptosis	Drooping of upper eyelid
Sclera	Outer covering of eye
Strabismus	Extraocular muscle deviation resulting in unequal visual axes
Tarsorrhaphy	Suturing together of eyelids
Tinnitus	Ringing in the ears
Transmastoid	Creates an opening in mastoid for drainage antrostomy
Tympanolysis	Freeing of adhesions of the tympanic membrane
Tympanometry	Test of the inner ear using air pressure
Tympanostomy	Insertion of ventilation tube into tympanum
Uveal	Vascular tissue of the choroid, ciliary body, and iris
Vertigo	Dizziness
Xanthelasma	Yellow plaque on eyelid (lipid disorder)

SENSES ANATOMY AND TERMINOLOGY QUIZ

1. The middle layer of the eye:
   a. sclera
   b. retina
   c. episclera
   d. choroid

2. The covering of the front of sclera and lining of eyelid:
   a. aqueous humor
   b. ossicles
   c. vitreous
   d. conjunctiva

3. Which of the following is NOT a bone of the middle ear?
   a. cochlea
   b. stapes
   c. malleus
   d. incus

4. This cranial nerve controls the sense of smell:
   a. I
   b. II
   c. III
   d. IV

5. Which of the following is NOT part of the inner ear?
   a. pinna
   b. vestibule
   c. semicircular canals
   d. cochlea

6. These receptors react to touch:
   a. nociceptors
   b. mechanoreceptors
   c. proprioceptors
   d. thermoreceptors

7. These react to position and orientation:
   a. nociceptors
   b. mechanoreceptors
   c. proprioceptors
   d. thermoreceptors

8. Combining form meaning eyelid:
   a. aque/o
   b. blephar/o
   c. optic/o
   d. uve/o

9. Combining form meaning eye lens:
   a. cor/o
   b. irid/o
   c. ocul/o
   d. phak/o

10. Abbreviation meaning the pupils are equal, round, and reactive to light and accommodation:
    a. PERRLA
    b. PERRL
    c. PERL
    d. PURL

SENSES—PATHOPHYSIOLOGY

Eye

Visual Disturbances

Astigmatism
Irregular curvature of refractive surfaces (cornea or lens) of eye

Can be congenital or acquired (as a result of disease or trauma)

Image is distorted

Treatment
    Corrected with cylindrical lens

Diplopia
Double vision

Amblyopia
Dimness of vision—impairment of vision without detectable organic lesion of eye

Hyperopia
Farsightedness

Shortened eyeball

- Can see objects in distance, not close up

Treatment
    Corrected with convex lens

Presbyopia
Age-related farsightedness

Treatment
    Magnification (reading glasses or bifocals)

Myopia
Nearsightedness

Elongated eyeball

- Can see objects up close, not in distance

Treatment
    Corrected with concave lens thicker at periphery

Nystagmus—unilateral or bilateral
Rapid, involuntary eye movements

Movements can be

- Vertical
- Horizontal
- Rotational
- Combination of above

Cause
> Brain tumor or inner ear disease

Normal in newborns

Due to underlying condition or adverse effect of drug

Various types, such as
- Vestibular nystagmus
- Rhythmic eye movements

Strabismus
Cross-eyed

Due to muscle weakness or neurologic defect

Forms of strabismus
- Hypotropia (downward deviation of one eye)
- Hypertropia (upward deviation of one eye)
- Estropia (one eye turns inward)
- Exotropia (one eye turns outward)

Treatment
- Eye exercises/patching of normal eye
- Surgery to establish muscle balance

Infections
Conjunctivitis (pink eye)
Inflammation of conjunctival lining of eyelid or covering of sclera

Due to
- Infection
- Allergy
- Irritation

Treatment
- Varies with cause
- Antibiotic eye drops

Hordeolum (stye)
Bacterial infection of eyelid hair follicle
- Usually *Staphylococci*

Results in mass on eyelid

Treatment
- Antibiotics
- Incision and drainage may be necessary

Keratitis
Corneal inflammation

Caused by herpes simplex virus

Causes tearing and photophobia

Macular Degeneration
Destruction of fovea centralis

- Fovea centralis is small pit in center of retina (fovea centralis retinae)

Usually age related—leading cause of blindness in elderly

Results from exposure to ultraviolet rays or drugs

- Also may have a genetic component

Central vision is lost

Two types of macular degeneration

- Wet—development of new vascularization and leaking blood vessels near macula
- Dry (85% of cases)—atrophy and degeneration of retinal cells and deposits of drusen (clumps of extracellular waste)

Treatment
None for "dry" macular degeneration

Surgical intervention with laser for "net" macular degeneration to coagulate leaking vessels; success is limited

Medications

Detached Retina
Retinal tear—two layers of retina separate from each other

- Vitreous humor then leaks behind retina
- Retina then pulls away from choroid

Results in increasing blind spot in visual field

Condition is painless

Pressure continues to build if left unattended

Final result is blindness

Treatment
Surgical intervention with laser to repair tear (emergency/urgency)—photocoagulation for small tears

Scleral buckle for large retinal detachments

Pneumatic retinopexy for medium to large retinal detachment. Gas bubble is injected to vitreous cavity; pressure to tear resulting in retinal reattachment.

Cataracts
Lens becomes opaque with protein aggregates

Classified by morphology
Size

Shape

Location

Also may be classified by etiology (cause) or time cataract occurs

UNIT I Anatomy, Terminology, and Pathophysiology

Examples of classification
Congenital cataract

- Bilateral opacity present at birth
- Also known as developmental cataract

Heat cataract

- Also known as glassblowers' cataract
- Caused by exposure to radiation

Traumatic cataract (Fig. 1–53)

- Result of injury to eye

Senile cataract

- Age related
- Usually forms on corneal area of lens

Symptoms
  Blurring of vision
  Halos around lights

Treatment
  Removal of cataract with intraocular lens implantation

If no intraocular lens implant, then glasses or contact lenses for refraction

Glaucoma
Excess accumulation of intraocular aqueous humor

- Results in decreased blood flow and edema
- Damages retinal cells and optic nerve

Narrow angle glaucoma
Acute type of glaucoma

Chronic glaucoma
  Also known as

  - Wide angle glaucoma
  - Open angle glaucoma

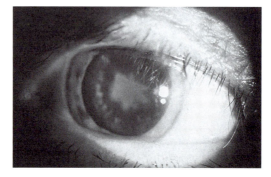

Figure **1-53** A concussion injury that resulted in a traumatic cataract. (From Yanoff M, Duker J: *Ophthalmology,* ed 2, St Louis, 2004, Mosby.)

Asymptomatic

Diagnosed in eye examination using tonometry to test anterior chamber pressure

Treatment
>Medications that decrease output of aqueous humor and decreased intraocular pressure (IOP)

>Laser treatment to provide drainage

Ear

■ Infections

Otitis Media
Infection or inflammation of middle ear cavity

Chronic infection produces adhesions
>Results in loss of hearing

Often occurs in children in combination with URI (upper respiratory infection)

Causes severe ear pain (otalgia)

Treatment
>Antibiotics

Surgical intervention with placement of tubes to allow for drainage
- Useful in patients with recurrent infection

Otitis Externa
Also known as swimmer's ear

Infection of external auditory canal and pinna (exterior ear)
>Caused by bacteria or fungus

>Results in pain and discharge

Treatment
>Antibiotic

Encouraged to keep ear dry

■ Hearing Loss

Conductive Hearing Loss
Due to a defect of sound-conducting apparatus
- Accumulation of wax
- Scar tissue on tympanic membrane

Also known as:
- Transmission hearing loss
- Conduction deafness

Treatment
- Hearing aids

Sensorineural

Due to a lesion of cochlea or central neural pathways

Also known as

- Perceptive deafness

May be divided into

- Cochlear hearing loss
  - Due to a defect in receptor or transducing mechanisms of cochlea
- Retrocochlear hearing loss
  - Due to defect located proximal to cochlea (vestibulocochlear nerve or auditory area of brain)

Presbycusis is age-related sensorineural hearing loss

Treatment
- Unknown

Ototoxic Hearing Loss

Due to ingestion of toxic substance

Also known as toxic deafness

Ménière's Disease

Inner ear disturbance

Also known as idiopathic endolymphatic hydrops

Cause unknown

Most common cause of vertigo (dizziness) of inner ear

Other symptoms include vertigo, hearing loss, and tinnitus

SENSES PATHOPHYSIOLOGY QUIZ

1. This condition can be acquired or congenital and results in an irregular curvature of the refractive surfaces of the eye:
    a. diplopia
    b. hyperopia
    c. nystagmus
    d. astigmatism

2. In this condition the eyeball is shorter than normal and results in being able to see objects in the distance but not close up:
    a. diplopia
    b. hyperopia
    c. nystagmus
    d. astigmatism

3. Rapid, involuntary eye movement is the predominant symptom of this condition:
    a. diplopia
    b. hyperopia
    c. nystagmus
    d. astigmatism

4. Age-related farsightedness is:
    a. presbyopia
    b. hyperopia
    c. diplopia
    d. myopia

5. Another name for a stye is:
    a. keratitis
    b. hordeolum
    c. hyperopia
    d. strabismus

6. An inflammation of the cornea that is caused by herpes simplex virus is:
    a. keratitis
    b. hordeolum
    c. hyperopia
    d. strabismus

7. In this condition there is destruction of the fovea centralis:
    a. macular degeneration
    b. detached retina
    c. glaucoma
    d. cataract

8. This is an infection that occurs in the middle ear cavity:
    a. otitis media
    b. otitis externa
    c. ototoxic
    d. retrocochlear

9. The hearing loss that can be due to a lesion on the cochlea is:
   a. conductive
   b. sensorineural
   c. ototoxic
   d. transmission

10. This condition is also known as perceptive deafness:
    a. conductive
    b. sensorineural
    c. otitis media
    d. transmission

UNIT I QUIZ ANSWERS

Integumentary System

Anatomy and Terminology Quiz
1. c
2. d
3. a
4. b
5. d
6. c
7. d
8. b
9. c
10. c

Pathophysiology Quiz
1. c
2. c
3. a
4. d
5. b
6. c
7. d
8. b
9. d
10. a

Musculoskeletal System

Anatomy and Terminology Quiz
1. b
2. c
3. a
4. c
5. a
6. d
7. b
8. d
9. a
10. c

Pathophysiology Quiz
1. d
2. c
3. b
4. a
5. d
6. d
7. a
8. c
9. b
10. d

UNIT I Anatomy, Terminology, and Pathophysiology

Respiratory System

Anatomy and Terminology Quiz
1. b
2. d
3. c
4. a
5. a
6. c
7. c
8. b
9. d
10. d

Pathophysiology Quiz
1. b
2. a
3. d
4. d
5. d
6. a
7. c
8. b
9. a
10. c

Cardiovascular System

Anatomy and Terminology Quiz
1. d
2. a
3. c
4. a
5. d
6. b
7. d
8. a
9. d
10. d
11. b
12. c

Pathophysiology Quiz
1. b
2. c
3. d
4. c
5. d
6. a
7. c
8. c
9. a
10. d

Female Genital System and Pregnancy

Anatomy and Terminology Quiz
1. d
2. a
3. a
4. b
5. c
6. a
7. b
8. b
9. c
10. d

Pathophysiology Quiz
1. b
2. d
3. a
4. c
5. b
6. a
7. a
8. c
9. b
10. c

Male Genital System

Anatomy and Terminology Quiz
1. c
2. a
3. d
4. b
5. a
6. a
7. a
8. d
9. d
10. b

Pathophysiology Quiz
1. a
2. b
3. d
4. a
5. c
6. b
7. d
8. b
9. a
10. b

UNIT I Anatomy, Terminology, and Pathophysiology

Urinary System

Anatomy and Terminology Quiz
1. c
2. d
3. a
4. c
5. b
6. d
7. c
8. b
9. d
10. a

Pathophysiology Quiz
1. c
2. d
3. d
4. c
5. b
6. c
7. a or c
8. c
9. b
10. c

Digestive System

Anatomy and Terminology Quiz
1. b
2. d
3. d
4. b
5. c
6. b
7. a
8. c
9. a
10. b

Pathophysiology Quiz
1. c
2. a
3. d
4. b
5. a
6. c
7. a
8. c
9. a
10. a

Mediastinum and Diaphragm

Anatomy and Terminology Quiz
1. a
2. b
3. d
4. c
5. c
6. b
7. a
8. b
9. a
10. d

Hemic and Lymphatic System

Anatomy and Terminology Quiz
1. b
2. d
3. a
4. d
5. c
6. c
7. a
8. d
9. b
10. d

Pathophysiology Quiz
1. c
2. a
3. b
4. d
5. b
6. c
7. a
8. a
9. c
10. b

Endocrine System

Anatomy and Terminology Quiz
1. c
2. d
3. b
4. a
5. d
6. a
7. d
8. a
9. b
10. d

Pathophysiology Quiz
1. a
2. b
3. c
4. a
5. d
6. b
7. a
8. d
9. a
10. c

UNIT I Anatomy, Terminology, and Pathophysiology

Nervous System

Anatomy and Terminology Quiz
1. b
2. a
3. a
4. b
5. b
6. c
7. a
8. d
9. b
10. a

Pathophysiology Quiz
1. a
2. c
3. b
4. d
5. a
6. b
7. a
8. b
9. b
10. c

Senses

Anatomy and Terminology Quiz
1. d
2. d
3. a
4. a
5. a
6. b
7. c
8. b
9. d
10. a

Pathophysiology Quiz
1. d
2. b
3. c
4. a
5. b
6. a
7. a
8. a
9. b
10. b

UNIT II

Reimbursement Issues

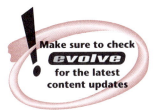

REIMBURSEMENT ISSUES

Your Responsibility

Ensure accurate coding based upon services provided and documented

Obtain correct reimbursement for services rendered

Upcoding (maximizing) or downcoding is never appropriate

Stay abreast of current and changing

- Reimbursement policies
- Coding guidelines
- HIPAA changes are based on various resources such as
  - Centers for Medicare and Medicaid Policy Manuals
  - National Correct Coding Guidelines

Population Changing = Reimbursement Change

Elderly fastest growing patient segment, due to "Baby Boomers"

By 2030, one elderly person for each person younger than 19 years

Medicare primarily for elderly

Medicare

Getting Bigger All the Time!

Over the next ten years, Medicare spending will total more than $3 trillion (http://www.cbo.gov/ftpdoc.cfm?index=308&type=0).

Health care will continue to expand to meet enormous future demands

- Job security for coders!

Those Covered

Originally established for those 65 and older

Later disabled and ESRD added

Persons covered are called "beneficiaries"

Basic Structure

Medicare program established in 1965

Part A: Hospital and Institutional Care Coverage

- This is the part that most inpatient coders will work with

Part B: Supplemental—nonhospital

   Example: Physician services and medical equipment

- This is the part that most outpatient coders will work with

Part C: Medicare Advantage plans—combines part A and B (added later)

Plans include

   Preferred Provider Organizations (PPO) plans

   Health Maintenance Organizations (HMO) plans

   Private Fee-for-Service (PPFS) plans

   Medical Savings Account (MSA) plans

   Special Needs plans

Part D: Prescription Drug Coverage (added January 1, 2006)

Plans include

    Medicare Advantage Plans (MA-PD)

    Private prescription drug plans (PDPs)

Officiating Office

Department of Health and Human Services (DHHS) (http://www.dhhs.gov)

Delegated to Centers for Medicare and Medicaid Services (CMS) (formerly HCFA)

- CMS runs Medicare and Medicaid
- CMS delegates daily operation to Medicare Administrative Contractors (MACs) or fiscal intermediaries (FIs)
- MACs/FIs are usually insurance companies
- The Medicare Prescription Drug Improvement and Modernization Act of 2003 allowed CMS to reduce the current 48 FIs to 19 Medicare Administrative Contractors (MACs)
  - Phased in with the final 19 MACs in place by 2011

Funding for Medicare

Social security taxes

Equal match from government

CMS sends money to MACs/FIs

MACs/FIs handle paperwork and pay claims

Medicare Covers

Medical necessity and frequency limitations

Defined in

- LCDs (Local Coverage Determination)
- NCDs (National Coverage Decisions)

Beneficiary pays

20% of Medicare-approved amount after deductible is met for Part B

Plus annual deductible

For Part A, patient pays deductible for service rendered

Medicare pays

80% of Medicare-allowed amount of covered services

For Part A, all covered costs except deductible

Participating Providers

Signed agreement with MACs/FIs and carrier

- Providers must report any change in practical within 60 days

Provider agrees to accept what MACs/FIs and carrier pays as payment in full

- Accepting assignment

Block 27 on CMS-1500 (Figure 2-1)

National Provider Identification (NPI)

10-digit number assigned to all covered healthcare providers

- Designed to provide one unique identifier for all providers as part of HIPAA

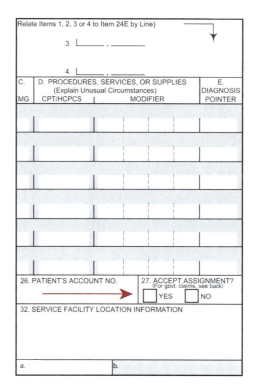

Figure **2-1** Block 27, Accept Assignment on the CMS-1500 (08-05) Health Insurance Claim Form. (Courtesy U.S. Department of Health and Human Services, Centers for Medicare and Medicaid Services.)

- Eliminates the need for additional numbers by other carriers
- Block 17b on CMS-1500

Good reasons to participate
MACs/FI usually do not reimburse non-QIO providers

- Significant decrease in reimbursed amount

Quality Improvement Organizations (QIO) providers receive 5% more from Medicare than non-QIO providers

Check sent directly from MACs/FIs to QIO providers

Faster claims processing

Provider names listed in QIO directory

- Sent to all beneficiaries

Part A, Hospital Inpatient
Hospitals submit charges on UB-04 form

ICD-9-CM codes primary basis for payment

Covered in-hospital expenses
Semiprivate room

Meals and special diets in hospital

All medically necessary services

Noncovered in-hospital expenses
Personal convenience items

> *Example:* Slippers, TV

Not medically necessary services or procedures

Types of covered expenses
Rehabilitation

Skilled nursing

Some personal convenience items for long-term illness or disabilities

Home health visits

Hospice care

Not automatically covered

- Must meet certain criteria

Part B, Supplemental
Part B pays services and supplies not covered under Part A

Not automatic

Beneficiaries purchase

- Pay monthly premiums

Types of items covered in part B
Physician services

Outpatient hospital services

Ambulatory surgical services

Home health care

Medically necessary supplies and equipment

Coding for Medicare Part B services
Three coding systems used to report Part B

- CPT
- HCPCS
- ICD-9-CM

NATIONAL CORRECT CODING INITIATIVE

Developed by the Centers for Medicare and Medicaid Services to

- Promote national correct coding methods
- Control improper coding that results in inappropriate payment of Part B claims (physician) and hospital outpatient claims

Unbundling

CMS defines unbundling as

- Billing multiple procedure codes for a group of procedures that are covered by a single comprehensive code

Example: Dividing one service into parts and coding for each part separately, such as:

    Reporting bilateral procedures unilaterally

        Reporting 31231, bilateral or unilateral diagnostic nasal endoscopy, with the -50 (bilateral procedure), rather than correctly as 31231

    Downcoding to use an additional code

        Reporting one of two lacerations of the same complexity and site with a lesser code to enable reporting two separate repairs

    Separating the surgical approach from the major surgical service

        Coding separately for a thoracic approach during an anterior spine procedure

FEDERAL REGISTER

Government publishes updates, revisions (changes), deletions in laws (Figure 2-2) (http://listserv.access.gpo.gov/)

November and December issues contain outpatient facility updates

QUALITY IMPROVEMENT ORGANIZATIONS (QIO)

Social Security Act (SSA) was amended to establish QIO

Purpose: Ensure hospitals adhere to payment system

PRO Reviews

Admission

Discharge

Quality of care

DRG validation

Coverage

Procedure

The Review

Begins with nurse who screens records based on PRO guidelines

Out-of-compliance cases forwarded to physician reviewer

Violations can result in severe sanctions

RESOURCE-BASED RELATIVE VALUE SCALE (RBRVS)

Physician payment reform implemented in 1992

Prior to reform, physicians were paid lowest of

- Physician's charge for service
- Physician's customary charge
- Prevailing charge in locality

UNIT II Reimbursement Issues

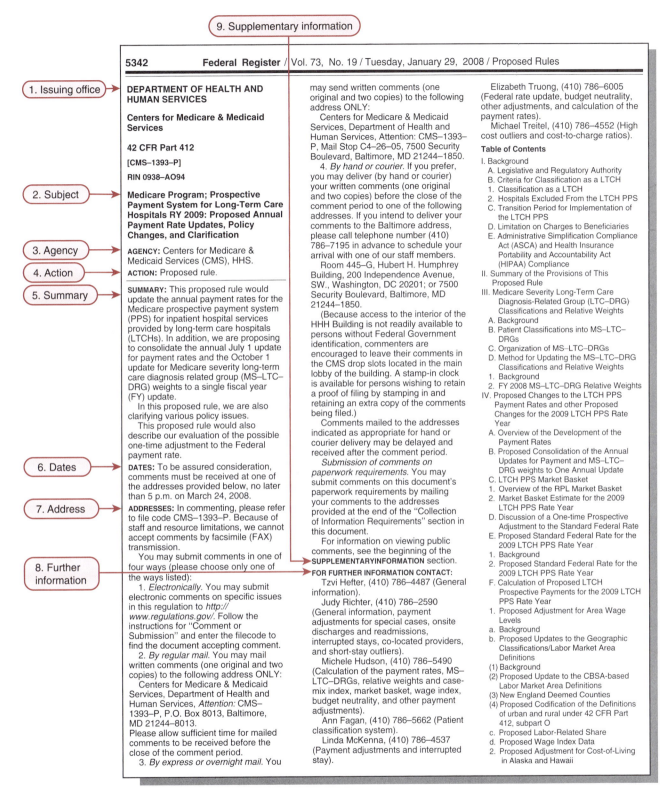

Figure 2-2 Example of page from the *Federal Register*. (From *Federal Register*, January 29, 2008, vol. 73, no. 19, Proposed Rules.)

National Fee Schedule (NFS)

Replaced RBRVS

Termed Medicare Fee Schedule (MFS)

Payment 80% of MFS, after patient deductible

Used for physicians and suppliers

Relative Value Units (RVUs)

Assigns national unit values to each CPT code

Local adjustments made

- Work and skill required
- Overhead costs
- Malpractice costs

Often referred to as fee schedule

Annually, CMS updates RVU based on national and local factors

MEDICARE FRAUD AND ABUSE

Program established by Medicare

- To decrease and eliminate fraud and abuse

Beneficiary signatures on file

- Service, charges submitted without need for patient signature

Presents opportunity for fraud

Fraud

Intentional deception to benefit

   Example: Submitting for services not provided

Anyone who submits for Medicare services can be violator

- Physicians
- Hospitals
- Laboratories
- Billing services
- YOU

Fraud Can Be

Billing for services not provided

Misrepresenting diagnosis or CPT/HCPCS codes

Kickbacks

Unbundling services

Falsifying medical necessity

Systematic waiver of copayment or deductible

Office of the Inspector General (OIG)

Develops and publishes work plan annually

Outlines Medicare monitoring program

FIs or MACs/carrier monitors those areas identified in plan

Complaints of Fraud or Abuse

Submitted orally or in writing to FIs or MACs or carrier

Allegations made by anyone against anyone

Allegations followed up by FIs or MACs or carrier (http://www.oig.hhs.gov/publications/workplan.htm#1)

Abuse

Generally involves
- Impropriety
- Lack of medical necessity for services reported

Review takes place after claim submitted
- FIs or MACs/carrier goes back and does historical review of claims

Kickbacks

Bribe or rebate for referring patient for any service covered by Medicare

Any personal gain kickback

A felony
- $25,000 fine or
- 5 years in jail or
- Both

Protect Yourself

Use your common sense

Submit only truthful and accurate claims
- Stay current with all coding changes

If you are unsure about charges, services, or procedures
- Check with physician or supervisor

MANAGED HEALTH CARE

Network health care providers that offer health care services under one organization

Group hospitals, physicians, or other providers

90% of people with health care coverage are covered by an organization (e.g., HMO, PPO, POS)

Managed Care Organizations

Responsible for health care services to an enrolled group or person

Coordinate various health care services

Negotiate with providers and groups

Preferred Provider Organization (PPO)

Providers form network to offer health care services as group

Enrollees who seek health care outside PPO pay more

Point of Service (POS)

In-network or out-of-network providers may be used

Benefits are paid at a higher rate to in-network providers

Subscribers are not limited to providers, but to amount covered by plan

Health Maintenance Organization (HMO)

Total package health care

Out-of-pocket expenses minimal

Assigned physician that acts as gatekeeper to refer patient outside organization

REIMBURSEMENT TERMINOLOGY

Advance Beneficiary Notice	ABN, notification in advance of services that Medicare probably will not pay for and the estimated cost to patient (Figure 2-3) (formerly WOL, waiver of liability)
Ancillary Service	A service that is supportive of care of a patient, such as laboratory services
Assignment	A legal agreement that allows the provider to receive direct payment from a payer and the provider to accept payment as payment in full for covered services
Attending Physician	The physician legally responsible for oversight of an inpatient's care (in residency programs, the teaching physician that monitors the resident's work)
Beneficiary	The person who benefits from insurance coverage; also known as subscriber, dependent, enrollee, member, or participant
Birthday Rule	When both parents have insurance coverage, the parent with the birthday earlier in the year carries the primary coverage for a dependent
Certified Registered Nurse Anesthetist	CRNA, an individual with specialized training and certification in nursing and anesthesia
"Clean Claim"	A properly completed CMS-1500 form submitted to a payer with all data boxes containing current and accurate information and submitted within the timely filing period required by the insurer

UNIT II   Reimbursement Issues

| Patient's Name: | Medicare # (HICN): |

ADVANCE BENEFICIARY NOTICE (ABN)

NOTE: You need to make a choice about receiving these health care items or services.

We expect that Medicare will not pay for the item(s) or service(s) that are described below. Medicare does not pay for all of your health care costs. Medicare only pays for covered items and services when Medicare rules are met. The fact that Medicare may not pay for a particular item or service does not mean that you should not receive it. There may be a good reason your doctor recommended it. Right now, in your case, **Medicare probably will not pay for –**

Items or Services:

Because:

The purpose of this form is to help you make an informed choice about whether or not you want to receive these items or services, knowing that you might have to pay for them yourself. Before you make a decision about your options, you should **read this entire notice carefully.**
- Ask us to explain, if you don't understand why Medicare probably won't pay.
- Ask us how much these items or services will cost you (**Estimated Cost: $_____**), in case you have to pay for them yourself or through other insurance.

PLEASE CHOOSE **ONE** OPTION. CHECK **ONE** BOX. **SIGN & DATE** YOUR CHOICE.

☐ **Option 1. YES.** I want to receive these items or services.
I understand that Medicare will not decide whether to pay unless I receive these items or services. Please submit my claim to Medicare. I understand that you may bill me for items or services and that I may have to pay the bill while Medicare is making its decision. If Medicare does pay, you will refund to me any payments I made to you that are due to me. If Medicare denies payment, I agree to be personally and fully responsible for payment. That is, I will pay personally, either out of pocket or through any other insurance that I have. I understand I can appeal Medicare's decision.

☐ **Option 2. NO.** I have decided not to receive these items or services.
I will not receive these items or services. I understand that you will not be able to submit a claim to Medicare and that I will not be able to appeal your opinion that Medicare won't pay.

_____   _____
Date   Signature of patient or person acting on patient's behalf

NOTE: Your health information will be kept confidential. Any information that we collect about you on this form will be kept confidential in our offices. If a claim is submitted to Medicare, your health information on this form may be shared with Medicare. Your health information which Medicare sees will be kept confidential by Medicare.

OMB Approval No. 0938-0566   Form No. CMS-R-131-G   (June 2002)

Figure **2-3** Centers for Medicare and Medicaid Services Advance Beneficiary Notice (ABN).

Coinsurance	Cost-sharing of covered services
Compliance Plan	Written strategy developed by medical facilities to ensure appropriate, consistent documentation within the medical record and ensure compliance with third-party payer guidelines and the Office of the Inspector General (OIG) Workplan guidelines
Concurrent Care	More than one physician providing care to a patient at the same time
Coordination of Benefits	COB, management of multiple third-party payments to ensure overpayment does not occur

UNIT II Reimbursement Issues

Co-payment	Cost-sharing between beneficiary and payer
Deductible	That portion of covered services paid by the beneficiary before third-party payment begins
Denial	Statement from a payer that coverage is denied
Documentation	Detailed chronology of facts and observations, procedures, services, and diagnoses relative to the patient's health
Durable Medical Equipment	DME, medically related equipment that is not disposable, such as wheelchairs, crutches, and vaporizers
Electronic Data Interchange	EDI, computerized submission of health care insurance information exchange
Employer Identification Number	EIN, an Internal Revenue Services (IRS)–issued identification number used on tax documents
Encounter Form Superbill	Medical document that contains information regarding a patient visit for health care services, can serve as a billing and/or coding document
Explanation of Benefits	EOB or EOMB, written, detailed listing of medical service payments by third-party payer to inform beneficiary and provider of payment
Fee Schedule	List of established payment for medical services arranged by CPT and HCPCS codes
Follow-up Days	FUD, established by third-party payers and listing the number of days after a procedure for which a provider must provide services to a patient for no fee. Also known as *global days*, *global package,* and *global period*
Group Provider Number	GPN, a numeric designation for a group of providers that is used instead of the individual provider number
HMO	Health Maintenance Organization
Invalid Claim	Claim that is missing necessary information and cannot be processed or paid
Medical Record	Documentation about the health care of a patient to include diagnoses, services, and procedures rendered
Noncovered Services	Any service not included by a third-party payer in the list of services for which payment is made
National Provider Identifier	NPI, 10-digit number assigned to provider by CMS and National Plan and Provider enumeration System (NPPES) and used for identification purposes when submitting services to third-party payers
Point of Service	POS, a plan in which either an in-network or out-of-network provider may be used with a higher rate paid to in-network providers
Preferred Provider Organization	PPO, providers form a network to offer health care services to a group

Prior Authorization	Also known as preauthorization, which is a requirement by the payer to receive written permission prior to patient services in order to be considered for payment by the payer
Provider Identification Number	PIN, or UPIN, is a number assigned by a third-party payer to providers to be used for identification purposes when submitting claims
Reimbursement	Payment from a third-party payer for services rendered to a patient covered by the payer's health care plan
Rejection/Denial	A claim that did not pass the edits and is returned to the provider as rejected
Resource-based Relative Value Scale	RBRVS, a list of physician services with assigned units of monetary value
State License Number	Identification number issued by a state to a physician who has been granted the right to practice in that state
UPIN	Unique provider identification number was replaced by the NPI
Usual, Customary, and Reasonable	UCR, used by some third-party payers to establish a payment rate for a service in an area with the usual (standard fee in area), customary (standard fee by the physician), and reasonable (as determined by payer) fee amounts

REIMBURSEMENT QUIZ

1. Any person who is identified as receiving life or medical benefits:
   a. primary
   b. beneficiary
   c. participant
   d. recipient

2. According to the Birthday Rule, if both parents are covered by an employer-provided health policy, the insurance policy that would be primary for reporting their child's health services is:
   a. parent with the birthday earlier in the year
   b. parent with the birthday later in the year
   c. either parent
   d. parent whose birthday is closer to the child's

3. Abbreviation for reusable medical equipment is:
   a. DRG
   b. CRN
   c. DME
   d. DIM

4. Management of multiple third-party payments to ensure that overpayment does not occur:
   a. PRO
   b. COB
   c. DME
   d. FUD

5. CMS delegates the daily operation of the Medicare program to:
   a. DHHS
   b. PRO
   c. RVU
   d. MACs or FIs

6. A QIO provider is one who:
   a. signs an agreement with the FIs or MACs
   b. submits charges directly to CMS
   c. receives 5% less than some other physicians
   d. can bill the patient the total remaining balance after payment from Medicare

7. This part of Medicare covers the inpatient portion of covered costs after the deductible has been paid:
   a. Part A
   b. Part B
   c. Part C
   d. Part D

8. This issue of the *Federal Register* contains outpatient facility changes for CMS programs for the coming year:
   a. October/November
   b. November/December
   c. December/October
   d. November/August

9. This replaced the RBRVS:
   a. RAI
   b. OPPS
   c. APC
   d. NFS

10. Entity responsible for development of the plan that outlines monitoring of the Medicare program:
    a. FIs or MACs
    b. OIG
    c. DHSS
    d. HEW

REIMBURSEMENT QUIZ ANSWERS

1. b
2. a
3. c
4. b
5. d
6. a
7. a
8. b
9. d
10. b

UNIT III

Overview of CPT, ICD-9-CM, and HCPCS Coding

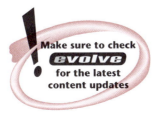

UNIT III Overview of CPT, ICD-9-CM, and HCPCS Coding

■ INTRODUCTION TO MEDICAL CODING

Translates services/procedures/supplies/drugs into CPT/HCPCS codes

Translates diagnosis(es) into ICD-9-CM codes

Three Levels of Service Codes

1. Level I CPT
2. Level II HCPCS, National Codes
3. Level III Local Codes—phased out with implementation of HIPAA code sets

Diagnosis Codes, ICD-9-CM

ICD-9-CM, Volumes 1 and 2, *International Classification of Diseases,* 9th ed., Clinical Modification

Volume 1, Tabular List

Volume 2, Alphabetic List

Volume 3, Index and Tabular of Procedures (hospital version)

- Classification system
- Translates diagnosis(es) (dx) into standardized codes that explain why service was provided
- Very specific in nature
- May be up to five numeric or alphanumeric places
- Example: Diabetes becomes 250.XX

■ CPT

Developed by the AMA in 1966

Five-digit codes to report services provided to patients

Updated each November for use January 1

Types of CPT Codes

- Medical
- Surgical
- Diagnostic services
- Anesthesia
- Evaluation and Management

CPT Codes

Allow communication that is both effective and efficient

Inform third-party payers of services/procedures provided

Used as a basis of payment

Incorrect Coding
Results in providers being paid inappropriately (either overpayment or underpayment)

Outpatient Physician (Non-Hospital) Services
Reported on standardized insurance form

CMS-1500 = universal form (Figure 3-1)

CPT Format

Symbols. Used to convey information

- Bullet = New code symbol

▲ Triangle = Revised Code

▶◀ Right and left triangles = Beginning and ending of text change

+ Plus = Add-on code
  - Full list in Appendix D of CPT

⊘ Circle with line = Modifier -51 exempt code
  - Modifier -51 cannot be used with these codes
  - Full list in Appendix E of CPT

⊙ Bullseye = Codes that include moderate (conscious) sedation
  - Such as 45391, flexible colonoscopy
  - Full list in Appendix G of CPT

⚡ Lightning bolt symbol = Codes for which the FDA status pending
  - Full list in Appendix K of CPT

CPT Sections
1. Evaluation & Management (E/M)
2. Anesthesia
3. Surgery
4. Radiology
5. Pathology and Laboratory
6. Medicine

TIP: During your examination, the front section of the CPT (Introduction and Illustrations) is an excellent resource on the format, definitions of terms, medical terms, and instructions in the CPT. Review these well before the examination to familiarize yourself with where to find the information that is contained in the front section.

Also, flag the different sections of the CPT for easy access during the examination—for example, the illustrations section, E/M Guidelines, Appendices, and other major sections of the manual.

Categorized by
Sections

Subsections

UNIT III Overview of CPT, ICD-9-CM, and HCPCS Coding

Figure 3-1 The CMS-1500 (08-05) Health Insurance Claim Form was revised from the CMS-1500 (12-90) form to accommodate reporting of the National Provider Identifier (NPI) number mandated for May 2007. The CMS-1500 (08-05) version was mandated for use on February 1, 2007. For more information: http://www.cms.hhs.gov/transmittals/downloads/R899CP.pdf. (Courtesy U.S. Department of Health and Human Services, Centers for Medicare and Medicaid Services.)

Subheadings

Categories

   Anatomy

      Knee or Shoulder

   Procedure

      Incision or Excision

   Condition

      Fracture or Dislocation

   Description

      Cast or Strap

   Surgical approach

      Anterior Cranial Fossa or Middle Cranial Fossa

Guidelines
Section-specific information begins each section

Provides instruction pertinent to entire section

Notes
Located throughout CPT

Provides instruction pertinent to specific subsection

Two Types of Code Descriptions

1. Stand-alone: Full description

   Example: 10080 Incision and drainage of pilonidal cyst; simple

2. Indented: Dependent on preceding stand-alone for meaning

   Example: 10080 Incision and drainage of pilonidal cyst; simple

        10081   complicated

Semicolon
- Description preceding semicolon is the common part of the description and applies to any indented codes under it
- You must return to stand-alone for full description

Modifiers Add Information

CPT Modifier
Added at the end of the CPT/HCPCS code

Some modifiers are informational; others affect reimbursement

   Example: 43820 gastrojejunostomy

- -62 two surgeons
- 43820-62 two surgeons performed a gastrojejunostomy
- Only used if both surgeons submit same CPT code

Level II HCPCS Modifiers

"-AS" physician's assistant

"-F1" Left hand, second digit

All modifiers used on CPT or HCPCS codes

All HCPCS modifiers begin with a letter

Modifiers are placed in 24D field on CMS-1500 (see Figure 3-1)

Unlisted Services

Codes end in "99" = "no specific code" in Category I or Category III

    99 Equals = Miscellaneous

Used when a more specific code can not be assigned

Written report must accompany claim form indicating

- Nature
- Extent
- Need
- Time
- Effort
- Equipment used

Category II Codes—Supplemental Tracking Codes

Used for performance measurements

    Optional unless practice participating in Physician Quality Improvement Reporting Initiative (PQRI)

These codes collect data concerning the quality of care and test results

Alphanumeric and end in the letter "F" (0005F)

Located after the Medicine section in CPT

Category III Codes—New Technology

Temporary codes—may be included in this section up to 3 years

Identify emerging technology, services, and procedures

Located after Category II codes

Alphanumeric and end in the letter "T" (0016T)

- May or may not receive future Category I code status
- Category I codes (00100-99607)
- Approved by AMA and the Food and Drug Administration (FDA)
- Proven clinical effectiveness (efficacy)
- Category III has not been approved and has no proven clinical effectiveness (efficacy)
- Use Category III code instead of unlisted code if no Category I code appropriate
- Use unlisted code if no Category III code exists

The Index

Used to locate service/procedure terms and codes

Speeds up code location

Uses dictionary format

- First entries and last entries on top of page
- Code display in index
  - Single code: 38115
  - Multiple codes: 26645, 26650
  - Range of codes: 22305-22325

Location Methods
Service/procedure: Repair, excision

Anatomic site: Medial nerve, elbow

Condition or disease: Cleft lip, clot

Synonym: Toe and interphalangeal joint

Eponym: Jones procedure, Heller operation

Abbreviation: ECG, PEEP (positive end-expiratory pressure)

"See" in index
Cross-reference terms: "Look here for code"

Index: Stem, Brain: *See* Brainstem

Appendices of CPT

Appendix A: Modifiers

Appendix B: Additions, Deletions, Revisions

Appendix C: Clinical Examples, E/M Codes

Appendix D: Add-On Codes

Appendix E: -51 Exempt Codes

Appendix F: -63 Exempt Codes

Appendix G: Conscious (Moderate) Sedation

Appendix H: Performance Measures, Category II Modifiers

Appendix I: Genetic Testing Modifiers

Appendix J: Electrodiagnostic Medicine Listing of Sensory, Motor, and Mixed Nerves

Appendix K: Products Pending FDA Approval

Appendix L: Vascular Families

Appendix M: Crosswalk to Deleted CPT Codes

Review information in the CPT appendices prior to examination

■ EVALUATION AND MANAGEMENT (E/M) SECTION (99201-99499)

> Your job is to code only from what is documented in medical record
> Optimize—never maximize
> Accurately report documented services
> Coding for services not provided is a punishable CRIME

Subsections by type of service

Types of service

- Consultation
- Office Services
- Hospital Services, etc.

Integral Factors When Selecting E/M Codes

1. Place of Service
Explains setting of service

- Office
- Emergency Department
- Nursing Home

2. Type of Service
Physicians provide many types of service

- Consultations
- Admissions
- Office visits

3. Patient Status
The four status types are

1. New patient
2. Established patient
3. Outpatient
4. Inpatient

New patient
Has not received any professional service in last 3 years from the same physician or another physician of the same specialty and in the same group

New patients are more labor-intensive for physician, medical staff, and clerical staff

Established patient
Has received professional services in last 3 years from the same physician or another physician of the same specialty in the same group

Medical record available with current, relevant information

Outpatient
One who has not been admitted to a health care facility

> *Example:* Patient receives services at clinic or same-day surgery center

Inpatient
One who has been formally admitted to a health care facility

> *Example:* Patient admitted to a hospital or nursing home

Physician dictates:

- Admission orders
- H&P (history and physical)
- Requests for consultations

Levels of E/M Service Based on

Skill required to provide service

Time spent

Level of knowledge necessary to treat the patient

Effort required

Responsibility required/assumed

E/M Levels Divided Based on

Key Components (KC)
- History (Hx)
- Physical examination (PE)
- Medical decision making (MDM)

Contributory Factors (CF)
- Counseling
- Coordination of care
- Nature of presenting problem

Every Encounter Contains Varying Amount of KC and CF
More extensive component/factor

- Higher level of service
  - Less extensive component/factor
- Lower level of service

KEY COMPONENTS

Four Elements of a History

1. Chief Complaint (CC)
2. History of Present Illness (HPI)
3. Review of Systems (ROS)
4. Past, Family, or Social History (PFSH)

Chief Complaint (CC)—Subjective

Reason for encounter or presenting problem: Patient's current complaint in patient's own words

Documented in medical record for each encounter

History of Present Illness (HPI)—Subjective

Description of development of current illness, e.g., date of onset

Patient describes HPI

Provider must personally document

PHYSICIAN AND PATIENT DIALOGUE

Development of a CC of Abdominal Pain (HPI):

"Started Thursday night and was mild. During the night, it got worse. Friday morning I went to work but had to leave because the pain got so bad."

Location. Specific source of pain

"Pain was in lower left-hand side, a little toward back."

Quality. Is pain sharp, intermittent, burning?

"Pain is really sharp and constant."

Severity. Is pain intense, moderate, mild?

"Pain is terrible, worst pain I have ever had." (intensity of pain/scale)

Duration. How long has pain been present?

"Pain has been going on now for 3 days."

Timing. Is pain constant or does it come and go?

"Pain just continues. It just doesn't go away."

Context. When does it hurt most?

"Pain is just there, it doesn't matter what I am doing."

Modifying factors. Does anything make it better or worse?

"Nothing I do makes it any better or any worse."

Associated signs and symptoms. Does anything else feel different when pain is present?

"Yes, I have nausea when pain is worst."

Review of Systems (ROS)—Subjective

Questions posed to the patient to identify signs and symptoms that have been or are being experienced relating to the HPI

Organ systems (OS), e.g., respiratory system, cardiovascular system

Extent of ROS depends on CC and patient status (new, established, inpatient, outpatient)

ROS Elements
Constitutional—General, Fever, Weight loss or gain

Eyes—Organ System (OS)

Ears, Nose, Mouth, Throat (OS)

Cardiovascular (OS)

Respiratory (OS)

Gastrointestinal (OS)

Genitourinary (OS)

Musculoskeletal (OS)

Integumentary (OS)

Neurologic (OS)

Psychiatric (OS)

Endocrine (OS)

Hematologic (OS)

Allergic/Immunologic (OS)

Past, Family, and Social History (PFSH)

Past. Contains relevant information about past illness, injury, or treatment, including

- Major illnesses/injuries
- Operations
- Hospitalizations
- Allergies
- Immunizations
- Dietary status
- Current medications

Family History
Health status or cause of death of family members

- Parents
- Siblings
- Children

Family history items related to CC

- Hereditary diseases

Social History
Review of past and current activities

- Marital status
- Employment
- Occupational history
- Use of drugs/alcohol
- Educational activities
- Sexual history
- Other relevant or contributory factors

Four History Levels

1. Problem Focused (PF)
2. Expanded Problem Focused (EPF)
3. Detailed (Det)
4. Comprehensive (Comp)

Problem Focused History
CC

Brief HPI

No ROS

No PFSH

Expanded Problem Focused History
CC

Brief HPI

Problem focused ROS

No PFSH

Detailed History
CC

Extended HPI

Problem pertinent ROS, extended to include a limited number of additional systems

Pertinent PFSH directly related to problem

Comprehensive History
CC

Extended HPI

Complete ROS directly related to CC, plus review of at least 8 additional systems

Complete PFSH

Summary of elements required for each level of history (Figure 3-2)

Evaluation and Management (E/M) Section

History Elements

Chief Complaint (CC)
  Reason for the encounter in the patient's words

History of Present Illness (HPI)
  Location
  Quality
  Severity
  Duration*
  Timing
  Context
  Modifying factors
  Associated signs and symptoms

Review of Systems (ROS)
  Constitutional symptoms (fever, weight loss, etc.)
  Ophthalmologic (eyes)
  Otolaryngologic (ears, nose, mouth, throat)
  Cardiovascular
  Respiratory
  Gastrointestinal
  Genitourinary
  Musculoskeletal
  Integumentary (skin and/or breast)
  Neurologic
  Psychiatric
  Endocrine
  Hematologic/Lymphatic
  Allergic/Immunologic

Past, Family, and/or Social History (PFSH)
  Past major illnesses, operations, injuries, and treatments
  Family medical history for heredity and risk
  Social activities, both past and current

Elements Required for Each Level of History

		Problem Focused	Expanded Problem Focused	Detailed	Comprehensive
History	HPI	Brief 1-3	Brief 1-3	Extended 4+	Extended 4+
	ROS	None	Problem-pertinent 1	Extended 2-9	Complete 10+
	PFSH	None	None	Pertinent 1	Complete 2-3

Figure **3-2** History elements required for each level of history.

Four Examination Levels (Objective)

Problem Focused Examination (1995 Documentation Guidelines [DG])
Limited examination of affected body area or organ system

Expanded Problem Focused Examination (1995 DG)
Limited examination of affected body area or organ system

Other related body area(s) or organ system(s)

Detailed Examination (1995 DG)
Extended examination of affected body area(s) and other symptomatic or related organ system(s)

Examination Elements

General
    Constitutional

Body Areas (BA)
    Head (including the face)
    Neck
    Chest (including breasts and axillae)
    Abdomen
    Genitalia, groin, buttocks
    Back
    Each extremity

Organ System (OS)
    Ophthalmologic (eyes)
    Otolaryngologic (ears, nose, mouth, throat)
    Cardiovascular
    Respiratory
    Gastrointestinal
    Genitourinary
    Musculoskeletal
    Integumentary
    Neurologic
    Psychiatric
    Hematologic/Lymphatic/Immunologic

Elements Required for Each Level of Examination

	Problem Focused	Expanded Problem Focused	Detailed	Comprehensive
Examination	Limited to affected BA or OS	Limited to affected BA or OS and other related OS(s)	Extended of affected BA(s) and other related OS(s)	General multi-system or complete single OS

Figure **3-3** Examination elements required for each level of examination.

Comprehensive Examination (1995 DG)

Complete single specialty or complete multisystem examination or 8 or more organ systems

Summary of elements required for each level of examination (Figure 3-3)

Medical Decision Making Complexity (MDM)

Management Options
Based on number of possible diagnoses

Levels: Minimal, limited, multiple, or extensive

Data Reviewed
Laboratory, radiology; any test/procedure results are documented along with the data reviewed and the identity of the reviewer in medical record

- "Hemoglobin within normal limits."
- "Chest x-ray, negative."

Old medical records (data) from others may be requested and reviewed

Levels: Minimal, limited, moderate, or extensive

Risks

Risks of morbidity (poor outcome), complications, or mortality (death) associated with problem, diagnostic procedure

Other diseases or factors (co-morbidities)

- Diabetes
- Extreme age

Urgency relates to risks

- Myocardial infarction
- Ruptured appendix

Levels: Minimal, low, moderate, or high

See Figure 3-4, CMS Table of Risk

Four Levels of MDM Complexity

1. Straightforward MDM
Number of diagnoses or management options: Minimal

Amount or complexity of data: Minimal/None

Risk of complications or death: Minimal

2. Low-complexity MDM
Number of diagnoses or management options: Limited

Amount or complexity of data: Limited

Risk of complications or death: Low

3. Moderate-Complexity MDM
Number of diagnoses or management options: Multiple

Amount or complexity of data: Moderate

Risk of complications or death: Moderate

4. High-Complexity MDM
Number of diagnoses or management options: Extensive

Amount or complexity of data: Extensive

Risk of complications or death: High

Summary of elements required for each level of MDM (Figure 3-5)

The diagnosis or management options, amount or complexity of data, and risk are totaled to arrive at the level of MDM

Only two of three categories must meet or exceed each other in any level to assign the MDM

Example: Moderate complexity for diagnosis or management options and moderate complexity of amount or complexity of data, but only a low risk would be assigned a moderate level MDM

Example: Low risk of death, moderate diagnosis or management options, and high amount or complexity of data: Assign the moderate level of MDM

TABLE OF RISK
(Total = highest risk in any one category)

Level of risk	Presenting problem(s)	Diagnostic procedure(s) ordered	Management options selected
Minimal	• One self-limited or minor problem, e.g., cold, insect bite, tinea corpus	• Laboratory tests requiring venipuncture • Chest x-rays • EKG/EEG • Urinalysis • Ultrasound, e.g., echo-cardiography • KOH prep	• Rest • Gargles • Elastic bandages • Superficial dressings
Low	• Two or more self-limited or minor problems • One stable chronic illness, e.g., well controlled hypertension or non-insulin dependent diabetes, cataract, BPH • Acute uncomplicated illness or injury, e.g., cystitis, allergic rhinitis, simple sprain	• Physiologic tests not under stress, e.g., pulmonary function tests • Non-cardiovascular imaging studies with contrast, e.g., barium enema • Superficial needle biopsies • Clinical laboratory tests requiring arterial puncture • Skin biopsies	• Over-the-counter drugs • Minor surgery with no identified risk factors • Physical therapy • IV fluids without additives
Moderate	• One or more chronic illnesses with mild exacerbation, progression, or side effects of treatment • Two or more stable chronic illnesses • Undiagnosed new problem with uncertain prognosis, e.g., lump in breast • Acute illness with systemic symptoms, e.g., pyelonephritis, pneumonitis, colitis • Acute complicated injury, e.g., head injury with brief loss of consciousness	• Physiologic tests under stress, e.g., cardiac stress test, fetal contraction stress test • Diagnostic endoscopies with no identified risk factors • Deep needle or incisional biopsy • Cardiovascular imaging studies with contrast and no identified risk factors, e.g., arteriogram, cardiac catheterization • Obtain fluid from body cavity, e.g., lumbar puncture, thora-centesis, culdocentesis	• Minor surgery with identified risk factors • Elective major surgery (open, percutaneous, or endoscopic) with no identified risk factors • Prescription drug management • Therapeutic nuclear medicine • IV fluids with additives • Closed treatment of fracture or dislocation without manipulation
High	• One or more chronic illnesses with severe exacerbation, progression, or side effects of treatment • Acute or chronic illnesses or injuries that pose a threat to life or bodily function, e.g., multiple trauma, acute MI, pulmonary embolus, severe respiratory distress, progressive severe rheumatoid arthritis • Psychiatric illness with potential threat to self or others • Peritonitis • Acute renal failure • An abrupt change in neurologic status, e.g., seizure, TIA, weakness, or sensory loss	• Cardiovascular imaging studies with contrast with identified risk factors • Cardiac electrophysiological tests • Diagnostic endoscopies with identified risk factors • Discography	• Elective major surgery (open, percutaneous, or endoscopic) with identified risk factors • Emergency major surgery (open, percutaneous or endoscopic) • Parenteral controlled substances • Drug therapy requiring intensive monitoring for toxicity • Decision not to resuscitate or to de-escalate care because of poor prognosis

Figure 3-4 Centers for Medicare and Medicaid Services (CMS) Table of Risk. (Courtesy U.S. Department of Health and Human Services, Centers for Medicare and Medicaid Services.)

Medical Decision-Making Elements

Number of Diagnoses or Management Options
Minimal
Limited
Multiple
Extensive

Amount or Complexity of Data to Review
Minimal/None
Limited
Moderate
Extensive

Risk of Complications or Death If Condition Goes Untreated
Minimal
Low
Moderate
High

Elements Required for Each Level of Medical Decision Making

	Straightforward	Low	Moderate	High
Number of diagnoses or management options	Minimal	Limited	Multiple	Extensive
Amount or complexity of data to review	Minimal/None	Limited	Moderate	Extensive
Risk	Minimal	Low	Moderate	High

Figure **3-5** Elements required for each level of medical decision making.

Contributory Factors

Counseling

Provided to patient or family members (synopsis must be stated in medical record)

Discussion of diagnosis, test results, impressions, recommendations, prognosis, risks/benefits of treatment options or lack thereof, and risk factor reduction

Coordination of Care
Work done on behalf of patient by physician to provide care

Nature of Presenting Problem
Type of problem patient presents to physician with or reason for encounter

Levels of Presenting Problem

Minimal Presenting Problem
May not require a physician

   Example: A dressing change or removal of an uncomplicated suture

Self-limiting or Minor Presenting Problem
Self-limiting problems are minor and with a good outcome and no complications predicted

Example: Sore throat or a slightly irritated skin tag

Low-Severity Presenting Problem
Without treatment, low risk

Example: A middle-aged, healthy male with an upper respiratory infection

Moderate-Severity Presenting Problem
Without treatment, moderate risk

Example: An elderly male with bacterial pneumonia

High-Severity Presenting Problem
Without treatment, high risk

Example: An elderly male in very poor health with diabetic ketoacidosis

Time
Direct face-to-face: Physician or NPP and patient together

Example: Clinic visit or at bedside in hospital

Calculated for code assignment beginning and ending times documented in medical record

Unit/Floor: Time spent by physician on patient's floor or unit, also at patient's bedside

Example: Reviewing patient records or at chart desk and then with patient

---

Over 50% of the total time should include counseling and/or coordination of care, and the documentation must reflect the total time of the visit and the time spent counseling and/or in coordination of care to qualify to assign the code based on time.

Use of E/M Code

Codes are grouped by type of service and place of service

- Consultation
- Office visit
- Hospital admission

Different codes are required for various levels of service assignment

New patient (99201-99205) services to new patient in office or other outpatient setting

Selection of Level of E/M Services

For the following categories/subcategories, all three of the key components must meet or exceed the level stated in the code description:

- Office or Other Outpatient Services, New Patient
- Hospital Observation Services
- Initial Hospital Care
- Office Consultation

- Inpatient Consultation
- Emergency Department Services
- Initial Nursing Facility Care
- Other Nursing Facility Services
- Domiciliary, Rest Home (e.g., Boarding Home), or Custodial Care Services, New Patient
- Home Services, New Patient

For the following categories/subcategories, two of the three key components must meet or exceed the level stated in the code description:

- Office or Other Outpatient Services, Established Patient
- Subsequent Hospital Care
- Subsequent Nursing Facility Care
- Domiciliary, Rest Home (e.g., Boarding Home), Established Patient
- Home Services, Established Patient

New Patient (99201-99205)
All new patients must be seen by physician

Established Patient (99211-99215)
99211 may not require a physician's presence

No such code in New Patient category; all new patients are seen by physician

Hospital Observation Status (99217-99220, 99234-99236)
Not officially admitted to "inpatient status"

Patient not ill enough to admit but is too ill not to be monitored or discharged

Read notes at beginning of subsection

Observation services are not codes for "inpatient" services

Observation admission can be reported only for first day of service

When patient admitted on observation status and discharged on same day:

- Use code from 99234-99236 (Observation or Inpatient Care Services category)

Patient in hospital overnight for observation but less than 48 hours:

- **First day:** 99218-99220 (Initial Observation Care)
- **Second day:** 99217 (Observation Care Discharge Services)

If observation stay longer than 48 hours:

- **First day:** 99218-99220 (Initial Observation Care)
- **Second day:** 99212-99215 (Established Patient, Office or other Outpatient)
- **Third day:** 99217 (Observation Care Discharge Services)

Initial Observation Care

- Beginning of observation care service
- Does not require a specific hospital unit; can be a regular bed on a floor or in emergency department (ED)
- Status specified as "observation"

E/M services immediately prior to admission bundled into observation service

Example: Office visit prior to observation, bundled into observation service

Hospital Inpatient Services (99221-99239)
Officially admitted to a hospital setting

Total (all day and night)

Partial (all day and no night, all night and no day, or a variation)

- Time in and out must be specified in medical record

Types of Physician Status
Attending: Primary or admitting physician

Consultant: Physician whose opinion and advice requested by attending physician

Referring: Physician requesting a consultation from another physician regarding a patient's health status

Types of Care
Concurrent care given to patient by more than one physician each of different specialities

Example: Pulmonologist and cardiologist both treating patient for different conditions at same time

Three Types of Hospital Inpatient Services
Initial Hospital Care (99221-99223)
First service includes admission

Initial paperwork

Initial treatment plans and orders

Used only once for each admission

- Only one admission by the attending or admitting physician billable per hospitalization

Subsequent Hospital Care (99231-99233)
After initial service

Physician reviews patient's progress using documentation, information received from nursing staff, examination of patient

- May be reported by multiple physicians of different specialities managing different conditions (concurrent care); only one per day per physician per speciality

Hospital Discharge Services (99238, 99239)
Final day of hospital stay when patient in hospital more than 1 day

Documentation indicates final patient status

Time based

- Total time

- Does not need to be continuous time

Beginning and ending time or total time spent must be documented to assign the extended discharge code or use lowest level code

Final Status of Patient
Summary of stay (Discharge)
Condition (final examination)

Medications

Plan for return (follow-up care) to physician

How hospital stay progressed

Discharged destination (to home, nursing facility, etc.)

Only attending physician can use discharge code (only one discharge per admission)

Code based on time spent in service

Beginning and ending time or total time spent must be documented to assign the extended discharge code or must use lowest level code

Consultation Services (99241-99255)
One physician or appropriate source requests another physician's opinion or advice

Either inpatient or outpatient; outpatient consultations include those provided in ED

Outpatient consultations (99241-99245)

Inpatient consultations (99251-99255)

Third-Party-Payer Consultations
Request consult for

- Past medical treatment
- Current condition
- Payers may request prior to approving procedure
- Report services with -32, mandated services

Emergency Department Services (99281-99285)
No distinction between new and established patients

Must be open 24 hours a day to qualify as ED (ER)

ED services often require additional codes from Critical Care Services

- Typically billed by ED physicians

Critical Care Services (99291, 99292)
Example: Multiple organ failure

Critical care services are provided to patients over 24 months of age in life-threatening (critically ill/injured) situations

Time-based codes

- Total time under 30 minutes reported with appropriate E/M code (e.g., ED)

Critical Care Services (99291, 99292)
Time must be documented in medical record to select from this code range; does not need to be continuous

- Over 24 months of age

99291 and 99292 used to report length of time a physician spends caring for critically ill patient

99291: 30-74 minutes

99292: Each additional 30 minutes

Nursing Facility Services (99304-99318)
Non-hospital settings with professional staff

- Provide continuous health care services to patients who are not acutely ill

Formerly known as Skilled Nursing Facility (SNF), Intermediate Care Facility (ICF), and Long-Term Care Facility (LTCF)

Various levels of nursing facility services

Initial Nursing Facility Assessment (99304-99306)
Provided at time of patient's initial admission/readmission

Subsequent Nursing Facility Care codes (99307-99310)
99307 stable, recovering, or improving

99308 not responding or minor complication

99309 significant complication or new problem

99310 significant new problem requiring immediate physician attention

Nursing Facility Discharge Services (99315, 99316)
For final discharge service

Time-based

- Total time, does not need to be continuous

Other Nursing Facility Services (99318)

Annual Nursing Facility Assessment

Domiciliary, Rest Home, or Custodial Care Services (99324-99337)
Health care services are not available on site

Types of services provided are lodging, meals, supervision, personal care, leisure activities

Residents cannot live independently

Codes for either new or established patients

Domiciliary, Rest Home, or Home Care Plan Oversight Services (99339, 99340)
Read notes at beginning of subsection

Reports individual physician supervision of patient in home or domiciliary rest home

Services not face-to-face

Time-based

99339 15-29 minutes

99340 30 minutes or more

Reported once per 30-day period

Home Services (99341-99350)
Care provided in patient's home

Services based on key components and contributory factors

Codes for new or established patients

Prolonged Services (99354-99359)
Time codes for direct face-to-face and without direct face-to-face contact

Report time beyond the usual service

- Must be documented in medical record

Codes for first 30-74 minutes and each additional 30 minutes thereafter

If less than 30 minutes, do not report service as prolonged

Standby Service (99360)
Physician not caring for other patient(s) to use these codes

Physician standing by only for that patient, if needed

Standby requested by another physician

- Must be documented in medical record

Report in 30-minute increments

Less than 30 minutes—do not report

Can report for subsequent 30 minutes only if a full 30 minutes

Carriers have strict policies regarding reimbursement for this service

Case Management Services (99363, 99364)
Anticoagulant Management Services, 99363 and 99364

- Anticoagulants are such as Warfarin
  - Thins the blood
- By physician or another qualified health care professional
- Provided in an outpatient setting
  - 60 days or more
  - 60 days or less is not reported

Medical Team Conferences (99366-99368)
Codes for with or without face-to-face patient/family contact

- Minimum of 3 health care professionals, different specialties/disciplines participate in team
- Each member must have performed face-to-face evaluation in past 60 days
- Documentation must reflect members contribution of information and treatment recommendation
- Note reported for organization or facility contracted services

Time-based

    Begins and ends at start and conclusion of review

Care Plan Oversight Services (99374-99380)
Used to report physician supervision of patient care in home health agency, hospice, domiciliary, or equivalent environment

Patient not present

Codes are time-based

- 15-29 minutes
- 30 minutes or more
- Must be documented in medical record

Reported once for each 30-day period

Preventive Medicine Services (99381-99397)
Used to report services when patient is not currently ill

Example: Annual checkup

Codes divided by new or established and age

If significant problem is encountered during preventive examination

- E/M code also reported, append modifier -25

Counseling Risk Factor Reduction and Behavior Change Intervention (99401-99429)
Patient is seen specifically to promote health and/or wellness

Example: Diet, exercise program

Patient without symptoms or an established diagnosis to use these codes

Codes based on

- Time
- Individual or group
- Physician review of assessment data

Non-Face-to-Face Physician Services (99441-99444)
Physician E/M services using telephone/internet

- 99441-99443 telephone E/M services

    Established patient, family member of the patient, or a guardian

- 99444 online E/M services

    Established patient, family member of the patient, or a guardian

Special E/M Services (99450-99456)
- 99450 is reported for services provided for insurance or disability assessments

Involves no treatment; any treatment provided would be coded separately

Codes divided

- 99455: Assessment by treating physician
- 99456: Assessment by nontreating physician

For new/established patients in any setting

- 99477: Initial hospital care neonate for intensive observation

Newborn Care and Neonatal/Pediatric Critical Care Services

Newborn Care (99460-99463)
Initial and subsequent care in/other than hospital or birthing center

    For normal newborn infant

    Per day, for E/M services

99463, initial hospital/birthing center when admission and discharge is same day

Delivery/Birthing Room Attendance (99464-99465)
99464, attendance at delivery

    Documented request by attending in medical record

    Provides initial stabilization

99465, resuscitation and ventilation

Neonatal and Pediatric Critical Care Services Subsection (99466-99480)
Pediatric Patient Transport

99466, 99467

First 30-74 minutes

    Each additional 30 minutes

Reports interfacility transport

    Face-to-face service

Critically ill or injured patient

    24 months or less

Inpatient Neonatal Critical Care Services
99468, 99469

Divided by

    Initial day

    Subsequent day

Critically ill neonate

    Age 28 days or less

Inpatient Pediatric Critical Care Services
99471-99476

Inpatient services

Divided by age

    29 days-24 months

    2-5 years

Subdivided by day

  Initial

  Subsequent

Initial and Continuing Intensive Care Services (99477-99480)
99477-99480

Hospital Care

99477 for neonate 28 days of age or less

99478-99480 divided by birth weight

  very low birth weight (VLBW) ≤1500 grams (≤3.3 pounds)

  low birth weight (LBW) 1500-2500 grams (3.3-5.5 pounds)

  normal birth weight 2501-5000 grams (5.51-11.01 pounds)

Subdivided on day

  Initial

  Subsequent

Other Evaluation and Management Services (99477-99499)

- 99499 reports unlisted E/M services

  Accompanied by a special report

ANESTHESIA SECTION (00100-01999)

Anesthesiologist

Doctor of medicine specializing in anesthesia

Usually outside practices, e.g., Anesthesia Associates, Inc., or Pain Clinic, Ltd.

Professional services reported separately

CRNA

Certified Registered Nurse Anesthetist

Uses of Anesthesia

Manage unconscious patients, life functions, and resuscitation

Analgesia

Relieve pain

Some Methods of Anesthesia

Endotracheal: Through mouth (general anesthesia)

Local: Application to area (injection or topical)

Epidural: Between vertebral spaces

Regional: Field or nerve block

MAC: monitored anesthesia care

Patient-Controlled Analgesia (PCA)

Patient self-administers drug

Used to relieve chronic pain or temporarily for severe pain following surgery

Moderate (Conscious) Sedation

99143-99145 used when surgeon administers sedation

99148-99150 used when physician other than surgeon administers sedation

- No anesthesia personnel are present

Decreased level of consciousness

Not reported by physician if provided in nonfacility setting

Anesthesia Formula

(B + T + M) × conversion factor = Anesthesia payment

B is for Base Units

Published in *Relative Value Guide (RVG)* by American Society of Anesthesiologists

National unit values for anesthesia services based on complexity of service

T is for Time
Patient record indicates time, e.g., 60 minutes

Usually, 15 or 30 minutes = 1 unit

   Example: 60 minutes = 2 units

Some payers may indicate 1 unit = 1 minute

Begins: Anesthesiologist begins to prepare patient for induction—preoperative

Continues throughout procedure—intraoperative

Ends: Patient no longer under care of anesthesiologist—postoperative

M is for Modifying Unit
Additional units based on physical status of patient (see modifiers that follow)

Physical Status Modifiers, P1-P6
Located in Anesthesia Guidelines

Not reported to Medicare

Help to show complexity of service

- P1 Normal healthy
- P2 Mild systemic disease
- P3 Severe systemic disease
- P4 Severe systemic disease is constant threat to life
- P5 Not expected to survive without the operation
- P6 Clinically brain dead

Qualifying Circumstances Codes (99100-99140)
Anesthesia services provided under difficult circumstances

Located in both Anesthesia Guidelines and Medicine section

Listed in addition to primary anesthesia code

More than one may be reported

Summing Up Formula
Base units (from *RVG*) based on CPT codes

Time units (usually 15 or 30 min is a unit)

- Total time ÷ 30 = time units

Modifiers [Qualifying Circumstances (99100-99140) and/or Physical Status (P1-P6)]

Conversion Factors
CMS anesthesia conversion factors

Sum of money allocated by payer, per unit for payment of anesthesia services

Anesthesia for Multiple Surgical Procedures
Once anesthetized, length of time, not number of procedures performed during session

Report highest relative value guide (RVG) valued CPT code

   Example: Two procedures during same session

- One, 10 units; the other, 5 units
- Report only 10 units and combined time for all procedures

CPT/HCPCS LEVEL I MODIFIERS (-21 to -99)

Alters CPT or HCPCS code

Full list, CPT, Appendix A

- Two separate lists
  - One for physician use
  - One for hospital outpatient use

Modifier Functions

Altered (i.e., increased or reduced service)

Bilateral

Multiple

Only portions of service (i.e., professional service only)

More than one surgeon

-21 Prolonged E/M Service

Used only with highest-level E/M codes (99205-99397)

Indicates extended service above highest level in category

-22 Increased Procedural Service

Indicates services significantly greater than usual

Accompanied by written report and supportive documentation

-23 Unusual Anesthesia

Use of general anesthesia where local or regional is norm

Example: Highly agitated senile patient

Used only with anesthesia codes

Written report with submission of modifier

-24 Unrelated E/M Services by Same Physician During a Postoperative Period

Service not related to surgery

If E/M provided during postoperative global period, no payment considered without -24

-25 Significant, Separately Identifiable E/M Service, Same Physician/and Day of Procedure/Service

Documentation must support service

Example: Patient seen for sinus congestion, physician performs H&P, prescribes decongestant, notes and removes lesion on back

Code: Procedure + E/M-25

-26 Professional Component

Professional component (physician, -26)

Technical component (technician + equipment, -TC)

-32 Mandated Service

Mandated by payer, worker's comp, or official body or court of law

Not request of patient, patient's family, or another physician

> **Example:** Worker's Compensation requests examination of person currently receiving disability benefits

-47 Anesthesia by Surgeon

Surgeon administers regional or general anesthesia

Physician acts as both surgeon and anesthesiologist

Used only with Surgery codes

-50 Bilateral Procedure

Body is bilateral

> **Example:** Procedure on hands

Caution: Some codes describe bilateral procedures

Typically not used on Integumentary System codes

-51 Multiple Procedure—Three Types

Same procedure, different sites

Multiple operation(s), same operative session

Procedure performed multiple times

List most resource-intense procedure first, then descending order of resource intensity

Next, other procedure(s) + -51 (unless code is -51 exempt or add-on code)

Usual procedure payment: 1st 100%, 2nd 50%, 3rd 25%-50%, depending on payer

-52 Reduced Services

Service reduced or not performed to the extent described in code description

There is no other code that accurately reflects the service actually provided

Physician directed reduction

Documentation substantiates reduction

Not to be used for patient unable to pay

Submit regular charge amount, payer will adjust

-53 Discontinued Procedure

Surgical/diagnostic procedures

Procedure started then stopped due to patient's condition

Does not apply to presurgical discontinuance

Submit regular charge, payer will adjust

DO NOT USE -53
- When patient cancels scheduled procedure
- With E/M codes
- With time-based code

-54 Surgical Care Only

Physician provides only procedure (intraoperative); other physician does preoperative and postoperative service

Documented patient transfer must be in record

Some payers require copy of transfer order

-55 Postoperative Management Only

Physician provides only the care after hospital discharge; report surgical code + modifier -55

If transferred while patient hospitalized, report postoperative management with subsequent hospital codes 99231-99233

Documentation of transfer in medical record

-56 Preoperative Management Only

Physician provided only preoperative care; report surgical code + modifier -56

Not acceptable for Medicare

Usual reimbursement for portions, surgical package
- 10% preoperative
- 70% intraoperative
- 20% postoperative

Each payer determines reimbursement for portions

-57 Decision for Surgery Used With

E/M, 99201-99499, 92002, 92004

Medicine, 92012 and 92014 ophthalmologic services

Medicare: Only for preoperative period of major surgery (day before or day of)

-58 Staged/Related by Same Physician During Postoperative Period

Subsequent procedure planned at time of initial surgery
- During postoperative period of previous surgery in series
    Example: Multiple skin grafts completed in several sessions
- Do not use when code describes total sessions
    Example: 67208 destruction of lesion of retina, one or more sessions

- More extensive than original procedure or
- For therapy following diagnostic procedure (e.g., breast biopsy and subsequent mastectomy)

-59 Distinct Procedural Service

Used to report services not normally reported together

Different session or encounter

Different procedure

Different site

Separate incision, excision, lesion, injury

> ***Example:*** Physician removes several lesions from patient's leg; also notes a suspicious lesion on torso and biopsies it

- Excision code for lesion removal + biopsy code for torso lesion with -59
- Indicates biopsy as distinct procedure, not part of lesion removal

-62 Two Surgeons

Both function as cosurgeons (equals)

Usually of different specialties

Each reports same code + -62

Each dictates operative/procedure note for their portion

Total reimbursement = 125%; each physician = $62\frac{1}{2}\%$

-63 Procedure Performed on Infants Less Than 4 kg

Kilogram: 2.2 pounds (4 kg = 8.8 lb)

Small size increases complexity

Use with all Surgery section codes except Integumentary System or directed otherwise (63700)

-66 Surgical Team

Team: Several physicians with various specialties plus technicians and other support personnel

Very complex procedures

Payers may increase payment up to 50%

- Each physician's service must be documented in the medical record

-76 Repeat Procedure/Service by Same Physician

Note: "Same Physician"

Used to indicate necessary service

> ***Example:*** X-rays before and after fracture repair

-77 Repeat Procedure/Service by Another Physician

Note: "Another Physician"

Performed by one physician, repeated by another physician

Submitted with written report to establish medical necessity and identity of performing physician

-78 Unplanned Return to Operating Room for a Related Procedure During Postoperative Period

For complication of first procedure

>   *Example:* Patient had outpatient procedure in morning; was returned to operating room in afternoon with severe hemorrhage

Indicates not typographical error

- Medical record must specifically document need for service provided

-79 Unrelated Procedure or Service by Same Physician During Postoperative Period

>   *Example:* Several days after discharge for procedure, patient returns for unrelated problem

Diagnosis code would also be different

-80 Assistant Surgeon

Reimbursed at 15% to 30%

Payers identify procedures for which they reimburse assistant at surgery

-81 Minimum Assistant Surgeon

Services at a level less than that described in -80

Reimbursed at 10% if services reported with the modifier are recognized by payer

-82 Assistant Surgeon

Teaching hospitals

- Have residents who assist as part of education
- Must demonstrate no qualified resident available to use -82
  - Unavailability must be documented in written report

-90 Reference (Outside) Laboratory

Physician has business relationship with outside lab

Physician pays lab

Physician bills payer for lab services

-91 Repeat Clinical Diagnostic Laboratory Test

Repeat same laboratory tests on same day for multiple test results

- e.g., serial troponin levels for acute MI confirmation

Not tests rerun to confirm or negate original test results

Not assigned for malfunction of equipment, loss of specimen, or technician error

-92 Alternative Laboratory Platform Testing

Used to report a laboratory test using portable instrument or kit

Usually single use

   86701-86703 HIV testing

-99 Multiple Modifiers

Used when service needs more than one modifier but payer allows for only one modifier with each code

The new CMS-1500 allows for multiple modifiers (Figure 3-6)

HCPCS Level II Modifiers

Examples of HCPCS Anatomical Modifiers

-LT   Left side

-RT   Right side

-E1   Upper left, eyelid

-E2   Lower left, eyelid

-E3   Upper right, eyelid

-E4   Lower right, eyelid

-FA   Left hand, thumb

-F1   Left hand, second digit

-F2   Left hand, third digit

-F3   Left hand, fourth digit

-F4   Left hand, fifth digit

-F5   Right hand, thumb

-F6   Right hand, second digit

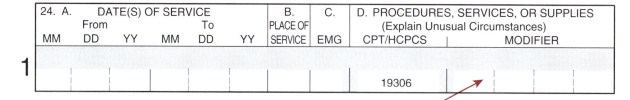

Figure 3-6 CMS-1500 (08-05) allows for multiple placement of modifiers. (Courtesy U.S. Department of Health and Human Services, Centers for Medicare and Medicaid Services.)

-F7 Right hand, third digit
-F8 Right hand, fourth digit
-F9 Right hand, fifth digit
-TA Left foot, great toe
-T1 Left foot, second digit
-T2 Left foot, third digit
-T3 Left foot, fourth digit
-T4 Left foot, fifth digit
-T5 Right foot, great toe
-T6 Right foot, second digit
-T7 Right foot, third digit
-T8 Right foot, fourth digit
-T9 Right foot, fifth digit
-LC Left circumflex, coronary artery
-LD Left anterior descending coronary artery
-RC Right coronary artery

Anatomical modifiers are not used with skin procedures

Example: Removal of skin tags, any area

Exception is with codes that indicate feet, hands, fingers, legs, arms, and eyelids

■ SURGERY SECTION (10021-69990)

Largest CPT Section

Section Format

Divided by subspecialty, e.g., Integumentary, Cardiovascular

Notes and Guidelines

Throughout section

Information varied and extensive

"Must" reading

Subsection notes apply to entire subsection

Subheading notes apply to entire subheading

Category notes apply to entire category

Parenthetical information (Figure 3-7)

Unlisted Procedure Codes

Used only when more specific code not found in Category I or Category III

Written report accompanies submission

Each unlisted code service paid on case-by-case basis

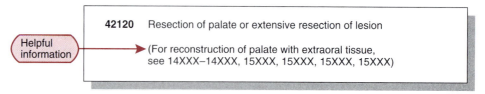

Figure 3-7 Parenthetical information in the CPT manual.

Separate Procedures

"(Separate procedure)" follows code description

Usually minor surgical procedure

Incidental to more major procedure:

- Breast biopsy before radical mastectomy would not be coded
- Appendectomy performed routinely when other abdominal surgery is performed

Separate procedures reported when

- Only procedure performed
- With another procedure
  - On different site
  - Unrelated to major procedure

Major Guideline of Surgical Packages

Usually include

- Preoperative (before, preop)
- E/M service subsequent to decision for surgery but prior to surgery date
- Intraoperative (during, intraop)
- Postoperative (after—also known as global period, postop)
  - Post-anesthesia recovery (PAR)
  - Follow-up office visits
- Local/topical anesthesia and digital block

To report these bundled services separately is "unbundling"

Remember to use modifiers during global period for unrelated E/M, return to OR, etc.

Supplies

Supplies that are beyond those typically included in the procedure are reported separately

Example: Report surgical tray with

- 99070 CPT, Medicine section
- A4550 HCPCS

Special Report

Submitting an unlisted service or one that is unusual, variable, or new may require a special report, as listed in Guidelines

Demonstrates medical necessity/appropriateness of service

Contains pertinent information describing service in terms of

- Nature
- Extent
- Need for procedure
- Time
- Effort
- Equipment necessary

May also include complexity of symptoms, final diagnosis, physical findings, procedures, concurrent problems, and follow-up care

GENERAL SUBSECTION (10021, 10022)

Fine needle aspirations with or without (w/wo) imaging guidance

Pathology 88172 and 88173 for evaluation of aspirate

INTEGUMENTARY SYSTEM SUBSECTION (10040-19499)

Often used in all specialties of medicine

Not just surgeons or dermatologists; wide range of physicians

Subheadings of Integumentary Subsection

- Skin, Subcutaneous, and Accessory Structures
- Nails
- Repair (Closure)
- Introduction
- Destruction
- Breast

Skin, Subcutaneous, and Accessory Structures (10040-11646)

Incision and Drainage (10040-10180)
I&D of abscess, carbuncle, boil, cyst, infection, hematoma, pilonidal cyst

- Lancing (cutting of skin)
- Aspiration (removal by puncturing lesion with a needle and withdrawing fluid)

Gauze or tube may be inserted for continued drainage

Pilonidal cyst
- Also known as a pilonidal abscess
- May be incised and drained (10080, 10081) or excised (11770-11772)

Excision—Debridement (11000-11044)
Dead tissue cut away and washed away with sterile saline

11000, 11001 Eczematous or infected skin

11004-11006 Debridement of infected area based on location and depth of necrotizing tissue (subcutaneous tissue, muscle, and fascia)

+11008 Removal of prosthetic material or mesh from abdominal wall

11010-11012 Foreign material with fracture or dislocation

11040-11044 Skin, subcutaneous muscle, bone

Paring or Cutting (11055-11057)
Removal by scraping or peeling (e.g., removal of corn or callus)

Codes indicate number: 1, 2-4, 4+

Biopsy (11100, 11101)
Skin, subcutaneous tissue, or mucous membrane biopsy

Not all of lesion removed

- All lesion removed = excision

Do not use modifier -51

Codes indicate number: 1 or each additional

Tissue removed during excision, shaving, etc., and submitted to pathology is NOT reported separately as a biopsy

- Rather, it is included in the code for the excision

Skin Tag Removal (11200, 11201)
Benign lesions

Removed with scissors, blade, chemicals, electrosurgery, etc.

Do not use -51

- Codes indicate number: Up to 15 and each additional 10 lesions or part thereof

Shaving of Lesions (11300-11313)
Removed by transverse incision or sliced horizontally

Based on

- Size (e.g., 1.1-2.0 cm)
- Location (e.g., arm, hand, nose)

Does not require suture closure

- Report most extensive lesion first with no modifier, then least extensive lesions with modifier -51

Benign/Malignant Lesions (11400-11646)
Codes divided: Benign or malignant

Physician assesses lesion as benign or malignant

Codes include local anesthesia and simple closure

Report each excised lesion separately

Lesion size

- Taken from physician's notes
- Includes greatest diameter plus margins (Figure 3-8)

  Example: A benign lesion measuring 0.5 cm at widest point is removed with 0.5-cm margin at narrowest point (each side, 0.5 + 0.5 = 1.0 cm). Reported as 1.5-cm lesion excision (11402)

  - Do not take size from pathology report—storage solution shrinks tissue
  - Margins (healthy tissue) are also taken for comparison with unhealthy tissue
  - Re-excisions following initial excision of malignant lesion coded as excision of malignant lesion

All excised tissue pathologically examined

Codes 11400-11646 report excision of lesion

Codes 17000-17286 report destruction

Destroyed lesions have no pathology samples

  Example: Laser or chemical

Lesion closure

- Simple or subcutaneous closure included in removal
- Reported separately
  - Layered or intermediate, 12031-12057 (Repair—Intermediate)
  - Complex, 13100-13153 (Repair—Complex)

Nails (11719-11765)

Includes toes and fingers

Types of services

- Trimming, debridement, removal, biopsy, repair

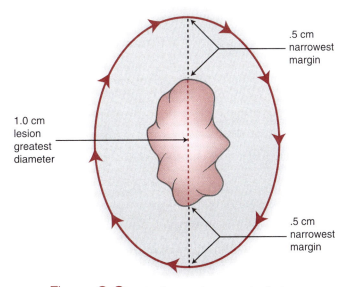

Figure **3-8** Calculating the size of a lesion.

Introduction (11900-11983)
Types of services
- Lesion injections (therapeutic or diagnostic), tattooing, tissue expansion, contraceptive insertion/removal, hormone implantation services, and insertion/removal of non-biodegradable drug delivery implant

Repair (12001-13160)

Repair Factors in Wound Repair
As types of wounds vary, types of wound repair also vary

Length, complexity (simple, intermediate, complex), and site must be documented

- Length measured in centimeters
- Measured prior to closure

Types of Wound Repair
Simple. Superficial, epidermis, dermis, or subcutaneous tissue
- One-layer closure
- Dermabond closure
- Medicare report Dermabond closure with G0168

Intermediate. Layered closure of deeper layers of subcutaneous tissue and superficial fascia with skin closure
- Single-layer closure can be coded as intermediate if extensive debridement required

Complex. Greater than layered; may include multiple layers of tissue and fascia or extensive debridement

   Example: Scar revision, complicated debridement, extensive undermining, stents, extensive retention sutures

Included in Wound Repair Codes
Simple ligation of vessels in an open wound

Simple exploration of nerves, blood vessels, and exposed tendons

Normal debridement
- Additional codes for debridement can be used when
  - Gross contamination requires prolonged cleaning
  - Appreciable amounts of devitalized/contaminated tissue are removed to expose healthy tissue
  - Debridement is provided without immediate primary closure

Grouping of Wound Repair
Add together lengths by
- **Complexity** of Wound
  - Simple, intermediate, complex
- **Location** of Wound
  - e.g., face, ears, eyelids, nose, lips

1 inch = 2.54 cm

Example: **Same complexity, same codes description location:**
Intermediate repairs of 2.9-cm laceration of leg and 1.1-cm laceration of buttocks. 2.9 + 1.1 = 4.0 cm (12032)

Example: **Different complexity:** Intermediate repair of 2.9-cm laceration of leg and simple repair of 1.1-cm laceration of buttocks. 2.9-cm intermediate repair (12032) and 1.1-cm simple repair (12001)

Example: **Same complexity, different code description locations:**
Intermediate repair of 2.9-cm laceration of leg and intermediate repair of 1.1-cm laceration of nose. 2.9-cm intermediate repair of leg (12032) and 1.1-cm intermediate repair of nose (12051)

Do not Group Wound Repairs that are
Different complexities

Example: Simple repair and complex repair

Different locations as stated in the code description

Example: Simple repairs of scalp (12001) and nose (12011)

Adjacent Tissue Transfer, Flaps, and Grafts

Information Needed to Code Graft
Type of graft—adjacent, free, flap, etc.

Donor site (from)

Recipient site (to)

Any repair to donor site

Size of graft

Adjacent Tissue Transfer/Rearrangement (14000-14350)
Includes lesion excision and/or repair (e.g., Z-plasty, W-plasty, V-plasty, Y-plasty, rotation flap, advancement flap)

Codes based on size and location of graft

Primary defect results from excision of lesion

Secondary defect results from formation of flap

To select code, add the size of the primary and secondary defects together

Skin Replacement Surgery and Skin Substitutes (15002-15431)
15002-15005 Site preparation based on size and site

15040 Harvest for tissue culture

15050-15431 Graft codes by type

Split-thickness: Epidermis and some dermis (Figure 3-9)

Full-thickness: Epidermis and all dermis

Grafts (15300-15431)
Bilaminate skin substitute

- Artificial skin, such as silicone-covered nylon mesh

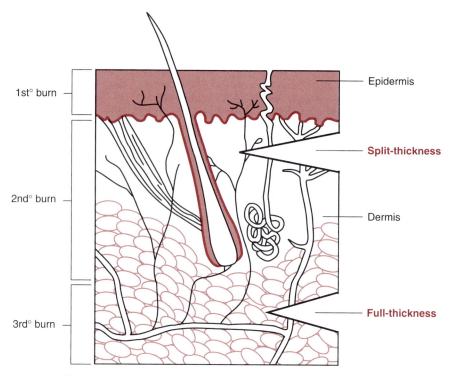

Figure 3-9 Split-thickness and full-thickness skin grafts.

Allograft: Donor graft

Xenograft: Nonhuman donor

Code is based on recipient site, not donor site

Flap (15570-15776)
Some skin left attached to blood supply

- Keeps flap viable

Donor site may be far from recipient site

Flaps may be in stages

Codes divided by location and size

Formation of flap (15570-15576)

- Based on recipient location: Trunk, scalp, nose, etc.

Transfer of flap (15650): Previously placed flap released from donor site

- Also known as walking or walk up of flap

Muscle, Myocutaneous, or Fasciocutaneous Flaps (15732-15738)

- Based on recipient location; head and neck, trunk, upper or lower extremity
- Repairs made with
  - Muscle
  - Muscle and skin
  - Fascia and skin
- Flaps rotated from donor to recipient site
- Includes closure donor site

Other Procedures (15780-15879)
Many cosmetic procedures including:

- Dermabrastion
- Chemical Peel
- Blepharoplasty
- Rhytidectomy
- Excessive skin excision

Pressure (Decubitus) Ulcers (15920-15999)
Excision and various closures

- Primary, skin flap, muscle, etc.

Many codes "with ostectomy"

- Bone removal

Locations

- Coccygeal (end of spine)
- Sacral (between hips)
- Ischial (lower hip)
- Trochanteric (outer hip)

Site preparation only: 15936, 15946, or 15956

- Defect repair of donor site reported separately

Burns Local Treatment (16000-16036)
Codes for small, medium, and large

Must calculate percentage of body burned using Rule of Nines for adults (Figure 3-10)

- <5% small
- 5% to 10% medium
- >10% large

Lund-Browder for children (Figure 3-11)

- Proportions of children differ from adults
- Heads are larger

Often require multiple debridements and redressing

Based on

- Initial treatment of 1st-degree burn (16000)
- Size

Report percent of burn and depth

Destruction (17000-17286)
Ablation (destruction) of tissue

- Laser, electrosurgery, cryosurgery, chemosurgery, etc.
- Benign/premalignant or malignant tissue
- Malignant tissue is based on location and size of lesion
- Benign/premalignant is based on the number of lesions destroyed

UNIT III   Overview of CPT, ICD-9-CM, and HCPCS Coding

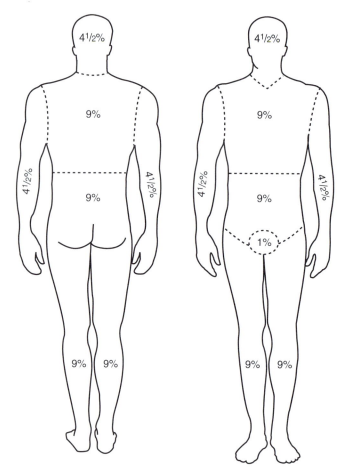

Figure 3-10 The Rule of Nines is used to calculate burn area on an adult.

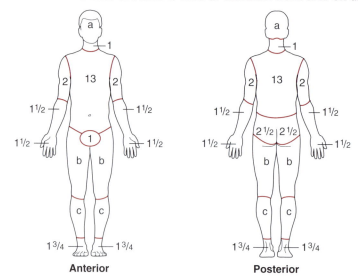

Figure 3-11 Lund-Browder chart for estimating the extent of burns on children.

Mohs' Micrographic Surgery (17311-17315)
Surgeon acts as pathologist and surgeon

Removes one layer of lesion at time

Continues until no malignant cells remain

Based on stages and number of specimens per stage indicated in medical record

Other Procedures (17340-17999)
Treatment of acne

- Cryotherapy
- Chemical exfoliation
- Electrolysis
- Unlisted procedures

Breast Procedures (19000-19499)
Divided based on procedure

- Incision
- Excision
- Introduction
- Mastectomy procedures
- Repair/Reconstruction

Use excision of lesion codes if entire lesion is removed during incisional biopsy

Use additional code for placement of radiological marker

Mastectomies based on extent of procedure

- Wide excision
- Removal of neoplasm, capsule, and surrounding margins
- Radical
- Wide excision and anatomical structure surrounding neoplasm

    Example: Muscle or fascia

- Conservative partial mastectomy in which lesion is removed with adequate margins (19301)
- Axillary dissection and partial mastectomy, 19302
- Radical and modified radical 19305, 19306, and 19307 based on extent

Confirm whether pectoral muscles, axillary, or internal lymph nodes were removed

19307 most common and includes breast and axillary lymph node removal

Code removal of lymph nodes separately unless included in code description

Bilateral procedures, use -50

Biopsy/Removal of Lesion
Incisional biopsy: Incision made into lesion and small portion of lesion removed

Excisional biopsy: Entire lesion removed

Open incisional biopsy most complex (19101)

Percutaneous core needle biopsy without imaging guidance (19100)

- Same procedure with imaging guidance is 19102

Automated vacuum assisted or rotating biopsy device described in 19103 is the use of advanced breast biopsy instrumentation

- Image guidance performed by physician reported separately
- Complete, simple removal of a mass is reported with 19120

Lesion may be preoperatively marked by placing thin wire (radiologic marker) down to lesion

- Wire placement reported separately (19290)
- Additional wires reported with 19291
- Metallic localization clips may be placed during biopsy operative session so the site can be located later, if necessary
- Placement of clip reported with 19295, once for each clip placed
- Image guidance performed by physician reported separately

MUSCULOSKELETAL SYSTEM SUBSECTION (20000-29999)

Subsection divided: Anatomic site, then service (e.g., excision)

Used extensively by orthopedic surgeons

- Many codes commonly used by variety of physicians

Extensive notes

Most common

- Fracture and dislocation treatments
- "General" subheading
- Arthroscopic procedures
- Casting and strapping

Eponyms are "things" named after "people"

> **Example:** Barr procedure is a tendon transfer of the lower leg (27690-27692), and Mitchell Chevron procedure is a complex metatarsal osteotomy (bunion correction) (28296)

- Procedures are often referred to with eponyms
- Check the index of the CPT manual for directions to eponym codes

Fracture Treatment

Type of treatment depends on type and severity of fracture

Diagnosis codes must support the procedure codes and document the medical necessity

Open: Surgically opened to view or remotely opened to place nail across fracture site

- Open reduction with internal fixation is ORIF

Closed: Not surgically opened

Percutaneous: Insertion of devices through skin or a remote site

Treatment terms should not be confused with **types** of fractures:

- Open fracture: Fractured bone penetrates skin
- Closed fracture: Fractured bone does not penetrate skin

Traction

- Application of force to align bone
- Force applied by internal device (e.g., wire, pin) inserted into bone (skeletal fixation)
- Application of force by means of adhesion to skin (skin traction)

Manipulation

Use of force to return bone back to normal alignment by manual manipulation (reduction) or temporary traction

Codes often divided based on whether manipulation was or was not used

Dislocation

Bone displaced from normal joint position

Treatment: Return bone to normal joint location

Subheading "General"

Begins "Incision" (20000, 20005)

Depth: Difference between Integumentary and Musculoskeletal incision codes

Musculoskeletal used when underlying bone or muscle is involved

Wound Exploration (20100-20103)

Traumatic penetrating wounds

Divided by wound location

Includes

- Enlargement
- Debridement
- Foreign body(ies) removal
- Ligation
- Repair of tissue and muscle

Use additional code for repair of major structures or blood vessels

Not used for integumentary repairs

- Unless the repair requires extension, enlargement, or exploration

Excision (20150-20251)

Biopsies for bone and muscle

Divided by

- Type of biopsy (bone/muscle)

- Depth
- Some by method

Can be percutaneous needle or excisional

Does not include tumor excision, which is coded separately

Biopsy with excision: Code only excision

Introduction or Removal (20500-20694)

Codes for
- Injections
- Aspirations
- Insertions
- Applications
- Removals
- Adjustments

Therapeutic sinus tract injection procedures
- Not nasal sinus
- Abscess or cyst with passage (sinus tract) to skin
- Antibiotic injected with use of radiographic guidance

Removal of foreign bodies lodged in muscle or tendon sheath

Integumentary removal codes for removal from skin

Injection into
- Tendon sheath
- Tendon origin
- Ligament
- Ganglion cyst
- Trigger points

Placement of needles or catheters into muscle and/or soft tissue
- For interstitial radioelement application

Arthrocentesis: Injection "and/or" aspiration of a joint
- Both aspiration and injection reported with one code (20600-20610)
- Codes based on joint size: Small, intermediate, major
- Do not unbundle and report aspiration/injection with two codes

External Fixation (20690-20694)

Device that holds bone in place
- Application, adjustment, removal under anesthesia

Code fracture treatment and external fixation device (EFD)
- Unless treatment and fixation both included in fracture care code description
- Adjustment to (20693) and removal of (20694) EFD are coded separately

Replantation (20802-20838)

Used to report reattachment of amputated limb

Code by body area

Grafts (20900-20938)

Autogenous Grafts

Used to report harvesting through separate incision of

- Bone
- Cartilage
- Tendon
- Fascia lata
- Tissue

Fascia lata grafts: From lower thigh where fascia is thickest

Some codes include obtaining grafting material (not coded separately)

Modifier -51 exempt

Other Procedures (20950-20999)

Monitoring muscle fluid pressure (interstitial for compartment syndrome, etc.)

- Pressure increases when blood supply decreases due to increased accumulation of fluids

Bone grafts identified by donor site

Free osseocutaneous flaps: Bone grafts

- Taken along with skin and tissue overlying bone

Electrical stimulation

- Used to speed bone healing
- Placement of stimulators externally or internally
- Ultrasound also used externally

Arthrodesis

Fixation of joint (arthro = joint, desis = fusion)

- Fixation with pins, wires, rods, etc. to immobilize the joint

Often performed with other procedure such as fracture repair

- Arthrodesis of the spine is also called spinal fusion

Subsequent Subheadings

After General subheading, divided by anatomic location

- Anatomic subheadings divided by type procedure

    Example: Subheading "Head" divided by procedure

- Incision
- Excision
- Manipulation
- Head prothesis
- Introduction or Removal
- Repair, Revision, and/or Reconstruction
- Other Procedures
- Fracture and/or Dislocation

Spinal Instrumentation and Fixation

Insertion of spinal instrumentation reported in addition to arthrodesis (fusion)

Many add-on codes reported in addition to definitive procedure

Spine (Vertebral Column), 22100-22899, divided by repair location

- Cervical (C1-C7)

    C1 = Atlas

    C2 = Axis

- Thoracic (T1-T12)
- Lumbar (L1-L5)
- Sacral (S1)

Coccyx (tailbone)

Vertebral segment: Single complete vertebral bone with articular processes and laminae

Vertebral interspace: Non-bony compartment between two vertebral bodies which contains the disk

Single level = two vertebrae and the disk that separates them

Percutaneous vertebroplasty

- Use of polymethylmethacrylate injected into the vertebral space
    - Polymethylmethacrylate is a type of bone cement/glue like silicone but not silicone
    - Adheres bone fragments together
    - Fills vertebral body defects

Types of spinal instrumentation

Segmental: Devices at each end of repair area + at least one other attachment

Nonsegmental: Devices at each end of defect only

Approach: Pay special attention to the approach used to perform the surgery

- Several different approaches to spine: Most common are anterior (front) and posterior (back)
- Most spinal instrumentation codes divided based on approach

Casting and Strapping (29000-29799)

Replacement procedure or initial placement to stabilize without additional restorative treatment

Example: Application of wrist splint or cast for wrist sprain

Initial fracture treatment includes placement and removal of first cast

- Subsequent cast applications coded separately
- Payers have strict individual reimbursement policies for subsequent casting

Application not coded when part of surgical procedure

Example: Application of wrist splint or cast for wrist sprain

Initial fracture treatment includes placement and removal of first cast

Elastic bandage application is not billed separately

Removal bundled into surgical procedure

Supplies reported separately

Endoscopy/Arthroscopy (29800-29999)
Surgical arthroscopy always includes diagnostic arthroscopy

Codes divided by joint

- Subdivided by procedure

Be aware of subterms and bundled procedures within code descriptions

Note: Parenthetical information following codes indicates codes to use if procedure was an open procedure

RESPIRATORY SYSTEM SUBSECTION (30000-32999)

Anatomic site arrangement

- Nose
- Larynx

Further subdivided by procedure

- Incision
- Excision

Endoscopy

Endoscopy in all subheadings except Nose

Each preceded by "Notes"

Endoscopy Rule One
Code full extent of endoscopic procedure performed

Example: Procedure begins at mouth and ends at bronchial tube

- Bronchial tube = full extent

Endoscopy Rule Two
Code correct approach

Example: For removal:

- Interior lung lesion via endoscopy inserted through mouth
- Exterior lung lesion via laparoscope inserted through skin

Incorrect approach = incorrect code = incorrect or no reimbursement

Endoscopy Rule Three
Diagnostic always included in surgical

Examples:

- Diagnostic bronchial endoscopy begins
- Identified foreign body
- Removed foreign body (surgical endoscopy)

Multiple Procedures

Frequent in respiratory coding

- **Watch for bundled services**

Sequence primary procedure first, no modifier

Sequence secondary procedures next, with -51

Bilateral procedures often performed, use -50

Format for reporting chosen by payer

> ***Example:*** Nasal lavage
> - 31000 × 2
> - 31000 and 31000-50
> - 31000-50
> - 31000-RT and 31000-LT

Nose (30000-30999)

Used extensively by otorhinolaryngologists (ear, nose, and throat [ENT] specialists)

Also used by wide variety of physicians in other specialties

Approach to nose

- External approach, use Integumentary System
- Internal approach, use Respiratory System

Incision (30000, 30020)

Bundled into Incision codes are drain or gauze insertion and removal

Supplies reported separately

Excision (30100-30160)

Contains intranasal biopsy codes

Polyp excision, coded by complexity

- Excision includes any method of destruction, even laser
- Use -50 (bilateral) for both sides

Turbinate excision and resection

- Three turbinates: Superior, middle, inferior
- Excision of inferior turbinate, 30130
- Excision of superior or middle turbinate, 30999
- Submucous resection of inferior turbinate, 30140
    - Reduction of inferior turbinates, 30140-52
- Submucous resection of superior or middle turbinate, 30999

Introduction (30200-30220)

Common procedures

Example: Injections to shrink nasal tissue or displacement therapy (saline flushes) to remove mucus

- Displacement therapy performed through nose

Removal of Foreign Body (30300-30320)
Distinguished by the site of removal, whether at office or hospital (requires general anesthesia)

Repair (30400-30630)
Many plastic procedures

- Rhinoplasty (reshaping nose internal and/or external)
- Septoplasty (rearrangement or plastic repair of nasal septum)

Destruction (30801, 30802)
Use of cauterization or ablation (removing by cutting)

Used for removal of excess nasal mucosa or to reduce turbinate inflammation

Based on intramural or superficial extent of destruction

- **Intramural:** Deeper mucosa
- **Superficial:** Outer layer of mucosa

Other Procedures (30901-30999)
Control of nasal hemorrhage

- Packing
- Ligation
- Cauterization
- The packing may be anterior or posterior

Accessory Sinuses, Incision, Excision, Endoscopy (31000-31294)

Codes for lavage (washing) of sinuses

- Cannula (hollow tube) placed into sinus
- Sterile saline solution flushed through

Procedures may involve multiple codes when multiple locations are accessed

Example: 31020, Sinusotomy, maxillary, can be coded with 31050 sinusotomy, sphenoid, and 31070 sinusotomy, frontal

Use -50 (bilateral) for both sides

Maxillary sinusotomy may use an external and intranasal approach to creating passage between sinus and nose

- Used to clear blocked or infected sinus
- Intranasal sinusotomy, 31020
- External sinusotomy, radical (such as Caldwell-Luc)

Access through mouth

Incision above eyetooth

Sinus is cleaned

New opening created or old opening enlarged

Repair of fractures occurring during procedure may be coded separately if not included in code description

Larynx (31300-31599)

Excision (31300-31420)
Laryngotomy: Open surgical procedure to expose larynx

- For removal procedure (e.g., tumor)

May be confused with Trachea/Bronchi codes for tracheostomy used to establish airflow

Introduction (31500-31502)
Used to establish, maintain, and protect air flow

Endotracheal intubation, establishment of airway

Based on planned (ventilation support) or emergency procedure

Laryngoscopic (Endoscopy) Procedures (31505-31579)
Uses terms *indirect* and *direct*

- **Indirect:** Tongue depressor with mirror used to view larynx
- **Direct:** Endoscopy passed into larynx; physician directly views vocal cords

Repair (31580-31590)
Several plastic procedures and fracture repairs

Laryngoplasty procedures based on purpose

Fracture codes based on whether manipulation used

Trachea and Bronchi (31600-31899)

Incision (31600-31614)
Most codes: Tracheostomy divided by

- Planned (ventilation support)
- Emergency

Divided by type

- Transtracheal or cricothyroid (location of incision)

Endoscopy (31615-31656)
Bronchoscope may be inserted into nose or mouth

Rigid endoscopy performed under general anesthesia

Flexible endoscopy usually performed under local or conscious (moderate) sedation

Introduction (31715-31730)
Catheterization

Instillation

Injection

Aspiration

Tracheal tube placement

Some include inhaled gas as contrast material

Excision, Repair (31750-31830)
Plastic repairs of tracheoplasty and bronchoplasty

Lungs and Pleura (32035-32999)

Incision (32035-32225)
Thoracotomy. Surgical opening of chest to expose to view.

Used for

- Biopsy
- Cyst
- Foreign body removal
- Cardiac massage, etc.

Excision/Removal (32310-32540)
Biopsy codes in both Excision and Incision categories

- Excisional biopsy with percutaneous needle
- Incisional biopsy with chest open

Also services of pleurectomy, pneumocentesis, and lung removal

- **Segmentectomy:** 1 segment
- **Lobectomy:** 1 lobe
- **Bilobectomy:** 2 lobes
- **Total Pneumonectomy:** 1 lung

Thoracentesis. Needle inserted into pleural space for aspiration (withdrawal) of fluid or air (32421, 32422)

Introduction (32550, 32551)
- Insertion of indwelling tunneled pleural catheter
- Tube thoracostomy

Destruction (32560)
- Chemical pleurodesis

CARDIOVASCULAR (CV) SYSTEM SUBSECTION (33010-37799)
CV coding may require codes from

- **Radiology:** Diagnostic studies
- **Medicine:** Nonsurgical and percutaneous
- **Surgery:** Open and percutaneous

Both Medicine and Surgery sections contain invasive procedures

Cardiology Coding Terminology

Invasive: Enters body

- Incisional

    Example: Opening chest for removal (i.e., tumor on heart)

- Percutaneously
    - Placement of catheter into artery or vein by means of wire threaded through needle and catheter slid over wire

    Example: PTCA (percutaneous transluminal coronary artery) procedure

- Cut down—small nick made and catheter inserted

    Example: Catheter inserted into femoral or brachial artery

Common catheters are:

- Broviac
- Hickman
- HydroCath
- Arrow multi-lumen
- Groshong
- Dual-lumen
- Triple-lumen

Noninvasive: Procedures that do not break skin

  Example: Electrocardiogram

Electrophysiology (EPS): Study of electrical system of heart

  Example: Study of irregular heartbeat (arrhythmia)

- EP studies are in Medicine section, 93600-93662
- Electrophysiologic Operative Procedures are in Surgery section, 33250-33266

Nuclear Cardiology: Diagnostic and treatment specialty; uses radioactive substances to diagnose cardiac conditions

  Example: MRI

■ Cardiovascular in Surgery Section

Codes for Procedures

Heart/Pericardium (33010-33999)

- Pacemakers, valve disorders

Arteries/Veins (34001-37799)

Heart/Pericardium (33010-33999)

Both percutaneous and open surgical

- Cardiologists often use percutaneous intervention; cardiovascular or thoracic surgeons often use open surgical procedures

Extensive notes throughout

Frequent changes with medical advances

Examples of categories of Heart/Pericardium subheading

- Pericardium
- Cardiac Tumor
- Pacemaker or Pacing Cardioverter-Defibrillator

Examples of services

- Pericardiocentesis: Percutaneous withdrawal of fluid from pericardial space (pericarditis)
- Cardiac Tumor: Open surgical procedure for removal of tumor on heart

Pacemakers and Cardioverter-Defibrillators (33202-33249)
Devices that assist heart in electrical function

- Differentiate between temporary and permanent devices
- Differentiate between one-chamber and dual-chamber devices

Divided by where pacer placed, approach, and type of service

Patient record indicates revision or replacement

- Pacemaker pulse generator is also called a battery
- Pacemaker leads are also called electrodes

Usual follow-up 90 days (global period)

Placed

Atrium (single chamber)

- Pulse generator and one electrode in atrium (single-chamber pacemaker)

Ventricle (single chamber)

- Pulse generator and one electrode in ventricle (single-chamber pacemaker)

Both (dual chamber)

- Pulse generator and one electrode in right ventricle and one electrode in right atrium

Biventricular, both ventricles and atrium (uses 3 leads)

- Pulse generator and one electrode in right ventricle, one electrode in right atrium, and one electrode in left ventricle via the coronary sinus

Approach

Epicardial: Open procedure to place on heart

Transvenous: Through vein to place in heart

Type of service

Initial placement or replacement of all or part of device

Number of leads placed is important in code selection

Electrophysiologic Operative Procedures (33250-33266)
Surgeon repairs defect causing abnormal rhythm

Chest opened to full view

- Cardiopulmonary (CP) bypass usually used

Endoscopy procedure

- Without cardiopulmonary bypass

Codes based on reason for procedure and if CP bypass used

Patient-Activated Event Recorder (33282, 33284)
Also known as cardiac event recorder or loop recorder

Internal surgical implantation required

Divided based on whether device is being implanted or removed

Cardiac Valves (33400-33496)
Divided by valve

- Aortic

- Mitral

- Tricuspid

- Pulmonary

Subdivided by whether replacement, repair, or excision is completed (all done with bypass machine)

Code descriptions are all similar, requiring careful reading

Coronary Artery Bypass Graft (CABG)
CABG performed for bypassing coronary arteries severely obstructed as in atherosclerosis or arteriosclerosis

Determine what was used in repair

- Vein (33510-33516)

- Artery (33533-33536)

- Both artery and vein (33517-33523 and 33533-33536)

Based on number of bypass grafts performed and if combined venous and arterial grafts are used

   Example: Three venous grafts

Venous Grafting Only for Coronary Artery Bypass (33510-33516)
Based on number of grafts being replaced

Combined Arterial-Venous Grafting (33517-33530)
Divided based on number of grafts and if procedure initial or reoperation

Procuring saphenous vein included, unless performed endoscopically

These codes are never used alone

- Arterial-Venous codes (33517-33523) report only **venous** graft portion of procedure

- Always used with Arterial Grafting codes (33533-33536)

   Example: 3 vein grafts and 2 arterial grafts = 33519 and 33534

Open procurement of saphenous vein is included in procedure (not coded separately)

Code harvesting of saphenous vein graft separately when endoscopic video-assisted procurement is performed (33508)

Code harvesting separately for upper extremity or femoral vein

Surgery Section (10021-69990)

Arterial Grafting for Coronary Artery Bypass (33533-33536)
Divided based on number of grafts

Obtaining artery for grafting included in codes, except

- Procuring upper-extremity artery (e.g., radial artery), coded separately

Several codes (33542-33548) for myocardial resection, repair of ventricular septal defect (VSD), and ventricular restoration

Endovascular Repair of Descending Thoracic Aorta (33880-33891)

Placement of an endovascular aortic prosthesis for repair of descending thoracic aorta

- Less invasive than traditional approach of chest or abdominal incision

Synthetic aortic prosthesis placed via catheter

- Report fluoroscopic guidance separately 75956-75959

    Includes diagnostic imaging prior to placement and intraprocedurally

Stent-graft (endoprosthesis) is deployed to reinforce weakened area

Arteries and Veins Subheading (34001-37799)

Only for noncoronary vessels

- Divided based on whether artery or vein involved

    Example: Different codes for embolectomy, depending on artery or vein

Catheters placed into vessels for monitoring, removal, repair

Nonselective or selective catheter placement

- Nonselective: Direct placement without further manipulation
- Selective: Place and then manipulate into further order(s)

Catheter Placement Example

- Nonselective: 36000 Introduction of needle into vein
- Selective: 36012 Placement of catheter into second-order venous system

Vascular Families Are Like a Tree
First-order (main) branch (tree trunk)

Second-order branch (tree limb)

Third-order branch (tree branch)

Brachiocephalic vascular family (Figure 3-12)

- Report farthest extent of catheter placement in a vascular family; labor intensity is increased with the extent of catheter placement

Embolectomy and Thrombectomy (34001-34490)
Embolus: Dislodged thrombus

Thrombus: Mass of material in vessel located in place of formation

- May be removed by dissection or balloon

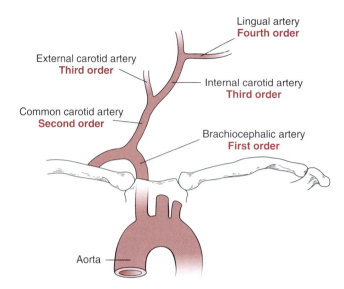

Figure 3-12 Brachiocephalic vascular family with first-, second-, third-, and fourth-order vessels.

Balloon: Threaded into vessel, inflated under mass, pulled out with mass

- Codes are divided by site of incision and whether artery or vein

Venous Reconstruction—CV Repairs (34501-34530)
Types of repairs
- Valve of the femoral vein
- Vena Cava
- Saphenopopliteal vein anastomosis

Aneurysm

Aneurysm: Weakened arterial wall causing a bulge or ballooning

Repair by removal, bypass, or coil placement

Endovascular repair (34800-34900) from inside vessel

Direct (35001-35152) from outside vessel

Endovascular Repair of Abdominal Aortic Aneurysm (34800-34834)
Fluoroscopic guidance use Radiology 75952 or 75953

Includes access, catheter manipulation, balloon angioplasty, stent placement, site closure

Reported separately; introduction of guideline and catheters

Other procedures performed at same time coded separately

Endovascular Repair of Iliac Aneurysm (34900)
Extensive notes preceding codes—"must" reading

Uses fluoroscopic guidance report Radiology 75954

Includes introduction, positioning, and deployment of graft, stent and balloon angioplasty

Reported separately: Introduction of guidewire and catheters

Repair Arteriovenous Fistula (35180-35190)

Abnormal passage from artery or vein

Divided based on fistula type

- Congenital
- Acquired/traumatic
- By site

Repair methods

- Autogenous graft—fistula created artery to vein
- Non-auto fistula—biocompatible tube connecting artery to vein

Angioplasty and Atherectomy (35450-35495)

Divided as open or percutaneous and by vessel

- **Transluminal:** By way of vessel
- **Transluminal Angioplasty:** Catheter passed into vessel and stretched
  - Placement of eluding or noneluding stents coded in addition to catheter placement
- **Transluminal Atherectomy:** Guide wire threaded into vessel and clots destroyed

Noncoronary Bypass Grafts (35500-35671)

Divided by

- Vein
- In Situ Vein (veins repaired in their original place)
- Other Than Vein

Code by type of graft and vessels being used to bypass

> ***Example:*** 35506 Bypass graft, with vein; carotid-subclavian

- Graft attached to carotid and to subclavian, bypassing defect of subclavian

Procurement of saphenous vein graft is included and not reported separately

Harvesting of upper-extremity vein or femoropopliteal vein is reported separately

Vascular Injection Procedures (36000-36522)

Divided into

- Intravenous
- Intra-arterial—Intra-aortic
- Venous

Used for many procedures, including

- Local anesthesia
- Introduction of needle
- Injection of contrast material
- Preoperative and postoperative care

> ***Example:*** Injection of opaque substance for venography (radiography of vein)

Central Venous Access (CVA) Procedures

Peripheral = long term, used for medication/chemotherapy administration

Central = short term, used for monitoring

Categories
1. Insertion
2. Repair
3. Replacement, partial or complete
4. Removal
5. Other central venous access
6. Guidance for vascular access

Insertion (36555-36571)
Insertion of newly established venous access

- Tunneled under skin (e.g., Hickman, Broviac, Groshong)
- Nontunneled (e.g., Hohn catheter, triple lumen, PICC)
- Central (e.g., subclavian, intrajugular, femoral, inferior vena cava)
- Peripheral (any other type of angiocatheter)

Codes divided by tunneled/non-tunneled, with/without port, central/peripheral, and age

Repair (36575, 36576)
Repair of malfunction without replacement

Repair of central venous access device

No differentiation between age of patient or central/peripheral insertion

Replacement (Partial or Complete) (36578-36585)
Partial (36578) is replacement of catheter only

Complete (36580-36585) is replacement through same venous access site

Differentiated by tunneled/non-tunneled, central/peripheral, and with or without subcutaneous port or pump

Removal (36589, 36590)
To be used for tunneled catheter

Removal of non-tunneled catheter is not reported separately

Other Central Venous Access (36591-36598)
Collection of blood specimen

Declotting of catheter by thrombolytic agent

Mechanical removal of obstructive material from catheter

Guidance for Vascular Access
77001, Fluoroscopic guidance for central venous access device placement, replacement, or removal

- Reported in addition to primary procedure

76937, Ultrasound guidance for vascular access

- Reported in addition to primary procedure

Transcatheter Procedures (37184-37216)
Arterial mechanical thrombectomy (37184-37186)

- Removal of thrombus by means of mechanical device
    From artery or arterial bypass graft

Venous mechanical thrombectomy (37187, 37188)

- Removal of a thrombus by means of a mechanical device

  From vein

Arterial and venous mechanical thrombectomy may be performed as primary procedure or add on

- Include

  Introduction of device into thrombus

  Thrombus removal

  Injection of thrombolytic drug(s), if used

  Fluoroscopic and contrast guidance

  Follow-up angiography

- Report separately

  Diagnostic angiography

  Catheter placement(s)

  Diagnostic studies

  Pharmacologic thrombolytic infusion before or after (37201, 75896)

  Other interventions

Other Procedures (37195-37216)

- Used to report a variety of transcatheter procedures

  Example: Transcatheter biopsy, therapy, infusion, retrieval, and intravascular stents

■ Cardiovascular in Medicine Section

Services can be

- Invasive or noninvasive
- Diagnostic or therapeutic

Subheadings

- Therapeutic Services
- Cardiography
- Echocardiography
- Cardiac Catheterization
- Intracardiac Electrophysiologic (EP) Procedures/Studies
- Peripheral Arterial Disease Rehabilitation
- Other Vascular Studies

Therapeutic Services (92950-92998)

Types of services

- Cardioversion
- Infusions
- Thrombolysis
- Catheter placement

Codes divided by
- Method (e.g., balloon, blade)
- Location (e.g., aortic or mitral valve)
- Number (e.g., single or multiple vessels)

Intracoronary Brachytherapy (92974)
New procedure; uses radioactive substances to destroy re-stenosis of coronary vessel

Patients have had stent placed in coronary vessel

Add-on code

Stent "re-stenosis" (re-formation of plaque)

Cardiologist: Places guide wire and catheter

Radiation oncologist: Places radioactive elements

Cardiography (93000-93278)
Types of services
- Stress tests
- Holter monitor
- Electrocardiogram

Separate codes for components of study, such as
- 93000 global
- 93005 tracing only
- 93010 interpretation and report only

Note: Coding structure eliminates use of modifiers -26 or -TC

Echocardiography (93303-93350)
Noninvasive diagnostic procedure. Ultrasound detects presence of cardiac or vascular disease

Codes divided by
- Approach
- Extent of study (e.g., limited, complete)
- Service provided (e.g., probe only, interpretation and report)

Cardiac Catheterization (93501-93572)
Used to identify valve disorders, abnormal blood flow

Many bundled services in catheterization codes

Examples:
- Introduction
- Positioning/Repositioning of catheter
- Pressure readings inside heart or vessels
- Blood samples
- Rest/Exercise studies
- Final evaluation and report
- Many codes are -51 exempt
- Many codes include conscious (moderate) sedation

Three components of coding cardiac catheterization
1. Placement of catheter (93501-93533)
2. Injection (93539-93545)
3. Imaging supervision, interpretation, and report (93555 or 93556)

Intracardiac Electrophysiologic Procedures/Studies (93600-93662)
Services to diagnose and treat conditions of electrical system of heart

- Arrhythmic induction
- Mapping
- Ablation

EP system of heart
Electrical conduction system

Electrical recording codes divided based on location of recording device

Example: Bundle of His or right ventricle

Pacing: Temporary pacing to stabilize beating of heart

Example: Intraventricular or intra-arterial pacing

Peripheral Arterial Disease (PAD) Rehabilitation (93668)
Rehabilitation sessions: 45-60 minutes

Use of motorized treadmill/track/bicycle to build patient's CV function

Supervised by exercise physiologist or nurse

If E/M is provided by physician, service is reported separately

Other Vascular Studies (93701-93790)
Category contains codes for services such as

- **Plethysmography:** Recordings of changes in size of body part when blood passes through it
- **Electronic Analysis:** Checks electronic function of devices, such as pacemakers
- **Ambulatory Blood Pressure Monitoring:** Outpatient basis over 24-hour period
- **Thermograms:** Visual recordings of body temperature

■ Cardiovascular in Radiology Section

Radiology section, Heart (75557-75564) and Aorta/Arteries (75600-75790) subsections

Prior to 1992, Radiology section contained codes for entire CV procedures

Major revision to CV radiology codes 1992

Divided complete procedures into two components: technical and professional

Example: Angiography

- Technical component angiography—remains in Radiology section
- Professional component injection—moved to Surgery section

Complete angiography requires radiology code and surgery code

Reflects common practice of cardiologist's performing injection and radiologist's performing angiography

Contrast Material

Often radiologic procedures use contrast material to improve image

Many codes have contrast material bundled into service

- "With contrast" or "with or without contrast"

Only injected contrast qualifies as with contrast

Contrast not included in description but used in procedure: Code contrast material and injection separately

- Specify site where service is received to differentiate between global, technical, and professional components of the procedure

Non-hospital-based (not employed by hospital) physician usually performs procedure in hospital outpatient department: Use -26 for professional component only

---

A COMPONENT CODING EXAMPLE

Two physicians (cardiologist and radiologist from same facility) perform angiography of third-order brachiocephalic artery with contrast

- Cardiologist places catheter (36217), Surgery section
- Radiologist performs angiography (75658), Radiology section
- Supply of contrast material (99070), Medicine section

HEMIC AND LYMPHATIC SYSTEM SUBSECTION (38100-38999)

Divisions

- Spleen
- General
- Lymph Nodes and Lymphatic Channels

Spleen Subheading (38100-38200)

Spleen easily ruptured, causing massive and potentially lethal hemorrhage

Excision:

- Splenectomy: Total or partial/open or laparoscopic

Often done as part of more major procedure

- Bundled into major procedure
- Repair
- Laparoscopy

General (38204-38242)

Bone Marrow
Codes divided based on

- Preservation
- Preparation
- Purification
- Aspiration

- Biopsy
- Harvesting
- Transplantation

Stem Cells

Immature blood cells originating in bone marrow

Used in treatment of leukemia

Types of stem cells
Allogenic: Same species

Autologous: Patient's own

Lymph Nodes and Lymphatic Channels Subheading (38300-38999)

Two types of lymphadenectomies:

1. **Limited:** Pelvic and para-aortic lymph nodes only for neoplasm staging
2. **Radical:** Aortic and/or splenic lymph nodes and surrounding tissue for neoplasm staging

Often bundled into more major procedure (e.g., prostatectomy)

Do not unbundle and report lymphadenectomy separately

MEDIASTINUM SUBSECTION (39000-39499)

Incision codes for foreign body removal, biopsy, or drainage

Excision codes for removal of cyst or tumor

DIAPHRAGM SUBSECTION (39501-39599)

Only category: Repair

Includes hernia or laceration repairs

DIGESTIVE SYSTEM SUBSECTION (40490-49999)

Divided by anatomic site from mouth to anus + organs that aid digestive process

   Example: Liver and gallbladder

Many bundled procedures

Endoscopy

Diagnostic procedure always bundled into surgical endoscopic

Code to furthest extent of procedure

Endoscopy Terminology
Notes define specific terminology

Code descriptions are specific regarding

- Technique and depth of scope
    Esophagoscopy: Esophagus only
    Esophagogastroscopy: Esophagus and past diaphragm
    Esophagogastroduodenoscopy: Esophagus and beyond pyloric channel

- Proctosigmoidoscopy: Rectum and sigmoid colon (6-25 cm)
- Sigmoidoscopy: Entire rectum, sigmoid colon, and may include part of descending colon (26-60 cm)
- Colonoscopy: Entire colon, rectum to cecum, and may include terminal ileum (greater than 60 cm)

Laparoscopy and Endoscopy

Some subheadings have both laparoscopy (outside) and endoscopy (inside) procedures

> ***Example:*** Subheading Esophagus

- Endoscopy views inside
- Laparoscopy inserted through umbilicus; views from outside

Hemorrhoidectomy and Fistulectomy Codes (46221-46320)

Divided by
- Complexity
  - Simple: No plastic procedure involved
  - Complex: Includes plastic procedure and fissurectomy
- Anatomy
  - Subcutaneous: No muscle involvement
  - Submuscular: sphincter muscle
- Complex fistulectomy involves excision/incision of multiple fistulas

Hernia Codes (49491-49659)

Divided by
- Type of hernia

  Example: Inguinal, femoral

- Initial or subsequent repair
- Age of patient determines code choice
- Clinical presentation
  - **Strangulated:** Blood supply cut off
  - **Incarcerated:** Cannot be returned to cavity (not reducible)

Additional code is used for implantation of mesh or prosthesis
- Laparoscopy surgical procedures

URINARY SYSTEM SUBSECTION (50010-53899)

Anatomic division
- Kidney
- Ureters
- Bladder
- Urethra

Further divided by procedure
- Incision
- Excision
- Introduction
- Repair
- Laparoscopy
- Endoscopy

Kidney Subheading (50010-50593)

Endoscopy codes are for procedure done through previously established stoma or incision

Caution: Codes may be unilateral or bilateral

Introduction Category (50382-50398)
Codes divided by renal pelvis catheter procedures or other introduction procedures

Renal pelvis catheters further divided; internal dwelling or externally accessible

Catheters for drainage and injections and for radiography

Aspirations

Insertion of guide wires

Tube changes

Usually reported with radiology component

Ureter Subheading (50600-50980)

Caution: Codes may be unilateral or bilateral

Divided by type of procedure
- Incision
- Excision
- Introduction
- Repair
- Laparoscopy
- Endoscopy

Bladder Subheading (51020-52700)

Includes codes for
- Incision
- Removal
- Excision
- Introduction
- Urodynamics
- Repair
- Laparoscopy

- Endoscopy
- Cystoscopy
- Urethroscopy
- Cystourethroscopy
- Transurethral surgery

Many bundled codes

Example: Urethral dilation is included with insertion of cystoscope

Read all descriptions carefully

Urodynamics (51725-51798)
Procedures relate to motion and flow of urine

Used to diagnose urine flow obstructions

Bundled: All usual, necessary instruments, equipment, supplies, and technical assistance

Vesical Neck and Prostate (52400-52700)
Contains codes for transurethral resection of the prostate (TURP)

Example: 52601 reports a complete transurethral electrosurgical resection of the prostate and includes vasectomy, meatotomy, cystourethroscopy, urethral calibration and/or dilation, internal urethrotomy, and control of any postoperative bleeding

Other approaches are reported with 55801-55845

Example: 55801 reports a removal of the prostate gland (prostatectomy) through an incision in the perineum and includes vasectomy, meatotomy, urethral calibration and/or dilation, internal urethrotomy, and control of any postoperative bleeding

MALE GENITAL SYSTEM SUBSECTION (54000-55899)

Penis

Testis

Epididymis

Tunica Vaginalis

Scrotum

Vas Deferens

Spermatic Cord

Seminal Vesicles

Prostate

Biopsy Codes
Located in anatomical subheading to which the codes refer

Example: Biopsy codes in subheadings
- Epididymis (Excision)
- Testis (Excision)

Penis (54000-54450)

Incision codes (54000-54015) differ from Integumentary System codes

- Penis incision codes used for deeper structures

Destruction (54050-54065)
Codes divided by

- Extent: Simple or extensive
- Method of destruction, e.g., chemical, cryosurgery

Extensive destruction can be by any method

Excision (54100-54164)
Commonly used codes biopsy and circumcision

Introduction (54200-54250)
Many procedures for corpora cavernosa (spongy bodies of penis)

- Injection procedures for Peyronie disease (toughening of corpora cavernosa)
- Treatments for erectile dysfunction (ED)

Repair (54300-54440)
Many plastic repairs

Some repairs are staged (more than one stage)

- Stage indicated in code description

REPRODUCTIVE SYSTEM PROCEDURES (55920)

Code 55920 reports the placement of catheters/needles into pelvic organs/genitalia

For subsequent interstitital radioelement application

INTERSEX SURGERY SUBSECTION (55970, 55980)

Only 2 codes within subsection

1. Male to female
2. Female to male

Complicated procedures completed over extended period of time

Performed by multiple physicians with extensive specialized training

FEMALE GENITAL SYSTEM SUBSECTION (56405-58999)

Anatomic division: From vulva to ovaries

- Many bundled services

Vulva, Perineum, and Introitus (56405-56821)

Skene's gland coded with Urinary System, Incision or Excision codes

- Group of small mucous glands, lower end of urethra
  - Paraurethral duct

Incision (56405-56442)
I&D of abscess. Vulva, perineal area, or Bartholin's gland

Marsupialization
Cyst incised

Drained

Edges sutured to sides to keep cyst open, creating a pouchlike repair

Destruction (56501, 56515)
Lesions destroyed by variety of methods

- Destruction = Eradication (not to be confused with excision; excision is removal)

Divided by simple or extensive destruction

- Complexity based on physician's judgment
- Stated in medical record

Destruction has no pathology report

Excision (56605-56740)
Biopsy includes

- Local anesthetic
- Biopsy
- Simple closure

Code based on number of lesions biopsied

Place number of lesions on CMS-1500 in Block 24-G (see Figure 3-1)

Vulvectomy. Surgical removal of portion of vulva (56620-56640)

Based on extent and size of area removed

Extent

- Simple: Skin and superficial subcutaneous tissues
- Radical: Skin and deep subcutaneous tissues

Size

- Partial: <80% vulvar area
- Complete: >80% vulvar area

Extent and size indicated in operative report

Repair (56800-56810)
Many plastic repairs

Read notes following category

- If repair procedure for wound of genitalia, use Integumentary System code

Endoscopy (56820-56821)
By means of a colposcopy with or without biopsy

Vagina (57000-57425)

Codes divided based on service, e.g., incision, excision

Introduction (57150-57180)
Includes vaginal irrigation, insertion of devices, diaphragm, cervical caps

Report device inserted separately

- 99070 or HCPCS National Level II codes, such as A4261 (cervical cap)

Repair (57200-57335)
For nonobstetric repairs

- Obstetric repairs, use Maternity Care and Delivery codes

Manipulation (57400-57415)
Dilation: Speculum inserted into vagina, which is enlarged by dilator

Endoscopy (57420-57425)
Colposcopy codes based on purpose

- e.g., biopsy, diagnostic

Includes code for laparoscopic approach for repair of paravaginal defect

Cervix Uteri (57452-57800)

Cervix uteri, narrow lower end of uterus

Services include endoscopy, excision, repair, manipulation

Excision (57500-57558)
Conization codes

Conization: Removal of cone of tissue from cervix

LEEP (loop electrocautery excision procedure) technology may be used for conizations or loop electrode biopsies

Corpus Uteri (58100-58579)

Many complex procedures

- Often very similar wording in code descriptions
- Requires careful reading and specific documentation in the medical record

Excision (58100-58294)
Dilation and curettage (D&C, 58120) of uterus

- After dilation, curette scrapes uterus
- Coded according to circumstances: Obstetrical or nonobstetrical

Do not report postpartum hemorrhage service with 58120

- Use 59160—Maternity and Delivery code

Many hysterectomy codes

- Based on approach (vaginal, abdominal) and extent (uterus, fallopian tubes, etc.)

Often secondary procedures performed with hysterectomy

Do not code secondary, related minor procedures separately

Introduction (58300-58356)
Common procedures

- e.g., insertion of an IUD

Report supply of device separately

Specialized services

- e.g., artificial insemination procedures

Used to report physician component of service

Component coding

- Necessary with catheter procedures for hysterosonography
- Notes following codes indicate radiology guidance component codes

Laparoscopy/Hysteroscopy (58541-58579)
Laparoscopic approach for:

- Removal of myomas
- Hysterectomies

Codes divided by tissue removed and weight

Oviduct/Ovary (58600-58770)

Oviduct. Fallopian tube
Incision category contains tubal ligations

- When during same hospitalization (but not at same session as delivery), is coded separately

Laparoscopy (58660-58679)
Through abdominal wall

Codes in the laparoscopy and hysteroscopy section are divided by approach

- Then by purpose of procedure, e.g., lysis, lesion removal

Caution: If only diagnostic laparoscopy

- Do not use Female Genital System codes
- Use 49320, Digestive System

Many codes can be reported separately with appropriate modifiers

> ***Example:*** 58660 Laparoscopy, surgical, with lysis of adhesions, can be coded with any of the indented codes that follow 58660 (58661, 58662, 58670)

Ovary (58800-58960)

Two categories only: Incision and Excision

Incision: Primarily for drainage of cysts and abscesses

- Divided by surgical approach

Excision: Biopsy, wedge resection, and oophorectomy

In Vitro Fertilization (58970-58976)

Specialized codes used by physicians trained in fertilization procedures

- Codes divided by type of procedure and method used

Surgery Section (10021-69990)

MATERNITY CARE AND DELIVERY SUBSECTION (59000-59899)

Divided by service

- Antepartum services, e.g.:

    Amniocentesis

    Fetal non-stress test

    Fetal monitoring during labor

- Type of delivery

    Vaginal delivery

    C-section

    Delivery after previous C-section

- Abortion

Gestation

Fetal gestation: Approximately 266 days (40 weeks)

EDD: Estimated Date of Delivery

- 280 days from last menstrual period (LMP)

Trimesters
First, LMP to Week 12

Second, Weeks 13-27

Third, Week 28 to EDD

Global Package and Delivery

Uncomplicated maternity care includes

- Antepartum care = Before birth
- Delivery
- Postpartum care = After birth

Antepartum Care Includes

Initial and subsequent H&P (history and physical)

Blood pressures

Weight

Routine urinalysis

Fetal heart tones

Monthly visits to 28 weeks

Twice-a-month visits, weeks 29 to 36

Weekly visits from week 37 to delivery

Listed in notes preceding 59000

- Services not related to antepartum care are reported separately

Example: Pregnant female with complaint of suspicious mole on left shoulder

- Visits OB/GYN physician, who provides antepartum care
- Service regarding mole, not antepartum care, requires good documentation in the maternity record and a specific diagnosis relative to the treatment provided

Delivery Includes
Admission to hospital with admitting H&P

Management of uncomplicated labor

Vaginal or cesarean section delivery

- Complications coded separately
- Listed in notes preceding 59000

Postpartum Care Includes
Normal follow-up care for 6 weeks after delivery

- Hospital visits, office visits
- Listed in notes preceding 59000

Antepartum (59000-59076)
Amniocentesis: Insertion of needle into pregnant uterus, withdrawal of fluid (59000, 59001)

- Ultrasound guidance with 59000 (76946)
- Ultrasound guidance included with 59001
- Component coding often part of services in subheading

Fetal services: Include stress tests, blood sampling, monitoring, and therapeutic procedures

Excision (59100-59160)
Postpartum curettage: Removes remaining pieces of placenta or clotted blood (59160)

Nonobstetric curettage: 58120 (Corpus Uteri, Excision)

Introduction (59200)
Insertion of cervical dilator: Used to prepare and soften the cervix for an abortive procedure or delivery (for abortive procedure, see 59855)

Cervical ripening agents may be introduced to prepare cervix

- Is a separate procedure and not reported when part of more major procedure

Repair (59300-59350)
Only for repairs during pregnancy

Repairs done as a result of delivery or during pregnancy

Episiotomy or vaginal repair by other than attending

Suture repair (cerclage) of cervix or uterus (hysterorrhaphy)

Routine Global Obstetric Care

59400, Vaginal delivery

59510, Cesarean delivery

59610, Vaginal delivery after previous cesarean delivery (VBAC)

59618, Cesarean delivery following attempted vaginal delivery after previous cesarean delivery

Note: Take care when assigning diagnosis codes for normal versus complicated delivery. ICD-9-CM states specific guidelines for a normal delivery.

Episiotomies and Use of Forceps
Included in delivery

Not reported separately

Physician Provides Only Portion of Global Routine Care, Delivery
59409, Vaginal delivery only

59514, Cesarean delivery only

59612, Vaginal delivery only, after previous cesarean delivery

59620, Cesarean delivery only, following attempted vaginal delivery after previous cesarean delivery

Delivery of Twins

Payers differ on reporting format

- -22 (Unusual Procedural Services)
- -51 (Multiple Procedures)

Abortion Services (59812-59857)

Spontaneous: Happens naturally (for a complete spontaneous abortion, report with a code from the E/M section)

Incomplete: Requires medical intervention

Missed: Fetus dies naturally but does not abort during first 22 weeks of pregnancy

Septic: Abortion with infection

Medical intervention

- Dilation and curettage or evacuation (suction removal)
- Intra-amniotic injections (saline or urea)
- Vaginal suppositories (prostaglandin)

ENDOCRINE SYSTEM SUBSECTION (60000-60699)

Nine glands in endocrine system; only four included in subsection

1. Thyroid
2. Parathyroid
3. Thymus
4. Adrenal

Pituitary and Pineal. See Nervous System subsection

Pancreas. Digestive System

Ovaries and Testes. Respective genital systems

Divided into two subheadings

- Thyroid Gland
- Parathyroid, Thymus, Adrenal Glands, and Carotid Body

Carotid Body. Refers to area adjacent to carotid artery

Can be site of tumors

Thyroid Gland, Excision Category (60100-60281)

- **Lobectomy:** Partial or subtotal (Something less than total)
- **Thyroidectomy:** Total (All)

Thyroid, 1 gland with 2 lobes

NERVOUS SYSTEM SUBSECTION (61000-64999)

Divided anatomically

- Skull, Meninges, and Brain
- Spine and Spinal Cord
- Extracranial Nerves, Peripheral Nerves, and Autonomic Nervous System

Skull, Meninges, and Brain (61000-62258)

Categories
Injection, Drainage, or Aspiration

Twist Drills, Burr Hole(s), or Trephine

Conditions that Require Openings Into Brain to
Relieve pressure

Insert monitoring devices

Place tubing

Inject contrast material

Craniectomy or Craniotomy (61304-61576)
Removal of portion of skull, usually as operative site, performed emergently to prevent herniation of brain into the brainstem

Codes divided by site and condition for which procedure is performed

Surgery of Skull Base (61580-61619)
Skull base: Area at base of cranium

- Lesion removal from this area very complex

Surgery of Skull Base Terminology

Approach procedure used to gain exposure of lesion

Definitive procedure is what is done to lesion

Repair/reconstruction procedure reported separately only if extensive repair

Surgery of Skull Base (61580-61619)

Approach procedure and definitive procedure coded separately

> ***Example:*** Removal of an intradural lesion using middle cranial fossa approach

- 61590 approach procedure, middle cranial fossa and
- 61608 definitive procedure of intradural resection of lesion

Cerebrospinal Fluid (CSF) Shunt (62180-62258)

Used to drain fluid

Codes describe placement of

- Devices
- Repair
- Replacement
- Removal of shunting devices

Spine and Spinal Cord (62263-63746)

Codes divided by condition and approach

Often used are

- Unilateral or bilateral procedures (-50)
- Multiple procedures (-51)
- Radiologic supervision and fluoroscopic guidance coded separately

Includes codes for

- Spinal anesthetic injections 62310-62319
- Intrathecal catheter placement/implantation 62350-62355

Introduction/Injection of Anesthetic Agent (Nerve Block), Diagnostic or Therapeutic Category (64400-64530)

Includes codes for

- Nerve blocks 64400-64450
- Facet joint injections 64470-64476
- Epidural injections 64479-64484
  - Used to provide pain relief
  - As compared with an epidural catheter placement used for anesthetic purposes

EYE AND OCULAR ADNEXA SUBSECTION (65091-68899)

Terminology extremely important

- Code descriptions often vary only slightly

Understanding of eye anatomy is necessary for proper coding in this subsection

Codes divided anatomically, e.g.,

- Eyeball
- Anterior segment
- Posterior segment
- Ocular adnexa
- Conjunctiva

Some codes specifically for previous surgery

Example: Insertion of ocular implant, secondary (65130)

Much bundling

Example: Subheading Posterior Segment, Prophylaxis category notes indicate:

- "The following descriptors (67141, 67145) are intended to include all sessions in defined treatment period."

Cataracts

Method used depends on type of cataract and surgeon preference

Nuclear cataract: Most common, center of lens (nucleus), due to aging process

Cortical cataract: Forms in lens of cortex and extends outward; frequent in diabetics

Subcapsular cataract: Forms at back of lens

Removal and lens replacement (66830-66986)

- Extracapsular cataract extraction (ECCE) is partial removal

  Removes hard nucleus in one piece

  Removes soft cortex in multiple pieces

- Intracapsular cataract extraction (ICCE) is total removal

  Removes lens and capsule in one piece

- Phacoemulsification

  Small incision into eye and introduction of probe

  High-frequency waves fragment cataract; then suctioned out

  Lens placed through same small incision

Eyelids (67700-67999)

Blepharotomy (67700)

- Incision into eyelid for drainage of abscess

Blepharoplasty

- Repair of eyelid
- Codes in Integumentary System (15820-15823)

- Codes in Eye and Ocular Adnexa (67916, 67917, 67923, 67924)
- These codes are strictly for entropion and ectropion repair
  Selection of code depends on technique used to repair eyelid
- Blepharoplasty codes with specific techniques, 67901-67908

AUDITORY SYSTEM SUBSECTION (69000-69979)

Codes divided by
- External Ear (69000-69399)
- Middle Ear (69400-69799)
- Internal Ear (69801-69949)
- Temporal Bone, Middle Fossa Approach (69950-69979)

Understanding of ear anatomy is necessary for proper coding in this subsection

External, middle, and internal ear further divided by procedure
- Incision
- Excision
- Removal
- Repair

Myringotomy and tympanostomy
- Eustachian tube connects middle ear to back of throat for drainage
- Fluid collects in middle ear when tube does not function properly
- Prevents air from entering middle ear and pressure builds
- Surgical intervention
  Myringotomy (incision into tympanic membrane)
  Tympanostomy (placement of PE tube [pressure equalization])

OPERATING MICROSCOPE SUBSECTION (+69990)

Employed with procedures using microsurgical techniques

Code in addition to primary procedure performed

Do not report separately when primary procedure description includes microsurgical techniques

Example: 15758 Free fascial flap with microvascular anastomosis

Note that following 15758 is the statement:

- "(Do not report code 69990 in addition to code 15758)" indicating to the coder not to report the use of the operating microscope separately

■ RADIOLOGY SECTION (70010-79999)

Radiology: Branch of medicine that uses radiant energy to diagnose and treat patients

Specialist in radiology: Radiologist (doctor of medicine)

Radiology Subsections

1. Diagnostic Radiology
2. Diagnostic Ultrasound
3. Radiologic Guidance
4. Breast Mammography
5. Bone/Joint Studies
6. Radiation Oncology
7. Nuclear Medicine

Procedures

Fluoroscopy views inside of body, projects onto television screen

Live images by which physician can view function, structure, and defects or anomalies within an organ

> *Example:* 71034 chest x-ray with fluoroscopy

Magnetic Resonance Imaging (MRI)

> *Example:* 72148 MRI of spinal canal

Tomography or Computed Axial Tomography (CAT or CT Scan)

> *Example:* 70450 tomographic scan of head or brain

Planes of Body (Figure 3-13)

Position and Projection

Position = method of positioning patients for examination

Projection path = pathway traveled by x-ray beam

Component Coding

Three component terms

1. Professional
2. Technical
3. Global

Professional Component

Physician portion of service, includes

- Supervision of technician
- Interpretation of results, including written report

Technical Component

- Technologist's services
- Equipment, film, and supplies

Global Procedure

Both professional and technical portions of radiology service

Radiology Section (70010-79999)

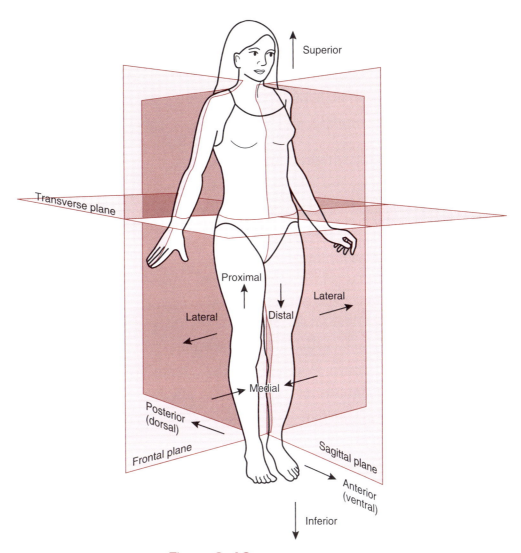

Figure 3-13 Planes of the body.

Component Modifiers

If only professional component of radiology service provided: -26 to code

If only technical component provided: -TC to code

- -TC HCPCS modifier used with CPT and HCPCS codes

If both professional and technical components of radiology service are provided by physician who owns equipment and facility, pays technician and supplies (global), no modifier is needed

Example: Chest x-ray

- Professional component: 71030-26 (supervision and final report)
- Technical component: 71030-TC (technician, supplies, equipment)
- Global procedure: 71030 (both professional and technical)

Third-party payers usually reimburse

- 40% professional component
- 60% technical component
- 100% global procedure

Contrast Material

Statement "with contrast" implies injection service included in code

Oral or rectal contrast does not qualify for "with contrast"

Notes indicate codes for components

> *Example:* 75801, Lymphangiography; see 38790 (Injection procedure)

Interventional Radiologist

Combination radiologist and surgeon

Provides total procedure for cystography with contrast

- Report 74430, x-ray portion
- 51600 for injection procedure
- Plus code for supply of contrast material (e.g., 99070)

DIAGNOSTIC RADIOLOGY SUBSECTION (70010-76499)

Most standard radiographic procedures

Codes often divided by whether contrast material used

Codes further divided by number of views

> *Example:* 71030, Chest x-ray, complete, minimum of 4 views

Used to:

- Diagnose disease
- Monitor disease process—progression or remission
- Therapeutic procedures (guidance)

Diagnostic Procedures Include

X-ray

Computerized axial tomography (CAT or CT scan)

Magnetic resonance imaging (MRI)

Angiography

Computed Axial Tomography (CAT or CT)
X-ray image taken in sections

Computer reconstructs and enhances image

Magnetic Resonance Imaging (MRI)
Uses magnetic fields to produce an image displayed on computer screen

Codes of same area (e.g., spine) divided by whether or not contrast material used

Angiography
Used to view vessel obstructions

Dye injected into vessel

Radiologist uses angiography to diagnose vascular conditions

Example:
- Malformation
- Stroke (cerebrovascular accident, CVA)
- Myocardial infarction (MI)

> **Remember**
> - If fewer than total number of views specified in code provided: Use -52, Reduced Service

DIAGNOSTIC ULTRASOUND SUBSECTION (76506-76999)

Uses high-frequency sound waves to image anatomic structures

Nine subheadings of Diagnostic Ultrasound

Primarily based on anatomy

A-mode (A = Amplitude)

Technique used to map structure outline in one-dimensional image

M-mode (M = Motion)

Technique used to display one-dimensional movement of structure

B-scan (B = Brightness)

Technique used to display two-dimensional movement of tissues and organs

Known as gray scale ultrasound

Real-Time Scan

Technique used to display both structure and motion with time of organ and tissues in a two-dimensional image

Extent of Study

Codes often divided on extent of study

Example: Extent of scan as follows

- **Complete:** Scans entire body or body region
- **Limited:** Scans part of body, e.g., one organ
- **Follow-up/repeat:** Limited study of part of body that was scanned previously

Three Locations for Ultrasound Services

76506-76999: Radiology codes for diagnostic ultrasound services

93875-93990: Medicine codes for non-invasive vascular studies

93303-93350: Medicine codes for echocardiography

RADIOLOGIC GUIDANCE SUBSECTION (77001-77032)

Guidance

- Fluoroscopic
- Computed tomography
- Magnetic resonance
- Other

BREAST MAMMOGRAPHY SUBSECTION (77051-77059)

Example: Computer-aided detection and screening

BONE/JOINT STUDIES SUBSECTION (77071-77084)

Example: Bone density, bone mineral density, and joint survey

RADIATION ONCOLOGY SUBSECTION (77261-77799)

Therapeutic use of radiation

Codes both professional and technical services

Subheading divided based on treatment

Initial consultation, prior to decision to treat, reported with E/M consultation code

- **Outpatient:** 99241-99245
- **Inpatient:** 99251-99255

Clinical Treatment Planning—Professional Component (77261-77299)

Includes

- Interpretation of special testing
- Tumor localization
- Determination of treatment volume
- Choice of treatment method
- Determination of number of treatment ports
- Selection of treatment devices
- Other necessary procedures

Clinical Treatment Planning consists of

- Planning
- Simulation

Three Levels of Planning (77261-77263, 77299)

1. **Simple:** One treatment area, one port, or one set of parallel ports
2. **Intermediate:** Three or more ports, two separate treatment areas, multiple blocking

3. **Complex:** Complex blocking, custom shielding blocks, tangential ports, special wedges, 3+ treatment areas, special beams

Simulation (77280-77295)

Determining placement of treatment areas/ports for radiation treatment

Does not include administration of radiation

Definitions of Simulation
1. **Simple:** 1 treatment area with 1 port or pair of ports
2. **Intermediate:** 3+ ports, 2 separate treatment areas, multiple blocking
3. **Complex:** Tangential ports, 3+ treatment areas, complex blocking
4. **Computer-generated 3-D** reconstruction of volume of tumor and critical structures

Medical Radiation, Physics, Dosimetry, Treatment Devices, and Special Services (77300-77370)

Decision making services of physicians

- Treatment types
- Dose calculation and placement (dosimetry)
- Development of treatment device

Stereotactic Radiation Treatment Delivery (77371-77373)

Delivers large radiation dose to discrete tumor sites

- Computer(s) map location
- Radiation delivered to one or more sites

Radiation Treatment Delivery (77401-77423, 77520-77525)

Technical component of actual delivery of radiation

Information Needed to Code Radiation Treatment Delivery
Amount of radiation delivered

Type of radiation—electron (most common), neutron, or proton

Number of

- Areas treated (single, two, three or more)
- Ports involved (single, three or more, tangential)
- Blocks used (none, multiple, custom)

Reporting Radiation Treatment Management (77427-77499)

Professional (physician) portion of services, including

- Review port films
- Review dosimetry, dose delivery, treatment parameters
- Treatment set-up
- Patient examination for medical E/M

Report in units of five fraction, unless last 3-4 fractions are at the end of the treatment; then you can count the last 3-4 as an additional fraction

Clinical Brachytherapy (77750-77799)

Placement of radioactive material into or around site of tumor

- Intracavitary (within body cavity)
- Interstitial (within tissues)

Source
Radioactive element delivers radiation dose over time

Example: Seeds, ribbons, or capsules

- **Ribbons:** Seeds embedded on tape and inserted into tissue
- Tape is cut to desired length, thereby controlling amount of radiation

Clinical Brachytherapy Codes Divided Based on
Number of sources applied

- Simple 1-4
- Intermediate 5-10
- Complex 11+

NUCLEAR MEDICINE SUBSECTION (78000-79999)

Placement of radioactive material into body and measurement of emissions

Used for both diagnosis and treatment

Codes divided primarily on organ system

- Except "Therapeutic," which is for radiopharmaceutical therapies

■ PATHOLOGY AND LABORATORY SECTION (80047-89356)

- Organ or Disease Oriented Panels
- Drug Testing
- Therapeutic Drug Assays
- Evocative/Suppression Testing
- Consultation (Clinical Pathology)
- Urinalysis
- Chemistry
- Hematology and Coagulation
- Immunology
- Transfusion Medicine
- Microbiology
- Anatomic Pathology
- Cytopathology
- Cytogenetic Studies

- Surgical Pathology
- Transcutaneous Procedures
- Other Procedures
- Reproductive Medicine Procedures

Pathology and Laboratory

Codes for laboratory test only

Specimen collection coded separately

Example: Venous blood draw reported 36415 (Surgery section)

Facility Indicators

Allow additional tests without physician written order

Example: Urinalysis positive for bacteria, built-in indicator for culture

Pathology/Laboratory Caution

Report second or subsequent tests without -51, multiple procedures

Organ or Disease Oriented Panels (80047-80076)

Groups of tests often ordered together

Examples:
- Basic Metabolic Panel
- General Health Panel
- Electrolyte Panel

Rules of Panels

All tests must have been conducted

Do not use -52, Reduced Service

Additional tests, over those in panel, reported separately

If all tests in panel not done

- List each test separately
- Do not use panel code

Drug Testing (80100-80103)

Identifies presence or absence of drug—qualitative analysis

Confirmation conducted to double-check results of positive drug test (80102)

Chromatography procedure in which multiple drugs identified (80100)

- Some machines identify all drugs present in 1 procedure
- Others require 2+ procedures to identify 2+ drugs

Code the number of procedures, not number of drugs tested for

Example:
- 2 procedures to identify 3 drugs = 80100 × 2
- 1 procedure to identify 3 drugs = 80100

Does not identify amount of drug present

- Only presence or absence

Therapeutic Drug Assays (80150-80299)

Reports the presence and amount (quantitative)

Material examined can be from any source

Drugs listed by generic names

Example: Amitriptyline, generic name for brand name Elavil

Evocative/Suppression Testing (80400-80440)

Measures stimulating (evocative) or suppressing agents

Codes report only technical component of service

Additional services reported

- Supplies and/or drugs used in testing (99070 or HCPCS code)

E/M code reported for physician monitoring of test

Consultations (Clinical Pathology) (80500, 80502)

At request of physician

Additional information about specimen

Consultant prepares written report

Levels

Limited without review of medical record

Comprehensive with review of medical record

More Consultation Codes (88321-88334)

Surgical Pathology

Used when pathologist either

- Reviews slides, material, or reports
- Provides consultation during surgery

Reported by number of specimens

Urinalysis (81000-81099)

Tests on Urine

Method of test

- e.g., tablet, reagent, or dipstick

Reason for test

- e.g., pregnancy

Constituents being tested for

- e.g., bilirubin, glucose

Equipment Used
Automated or nonautomated

With or without microscope

Chemistry (82000-84999)
Specific tests on any bodily substances

- Urine
- Blood
- Breath
- Feces
- Sputum

Most are for quantitative (amount of) screenings only

Few report qualitative (presence of) screenings

Samples from different sources reported separately, e.g., blood, feces

Samples taken different times of day reported separately

Hematology and Coagulation (85002-85999)

Laboratory procedures on blood

Example:

- Complete blood count (CBC)
- White blood cell count (WBC)

Codes divided based on method of

- Blood draw
- Test being conducted

Immunology (86000-86804)

Identifying immune system conditions caused by antibodies and antigens

Example: Hepatitis C antibody screening

Tissue Typing (86805-86849)

Compatibility test on tissue

- Match donor to recipient
- Measure/monitor cytotoxic reactions

Transfusion Medicine (86850-86999)

Blood bank codes

Tests performed on blood or blood products

Identifies

- Collection
- Processing
- Typing

Microbiology (87001-87999)

Study of Microorganisms
Identification of organism

Sensitivities of organism to antibiotics

> **Microbiology Caution:** Many code descriptions similar to those in Immunology (86000-86849), with only difference **technique** used

Anatomic Pathology (88000-88099)

Postmortem examinations

- Autopsies

Reports only physician service

Codes divided on extent of exam and type of examination—gross versus gross and microscopic

  Example: Gross examination without central nervous system (88000)

Cytopathology (88104-88199)

Identifies cellular changes

Common laboratory procedures, e.g., Pap smear

Codes divided by

- Type of procedure
- Technique used

Cytogenetic Studies (88230-88299)

Branch of genetics concerned with cellular abnormalities and pathologic conditions

  Example: Chromosomes

Surgical Pathology (88300-88399)

Pathology Terminology
Specimen sample of tissue of suspect area

- Basis of reporting determined by number of labeled specimens

Block: Frozen piece of specimen

Section is a slice of frozen block

Evaluation of Specimens to Determine Disease Pathology
All tissue removed during procedures undergoes pathology evaluation

Operative report usually coded after pathology report received

Pathology reports usually coded with operative report

Unit of measure (88300-88309), specimen

- 2 separately identifiable anus tags, each examined, 88304 × 2
- 1 anus tag examined in 2 different areas of tag, 88304

Types of Pathologic Examination
Microscopic: With microscope

Gross: Without microscope

- 88300, only gross exam code
- Other codes are gross and microscopic

Six levels of surgical pathology
Based on specimen examined, e.g., breast, prostate, lung, and reason for evaluation, e.g., radical procedure for suspected carcinoma

Levels divided on complexity of examination

Example:

88305, Colon, Biopsy

88307, Colon, Segmental Resection, Other than for Tumor

88309, Colon, Total Resection

Level I
- Specimen can be accurately diagnosed without microscopic examination

Level II
- Gross and microscopic examination is performed on the specimen

Levels III, IV, V, and VI
- Include gross and microscopic examination and additional ascending levels of physician work (increasing difficulty)

Based upon method of or need for removal

Same anatomical site can be listed in each level

Additional service codes 88311-88399 are not included in codes 88300-88309

Example: Special stains (88312)

MEDICINE SECTION (90281-99607)

Most procedures noninvasive (not entering body)

Contains invasive procedures

Example: 92973, Percutaneous thrombectomy

Many specialized tests

Example: Audiology and biofeedback

Special icon lightning bolt (⚡)

- Indicates substances pending FDA (Food and Drug Administration) approval

Immunizations

Often used

Two types of immunizations

- Active and passive

Correct coding includes

- Supply injected
- Administration of injection

Active—Bacteria or Virus
Bacteria that cause disease made nontoxic (toxoid)

- Injected to build immunity

Small dose active virus injected (vaccine)

- Injected to build immunity

Example: Poliovirus

Passive Immunization
Does not cause immune response

Contains antibodies against certain diseases—immune globulins

Immune Globulins (90281-90399)

Identifies immune globulin product

Example: Botulism antitoxin

Report administration separately

Immune Globulin Codes Divided by
Type
e.g., rabies, hepatitis B

Method
e.g., intramuscular, intravenous, subcutaneous

Dose
e.g., full dose, minidose

Immunization Administration (90465-90474)

Administration (giving of substance)

- Reported in addition to substance given
- 90465-90468 Patients under 8 years of age when physician counsels regarding immunization

- 90465, +90466 = Percutaneous, intradermal, subcutaneous, or intramuscular injection
- 90467, +90468 = Oral or intranasal
- 90471-90474 Patients 8 years of age or over

    Patients of all ages, including under 8 years of age, when physician does not counsel regarding immunization
- 90471, +90472 = Percutaneous, intradermal, subcutaneous, or intramuscular injection
- 90473, +90474 = Oral or intranasal

Methods of Administration
- Percutaneous
- Intradermal
- Subcutaneous
- Intramuscular
- Intranasal
- Oral

Report Administration for Each Dose—Single or Combination

Example: 10-year-old patient receives 3 separate injections
- 90471 administration tetanus
- 90472 administration rubella
- 90472 administration diphtheria

OR depending on payer:
- 90471 administration tetanus
- 90472 × 2 administration rubella and diphtheria

Vaccines, Toxoids (Vaccine Product Codes) (90476-90749)

Many codes age-specific

Example: 90658, influenza vaccine, for ages 3 and over

Codes for products for single diseases

Example: 90703, tetanus

Codes for combination diseases

Example: 90701, diphtheria, tetanus, and whole cell pertussis (DTP)

Some vaccines given on schedule

Example: 90633, 2-dose hepatitis A vaccine
- 1st dose, 1st visit
- 2nd dose, 2nd visit

Caution: There are Multiple Diphtheria Codes

- 90696-90702, 90719-90723 diphtheria and diphtheria with other substances

    Example: 90719, diphtheria for IM use

    Example: 90698, diphtheria, tetanus toxoids, and acellular pertussis (synthetic form of pertussis) (DTaP), *Haemophilus influenza* Type B (HiB), and inactivated poliovirus (IPV) for IM use

> **Remember**
> Third party payers do not usually require modifier -51 used with Vaccine/Toxoid codes
> Rather, depending on payer:
> - List each code multiple times or
> - Use times (×) symbol and indicate number

Important Reporting Rule. If vaccine administered during an office visit that was not related to the E/M

- Report E/M service (with modifier -25) + Vaccine + administration

Office visit for vaccine only: Code only vaccine and the administration (no E/M service)

Routine Vaccinations
Influenza
Substance (vaccine) 90655-90663

Administration for patients 8 or over

- G0008 HCPCS National Level II for Medicare patients
- 90471/90472

Pneumococcal
Substance (vaccine) 90732

Administration

- G0009 HCPCS National Level II for Medicare
- 90471/90472 administration

Psychiatry (90801-90899)

Psychiatric treatment at same time as E/M service, report

- One code for psychotherapy with E/M

Time major billing factor

- Record indicates session time

Many services provided in partial hospital settings

- Patient in hospital during day, returns home for evenings and weekends

Codes Divided Based on
Interactive or insight-oriented psychotherapy

Inpatient or outpatient

With or without E/M service

Individual or group

Biofeedback (90901, 90911)

Used to help patients gain control over body processes

Example: Elevated BP (blood pressure) or manage chronic pain

Patient training in biofeedback by professional

- Continues on own

Services often part psychophysiologic (mind/body) therapy

Dialysis (90935-90999)

Cleanses blood

- Temporary (non-ESRD [end-stage renal disease])
- Permanent (ESRD)

Two parts to report ESRD dialysis services

- Physician service
- Hemodialysis procedure

Hemodialysis Service (90935-90940)

Hemodialysis is the procedure

Used for ESRD and non-ESRD

Billed per day for inpatients receiving hemodialysis and also for outpatient non-ESRD

Includes all physician E/M services related to procedure

- Use modifier -25 if separate E/M service provided

Miscellaneous Dialysis Procedures (90945-90947)

Describes other dialysis procedures

Example: Peritoneal dialysis in which toxins are passively absorbed into dialysis fluid

Peritoneal Dialysis (90945-90947)

Services billed on per-day basis for inpatient ESRD patients

ESRD Physician Services (90951-90970)

Include

- Establishment of dialyzing cycle
- Physician services
- E/M outpatient dialysis visits
- Telephone calls
- Patient management during dialysis

Reported per month: 90951-90966

Month is defined as 30 days

Less than full month of service 90967-90970 per day

Codes divided by age and number of encounters

Codes are used to report outpatient dialysis services for ESRD patients

Other Diagnosis Procedures (90989-90999)
Patients can receive training in self-dialysis (90989, 90993)

Codes divided by complete or partial training program

Gastroenterology (91000-91299)

For tests and treatments of esophagus, stomach, and intestine

Codes usually reported with E/M or consultation service code

- **Caution:** Many bundled services

Ophthalmology (92002-92499)

Contains E/M "eye" codes

Definitions for new and established patients same as for E/M section

Codes are for bilateral services

- If only one eye, use modifier -52 (reduced service)

Special Ophthalmologic Services (92015-92371)

For special evaluations of visual system

Goes beyond those usually provided in evaluation

May be reported in addition to basic visual service

Special Otorhinolaryngologic Services (92502-92700)

Special treatments and diagnostic services

 Example: Nasal function tests (rhinomanometry) or audiometric tests

All hearing tests bilateral unless one ear indicated in description

Cardiovascular in Medicine Section

Services can be

- Invasive or noninvasive
- Diagnostic or therapeutic

Subheadings

- Therapeutic Services
- Cardiography
- Echocardiography
- Cardiac Catheterization

- Intracardiac Electrophysiologic (EP) Procedures/Studies
- Peripheral Arterial Disease Rehabilitation
- Other Vascular Studies

Noninvasive Vascular Diagnostic Studies (93875-93990)

Vascular codes for procedures on noncoronary veins and arteries

Include

- Patient care
- Supervision and interpretation (S&I)
- Copy of results

Pulmonary (94002-94799)

For ventilation management therapies and diagnostic tests

Includes procedure and interpretation of test results

- Additional E/M service reported separately

Allergy and Clinical Immunology (95004-95199)

Divided into two subheadings

1. Allergy Testing (95004-95075)
2. Allergen Immunotherapy (95115-95199)

Allergy Testing (95004-95075)
Sensitivity testing using various types of tests

Example: Percutaneous, intracutaneous, inhalation

Tests use numerous substances

Example: Extracts, venoms, biologics, and foods

Type and number of tests based on physician's judgment

Coding allergy testing
Medical record will indicate

- Number of tests
- Type of test
- Method testing

Allergen Immunotherapy (95115-95199)
Codes divided into three types of services:

1. Injection only
2. Prescription and injection
3. Provision of antigen (substance) only

Physician service bundled into immunotherapy codes

If separate E/M service provided, report separately

Neurology and Neuromuscular Procedures (95805-96020)

Contains codes to report tests, such as

- Sleep tests
- Muscle tests (electromyography)
- Range-of-motion measurements
- Electroencephalogram (EEG)

Analysis and programming of neurostimulators

- Motion analysis
- Functional brain mapping

Many bundled services

Services usually provided in addition to E/M service

Medical Genetics and Genetic Counseling Services (96040)

Trained genetic counselors assess risk of genetic defects in offspring

Includes

- Pedigree construction
- Obtaining structured genetic history
- Analysis of risk
- Counseling

Central Nervous System (CNS) Assessments/Tests (96101-96125)

Used to report

- Psychological tests
- Speech/Language assessments
- Developmental progress assessments
- Thinking/Reasoning examinations

Standardized cognitive performance testing

Codes based on per-hour basis

- Includes written report of results

Health and Behavior Assessment/Intervention (96150-96155)

- Identify psycological behavior, emotional, cognitive, or social factors important to treatment or management of physical health problems

Hydration (96360, 96361)

Infusion: Therapeutic procedure to introduce fluid into body

Hydration: Infusion for purpose of rehydration; includes prepackaged fluid

Medicine Section (90281-99607)

Injection: Subcutaneous (Sub-Q), intramuscular (IM), intra-arterial (IA), and intravenous (IV)

Codes report the physician work related to the infusion, hydration, or injection

- Affirmation of treatment plan
- Direct supervision of staff
- Significant, separately identifiable E/M is reported with -25

Codes include

- Local anesthesia
- Intravenous start
- Access to indwelling intravenous catheter or port
- Flush at conclusion
- Standard tubing, syringes, and supplies

Multiple drug administrations in same session are reported separately

Use only one initial code to report multiple infusions or injections or combinations

> Assign initial code based on primary reason for encounter
>
> The secondary infusion/injection is reported with a subsequent or concurrent code, unless the protocol requires two separate IV sites
>
> ***Example:*** If three different agents were administered in the same session, report one initial code and two additional sequential codes
>
> Determination of initial code is based on primary reason for encounter

Some codes are time based, so medical documentation must indicate time infusion begins and ends

Time is defined as the actual time used to administer the drug/substance

96360, 96361 report IV infusion for hydration and includes prepackaged fluid/electrolytes

- 96360 IV infusion for hydration up to 1 hour
- 96361 IV infusion for hydration, each additional hour
  - Report for hydration intervals greater than 30 minutes beyond 1 hour
  - Start infusion time over if a different bag is started
  - Do not report hydration codes when the fluid is used to administer a drug
  - Do not report hydration codes for infusion of <30 minutes

96365-96368 report therapeutic, prophylactic, or diagnostic IV infusions, other than hydration and chemotherapy

- Typically require direct physician supervision
- Special consideration for preparing, dosing, or disposing
- Trained staff who administer infusion
- Monitoring of vital signs during infusion

Therapeutic, Prophylactic, and Diagnostic Injections and Infusions (Excludes Chemotherapy and Other Highly Complex Drug or Highly Complex Biologic Agent Administration) (96365-96379)

Types of drug administration

- Therapeutic
- Prophylactic
- Diagnostic

Codes divided by administration method

- Subcutaneous
- Intramuscular
- Intra-arterial
- Intravenous push

A push is defined as when a health care professional is needed to administer the drug/substance and monitor the patient or an infusion that takes 15 minutes or less to administer

Also report the substance administered

Chemotherapy Administration (96401-96549)

Represents only preparation and administration of chemotherapy

- If separate E/M service provided, report E/M code + -25

Report all drugs/substances separately

Codes are not limited to patients with diagnosis of cancer

Codes also include infusion of anti-neoplastic agents, monoclonal antibody agents, and biological response modifiers for treatment of noncancer diagnoses

Chemical can be administered (injected) into

- Lesion
- Vein
- Tissue
- Muscle
- Artery
- Cavity
- Nerve

Intravenously injected chemicals: Two methods of delivery of chemical

1. IV push quickly puts into vein (15 minutes or less)
2. IV infusion delivers over longer period of time

Codes often divided by time the infusion/injection procedure takes

Example: 96413 chemotherapy administration, intravenous, infusion up to 1 hour

Medicine Section (90281-99607)

Report the initial code that represents the main reason why the patient was being treated, even though it might not be the first drug/substance infused

Example: Patient received 1 hour of hydration first, then 2 hours of chemotherapy intravenously. Code the initial chemotherapy infusion, 96413 for the first hour of chemo, 96415 for the second hour, then code 96360 for the hydration

Special supplies (e.g., special needles) reported separately using 99070 or HCPCS National Level II code

Report any intra-arterial catheter placement with 36620-36640

Injections with chemotherapy

- Report separately any analgesic or antiemetic (for vomiting)
- Given before or after chemotherapy

> Use codes J0881 to report injection of darbepoetin alfa and J0885 to report injection of epoetin alfa

Photodynamic Therapy (96567-96571)

Used in addition to bronchoscopy or endoscopy codes

Injected agent remains in cancerous cells longer than normal cells

- After agent dissipates from normal cells, patient exposed to laser light
- Agent absorbs light
- Light produces oxygen and cancer cell destroyed

Special Dermatologic Procedures (96900-96999)

Usually specialized procedures provided on consultation basis

- Separate E/M consultation code would then be appropriate

Treatment of skin conditions:

Actinotherapy—with ultraviolet light

Photochemotherapy—with light-sensitive chemicals and light rays

Physical Medicine & Rehabilitation (97001-97799)

Used by physicians and therapists to report a variety of services

Treatments
Traction

Electrical stimulation (used to help heal fractures)

Therapeutic procedures

Patient Training
Gait training

Functional activities

Codes often have time components

Example: 97761 reports prosthetic training, extremity, each 15 minutes

Active Wound Care Management (97597-97606)

Debridement

Selective debridement without anesthesia with removal of devitalized tissue by different techniques, such as sharp selective debridement with scissors, scalpel, and forceps

97597 and 97598 include total surface area of all wounds

Codes based on centimeters treated

Nonselective debridement (97602): Healthy tissue removed along with necrotic tissue, with wet-to-moist dressings, enzymatic or abrasive methods

Negative pressure wound therapy (NPWT) (97605, 97606)

- Vacuuming of drainage and tissue from wound
  - Then negative pressure draws the edges of the wound together
- Application of topical medications/ointments
- Assessment of wound
- Directions to patient on continued care of wound
- Each code for ongoing care reported on per-session basis

Osteopathic and Chiropractic Services (98925-98943)

Both inpatient and outpatient settings

Physician services bundled into codes

Codes divided by body area

Education and Training for Patient Self Management (98960-98962)

- Use of standardized curriculum for education to individual or group for management of illness

Non-Face-to-Face Nonphysician Services (98966-98969)

Reports nonphysician E/M services using telephone/internet

Established patient, family member of the patient, or a guardian

98966-98968 telephone E/M services

98969 online E/M services

To report physician services, see 99441-99443

Special Services, Procedures, and Reports (99000-99091)

Handling and conveyance of laboratory specimens
- 99000-99002

Postoperative follow-up visits included in surgical package
- 99024

Office visits after posted hours or in locations other than office

- 99050-99060

Supplies and materials

- 99070

Hospital mandated on-call services

- 99026, 99027

Moderate (Conscious) Sedation (99143-99150)

Type of sedation in which the patient can respond to verbal commands

- Appendix G contains summary of codes that include moderate (conscious) sedation

The bullseye symbol ⊙ indicates these codes in the CPT manual

Do not report sedation services with codes marked with bullseye when sedation is provided by same physician performing procedure

- Second physician provides sedation, report with 99148-99150

Included in service is:

- Patient assessment
- IV establishment
- Administration of agent
- Maintenance of sedation
- Monitoring of vital signs
- Recovery

Codes divided based on patient age (under 5 and 5 and over) and time (30 minutes and each 15 minutes over)

HCPCS CODING

Developed by Centers for Medicare and Medicaid Services (CMS)

- Formerly HCFA

HCPCS developed, 1983
CPT did not contain all codes necessary for Medicare services reporting

---

One of Two Levels of Codes

1. Level I, CPT
2. Level II, HCPCS, also known as national codes

Phased Out Level III, Local Codes
Developed by Medicare and other carriers for use at local level

Varied by locale

Discontinued October 2002 due to HIPAA code set regulations

Some codes incorporated into HCPCS Level I and Level II

Level II, National Codes
Codes for wide variety of providers

- Physicians
- Dentists
- Orthodontists

Codes for wide variety of services

- Specific drugs
- Durable medical equipment (DME)
- Ambulance services

Code book published every January, but codes are added and deleted throughout the year and providers are notified through carrier bulletins

Format
Begins with letter, followed by four digits

Example: E0605, vaporizer, room type

Each letter represents group codes

Example: "J" codes used to report drugs, J0585, Botox, per unit

Temporary Codes
Certain letters indicate temporary codes

Example: K0552, Supplies for external drug infusion pump

- K codes are temporary codes

HCPCS National Level II Index
Directs coder to specific codes

Do not code directly from index

Reference main portion of text before assigning code

Alphabetical order

Table of Drugs
Listed by generic name, not brand name

AN OVERVIEW OF THE ICD-9-CM

INTRODUCTION

Morbidity (illness)

Mortality (death)

CM = Clinical Modification

Provides continuity of data

World Health Organization's (WHO) ICD-9 used globally; many countries already use ICD-10

1977: U.S. develops ICD-9 version

- Has more code subsets
- Data collapse back to ICD-9 for uniformity of data

Medicare

Medicare Catastrophic Act of 1988

Required use of ICD-9-CM codes for outpatient claims

Act abolished but codes still used

Uses of ICD-9-CM

Facilities track patient use through codes

Fiscal entities track health care costs

Research

- Health care quality
- Future needs
- Newer cancer center built if patient use warrants

ICD-9-CM on Insurance Forms

Diagnoses establish medical necessity

Services and diagnoses must correlate

CMS-1500 in Block 21 and 24E (Figure 3-14)

Office visit: croup, 464.4, Block 21, 1; 1 placed in Block 24E, Line 1

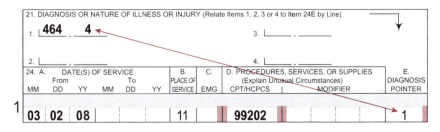

Figure **3-14** Diagnosis code and service must correlate.

UNIT III Overview of CPT, ICD-9-CM, and HCPCS Coding

> **Ethics**
> Documentation must support diagnosis and match procedures or service performed
>
> **Example:**
> - Services provided
> - Diagnosis justifies services
>
> If in doubt, check it out; don't make assumptions
>
> **Your Job:** Translate documentation into ICD-9-CM codes

FORMAT OF ICD-9-CM

Volume 1, Diseases, Tabular List

Volume 2, Diseases, Alphabetic Index

Volume 1, Diseases, Tabular List

Contains code numbers

001.0-999.9 Diagnosis codes describe condition

V & E codes = supplemental information

Volume 2, Diseases, Alphabetic Index

Appears first in book

Refers coder to code numbers in Volume 1

Never code directly from Index!

ICD-9-CM CONVENTIONS

Symbols, abbreviations, punctuation, and notations

NEC: Not elsewhere classifiable

- No more-specific code exists

NOS: Not otherwise specified

- Unspecified in documentation

[ ] Brackets

Enclose synonyms, alternative wording, or explanatory phrases

Helpful, additional information

Can affect code

Found in Tabular List (001.0-999.9)

( ) Parentheses

Contain nonessential modifiers

- Take them or leave them

Found in Tabular List and Index

Do not affect code assignment

Colon & Brace

: **Colon:** Tabular List, completes statement with one or more modifiers

} **Brace:** Tabular List, modifying statements to right of brace

Lozenge, Section Mark, & Bold Type

◇ **Lozenge:** Can indicate code unique to ICD-9-CM

§ **Section:** Can be footnote indicator

Bold type: Codes and code titles in Tabular List, Volume 1

Italicized Type

All excludes notes

Codes NOT used as principal diagnosis

Slanted Brackets [ ]

Enclose manifestations of underlying condition

Code underlying condition first

Includes, Excludes, Use Additional Code

Includes notes: In chapter, section, or category

Excludes notes: Conditions are coded elsewhere

Use Additional Code: Assignment of other code(s) is necessary

And/With

And: Means and/or

With: One condition with (in addition to) another condition

Code, if Applicable, any Causal Condition First

May be first-listed diagnosis if no causal condition applicable or known

  Example: 707.1X, Ulcer of lower limb, except decubitus; states
  - Chronic venous hypertension with ulcer (459.31)

If ulcer caused by chronic venous hypertension

- **First:** 459.31 chronic venous hypertension
- **Second:** 707.10 ulcer of lower limb

VOLUME 2, ALPHABETIC INDEX

Nonessential Modifiers: Have no effect on code selection

Enclosed in parentheses

Clarify diagnosis

  Example: Ileus (adynamic) (bowel) . . .

Terms

Main terms (bold typeface)

- Subterms
- Indented two spaces to right
- Not bold

Cross References

Directs you: *see, see also*

- "*see*" directs you to specific term

    Example: Panotitis—*see* Otitis media

- "*see also*" directs you to another term for more information

    Example: Perivaginitis (*see also* Vesiculitis)

- "*see category*" Volume 1, Tabular List, specific information about use of code

    Example: Mesencephalitis (*see also* Encephalitis) 323.9; late effect—*see* category 326

Notes

Define terms

Give further coding instructions

   Example: Index: "Melanoma"

   Note: "Except where otherwise indicated..."

Mandatory fifth digits also appear as notes (one reason to never code from Index)

Eponyms

Disease or syndrome named for person

   Example: Arnold-Chiari (*see also* Spina bifida)

Etiology and Manifestation of Disease

Etiology = cause of disease

Manifestation = symptom

Combination codes = etiology and manifestation in one code

Neoplasm

In Volume 2, Index, locate Neoplasm Table under the alphabetic entry "N"

SECTIONS

Section 1, Index to Diseases

Section 2, Table of Drugs and Chemicals

Section 3, Index to External Causes of Injuries and Poisonings (E Codes)

An Overview of the ICD-9-CM

Section 1, Index to Diseases

Largest part of Volume 2—Index

First step in coding, locate main term in Index

Subterms indented two spaces to right

May have more than one subterm

Section 2, Table of Drugs and Chemicals

Located after the Index to Diseases

Contains classification of drugs and substances to identify poisoning and adverse effects

- Adverse effect occurs when substance is taken correctly but patient has a negative reaction to substance

  Condition E-code for drug found under therapeutic column

- Poisoning occurs when substance is incorrectly taken

  Example: Amoxicillin prescribed for bronchitis causes rash (adverse effect). Rather than one tablet of prescribed amoxicillin, patient takes 4 tablets and nausea results (poisoning)

Drug name placed alphabetically on left under heading "Substance" (Figure 3-15)

First column: "Poisoning" code for substance involved if not related to an adverse effect

E codes identify how poisoning occurred

Example: If Alkaline antiseptic solution poisoning occurred by accident, E858.7

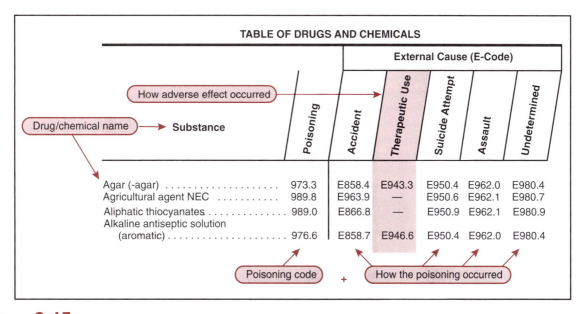

Figure **3-15** Section 2, Table of Drugs and Chemicals. (From *International Classification of Diseases*, 9th Revision. U.S. Department of Health and Human Services, Public Health Service, Center for Medicare and Medicaid Services.)

UNIT III Overview of CPT, ICD-9-CM, and HCPCS Coding

- Accidental poisoning by alkaline antiseptic solution: 976.6 (substance) and E858.7 (how it occurred)
- Identify agent condition E code for occurrence
- Code any resulting condition (e.g., coma)

Headings
Accident: Unintentional

Therapeutic: Correct dosage, correctly administered, with adverse effects

Suicide attempt: Self-inflicted

Assault: Intentionally inflicted by another person

Undetermined: Unknown cause

Section 3, E Codes

Alphabetic Index to External Causes of Injuries and Poisonings

Provides additional information about the nature of the injury/poisoning and locality

Never principal (inpatient), sole, or primary (outpatient) diagnosis

Separate Index to External Causes

- Alphabetical, main terms in bold
- Subterms are indented 2 spaces to right under main term

A Word of Caution about the Alphabetic Index

Some words in Index do not appear in Tabular—saves space

Exact word may not be in code description in Tabular

- Usually found in Alphabetic Index
- Must locate the term in the Index, then locate in Tabular
- Additional coding instructions found in Tabular

VOLUME 1, TABULAR LIST

Two Major Divisions

1. Classification of Diseases and Injuries (codes 001.0-999.9)
2. Supplementary Classification (V codes and E codes)

Classification of Diseases and Injuries

Main portion of ICD-9-CM

Codes from 001.0 to 999.9

Most chapters are body systems

   Example:
   - Digestive System
   - Respiratory System

Divisions of Classification of Diseases and Injuries

Chapters 1 through 17

- *Section:* A group of related conditions
- *Category:* Represents single disease/condition
- *Subcategory:* More specific
- *Subclassification:* Most specific

> **Remember**
> Assign to highest level of specificity, based on documentation
> If 4-digit code exists, do not report 3-digit code
> If 5-digit code exists, do not report 4-digit code

■ USING THE ICD-9-CM

Guidelines developed by Cooperating Parties

- American Hospital Association (AHA)
- American Health Information Management Association (AHIMA)
- Centers for Medicare and Medicaid Services (CMS)
- National Center for Health Statistics (NCHS)

GENERAL GUIDELINES

Appendix A of this text contains *Official Guidelines for Coding and Reporting*

You must know and follow the Guidelines when assigning diagnoses codes

- All certification examinations adhere to the Guidelines
- As you review this ICD-9-CM material, locate the information in the Guidelines of your ICD-9-CM
- In this way, you will become familiar with the location of Guidelines content to be able to quickly reference the Guidelines during the examination

Outpatient coders primarily use Sections I and IV

Diagnostic Coding and Reporting Guidelines do NOT cover all situations

- Outpatient coders also use many Section II and III guidelines

STEPS TO DIAGNOSIS CODING

Identify MAIN term(s) in diagnosis

Locate MAIN term(s) in Index

Review subterms

Follow cross-reference instructions (e.g., *see, see also*)

Verify code(s) in Tabular

- Read Tabular notes
- Code to highest specificity
- Never code from index!

Level of Detail in Coding

Assign diagnosis (dx) to highest level of specificity

Do NOT use 3-digit code if there is 4th

Do NOT use 4-digit code if there is 5th

Acute and Chronic Conditions

Exists alone or together

May be separate or combination codes

If two codes, code acute first

Example: acute (577.0) and chronic (577.1) pancreatitis

Combination code: Both acute and chronic condition

- Diarrhea (acute) (chronic) 787.91, Acute and subacute bacterial endocarditis 421.0
- Otitis acute and subacute 382.9

Combination Code

Always use combination code if one exists

Example: encephalomyelitis (dx) due to rubella (manifestation), 056.01

Multiple Coding for Single Condition

Etiology (cause)

Manifestation (symptom)

- Slanted brackets [ ]

    Example: Retinopathy, diabetic 250.5 *[362.01]*

- Must check Tabular notes to assign correct 5th digit for diabetes
- Tabular: 362.0, Diabetic retinopathy, instructs to "Code first diabetes 249.5, 250.5"

SELECTION OF PRIMARY DIAGNOSIS

Condition for encounter

Documented in medical record

Condition that is responsible for services provided

Also list coexisting condition(s) or comorbidity(ies)

Diagnosis and procedure MUST correlate

- Medical necessity established
- No correlation = no reimbursement

Codes in Brackets

Never sequence as principal dx

Always sequence in order listed in Index

Example:

- Index lists: Diabetes, gangrene 250.7 *[785.4]*
- 785.4 = gangrene
- Tabular, 785.4 indicates "Code first any associated underlying condition: diabetes (250.7X) . . ."
- Code first diabetes, then gangrene
- 250.7X = diabetes (X = 5th digit)
- 785.4 = gangrene

Two or More Interrelated Conditions

When two or more interrelated conditions exist and either could be principal dx, either may be sequenced first

Example: Patient with mitral valve stenosis and coronary artery disease (two interrelated conditions)

- Either can be principal dx and sequenced first
- Resource intensiveness affects choice

V CODES

Located after 999.9 in Tabular

Two digits before decimal (e.g., V10.10)

Index for V codes, Alphabetic Index to Diseases

Main terms: contraception, counseling, dialysis, status, examination

Uses of V Codes

Not sick BUT receives health care (e.g., vaccination)

Services for known disease/injury (e.g., chemotherapy)

A circumstance/problem that influences patient's health BUT NOT current illness/injury

Example: Organ transplant status

Example: Birth status and outcome of delivery (newborn)

Section I.18.e of Guidelines contains the V Code Table

- Identifies how V codes are listed (first, first/additional, additional only)

> **Special Note about "History of"**
> Index to Disease, MAIN term "History"
> Entries between "family" and "visual loss V19.0" = "Family history of"
> Entries before "family" and after "visual loss V19.0" = "Personal history of"

History V Code Categories in Tabular

V10 Personal history of malignant neoplasm

V12 Personal history of certain other diseases

V13 Personal history of other diseases

Except: V13.4 Personal history of arthritis, and V13.6 Personal history of congenital malformations. These conditions are life-long so are not true history codes

V14 Personal history of allergy to medicinal agents

V15.8 Other personal history presenting hazards to health

Except: V15.7 Personal history of contraception

V16 Family history of malignant neoplasm

V17 Family history of certain chronic disabling diseases

V18 Family history of certain other specific diseases

V19 Family history of other conditions

LATE EFFECTS

Late effect residual of (remaining from) previous illness/injury, e.g., burn that leaves scar

Residual coded first (scar)

Cause (burn) coded second

Late effect codes are not in a separate chapter; rather, throughout Tabular

Reference the term "Late" in the Index

There is no time limit on developing a residual

There may be more than one residual

> ***Example:*** Patient has a stroke (434.91) and develops paralysis on dominant side (hemiparesis, 438.21) and loss of ability to communicate (aphasia, 438.11)

DIAGNOSTIC CODING AND REPORTING GUIDELINES FOR OUTPATIENT SERVICES

Physician's office

Hospital-based outpatient services

Part of *Official Guidelines for Coding and Reporting*, Section IV

Using the ICD-9-CM

Guideline A

The term *first-listed diagnosis* is used rather than *principal diagnosis*

Outpatient Surgery: Reason for surgery

Observation Stay: Medical condition that occasioned admission

Guideline B

Use codes 001.0 through V86.1 to code dx, symptoms, conditions, problems, complaints, or other reason(s) for visit

Guideline C

Documentation should describe patient's condition, using terminology that includes specific diagnoses as well as symptoms, problems, or reasons for encounter

Guideline D

Selection of codes 001.0 through 999.9 (Chapters 1-17) will frequently be used to describe reason for encounter

Guideline E

Codes that describe symptoms and signs, as opposed to diagnoses, acceptable for reporting purposes when an established dx has NOT been confirmed by physician

Guideline F

V codes deal with encounters for circumstances other than disease or injury

 Example: Well-baby checkup (V20.2)

Guideline G

Codes have either three, four, or five digits

4th and/or 5th digit codes provide greater specificity

Three-digit code used ONLY if there is NO 4th or 5th digit

Where 4th and/or 5th digits provided, must be assigned

Diagnoses NOT coded to full digits available are invalid

Guideline H

List first code for dx, condition, problem, or other reason for encounter/visit shown in medical record to be chiefly responsible for services provided

List additional codes that describe any coexisting conditions

Guideline I

Do NOT code diagnoses documented as probable, suspected, questionable, ruled out, or working diagnoses

Rather, code condition(s) to highest degree of certainty for that encounter/visit, such as symptoms, signs, abnormal test results, or other reason for visit

> ***Example:*** Cough and fever, probably pneumonia

- Code as cough (786.2) and fever (780.6X) (in this order)

Guideline J

Chronic diseases treated on an ongoing basis may be coded and reported as many times as patient receives treatment and care for condition(s)

Guideline K

Code all documented conditions that coexist at time of visit, that require or affect patient care, treatment, or management

Do NOT code conditions previously treated, no longer existing

"History of" codes (V10-V19) may be used as secondary codes if

- Impacts current care or treatment

Guidelines L and M

For patients receiving diagnostic or therapeutic services ONLY

Sequence first

- Diagnosis,
- Condition,
- Problem, or
- Other reason shown in medical record to be chiefly responsible for encounter

Codes for other diagnoses (e.g., chronic conditions)

- May be sequenced as secondary diagnoses

> **Exception:**

Patients receiving chemotherapy (V58.11), radiation therapy (V58.0), or rehabilitation (code depends on type)

- V code first; dx or problem for which service being performed second

Guideline N

For patients receiving preoperative evaluations ONLY

- Code from category V72.8 (Other specified examinations)
- Assign secondary code for reason for surgery
- Code also any findings related to preoperative evaluation

Guideline O

Code dx which required ambulatory surgery

If postoperative dx different

- Code postoperative dx

Guideline P

Code routine prenatal visits with no complications

- V22.0 (Supervision of normal first pregnancy)
- V22.1 (Supervision of other normal pregnancy)
- Do NOT use these codes with pregnancy complication codes

ICD-9-CM, CHAPTER 1, INFECTIOUS AND PARASITIC DISEASES

Divided based on etiology (cause of disease)

Many Combination Codes

Example: 112.0 candidiasis infection of mouth, which reports both organism and condition with one code

Multiple Codes

Sequencing must be considered

- UTI due to *Escherichia coli*
- 599.0 (UTI) etiology
- 041.4 *(E. coli)* organism (in this order)

Human Immunodeficiency Virus

Code HIV or HIV-related illness ONLY if stated as confirmed in diagnostic statement

- 042 HIV or HIV-related illness
- V08 Asymptomatic HIV status
- 795.71 Nonspecific HIV serology

Previously Diagnosed HIV-Related Illness

Code prior dx HIV-related disease 042 (HIV)

NEVER assign these patients to

- V08 (Asymptomatic) or
- 795.71 (Nonspecific serologic evidence of HIV)

Patient with HIV admitted for unrelated condition

HIV Sequencing

Sequence first that reason most responsible for encounter, if HIV (042)

Followed by secondary dx that affects encounter or patient care

HIV and Pregnancy

This is an exception to HIV sequencing

During pregnancy, childbirth, or puerperium, code

- 647.6X (Other specified infectious and parasitic diseases), followed by 042 (HIV)

Asymptomatic HIV during pregnancy, childbirth, or puerperium

- 647.6X (Other specified infections and parasitic diseases) and
- V08 (Asymptomatic HIV infection status)
- Reporting asymptomatic HIV varies by state
  - Check the state's reporting laws

Inconclusive Laboratory Test for HIV

795.71 (Inconclusive serologic test for HIV)

- Reporting inconclusive laboratory HIV tests varies by state
  - Check the state's reporting laws

HIV Screening

Code V73.89 (Screening for other specified viral disease)

- Patient in high-risk group for HIV
- V69.8 (Other problems related to lifestyle)

Patients returning for HIV screening results = V65.44 (HIV counseling)

Caution
Incorrectly applying these HIV coding rules can cause patient hardship and may be a violation of law

- Insurance claims for patients with HIV usually need patient's written agreement to disclosure

---

Section I.C.1.b. Septicemia, Systemic Inflammatory Response Syndrome (SIRS), Sepsis, Severe Sepsis, and Septic Shock

Sepsis: Assign systemic infection code as first listed when sepsis is present

- Assign a sepsis code as secondary when sepsis develops during encounter

Septicemia/Sepsis: Usually a 038 septicemia code and a 995.9x SIRS code (in this order)

- Code the organ system dysfunction followed by the SIRS (e.g., 518.81 respiratory failure followed by 995.92)

Septic Shock: Organ dysfunction associated with severe sepsis

- Code underlying systemic infection (e.g., 038.xx) followed by the SIRS code (995.92)

ICD-9-CM, CHAPTER 2, NEOPLASMS

Two steps for coding neoplasms

- Incorrectly applying these neoplasm codes can also cause patient hardship

Index

1. Locate histologic type of neoplasm (e.g., sarcoma, melanoma)
   - Review all instructions
2. Locate code identified by body site
   - Usually in Neoplasm Table in Index under "N"
   - Neoplasm Table divided into columns:
     - Malignant (primary, secondary, ca in situ)
     - Benign
     - Uncertain behavior
     - Unspecified

Example: Pathology report confirmed diagnosis stated in operative report of primary malignant neoplasm of the bladder neck. ICD-9-CM Index, Neoplasm Table, bladder, neck, under Primary column, 188.5. Code then referenced in Tabular to ensure accurate assignment.

Treatment directed at malignancy: Neoplasm is principal dx

Except for Chemotherapy or Radiotherapy:
- Therapy (treatment) followed by neoplasm code
  - Chemotherapy: V58.11
  - Radiotherapy: V58.0

Surgical removal of neoplasm and subsequent chemotherapy or radiotherapy
- Code malignancy as principal dx

Surgery to determine extent of malignancy
- Code malignancy as principal dx
  - V10, "Personal history of malignant neoplasm" if
    - Neoplasm was previously destroyed
    - No longer being treated

If patient receives treatment for secondary neoplasm (metastasis)
- Secondary neoplasm is documented principal dx
- Even though primary is still present

Patient treated for anemia or dehydration due to neoplasm or therapy code
- Anemia or dehydration followed by neoplasm

Patient admitted to repair complication of surgery for an intestinal malignancy
- Complication principal dx
- Complication is reason for encounter
- Malignancy secondary dx

Patient receiving chemotherapy or radiotherapy post-op removal of neoplasm
- Code: Therapy followed by active neoplasm
- Do NOT report H/O (history of) neoplasm

ICD-9-CM, CHAPTER 3, ENDOCRINE, NUTRITIONAL, AND METABOLIC DISEASES AND IMMUNITY DISORDERS

Disorders of Other Endocrine Glands

Diabetes Mellitus 250 coded frequently

Subterms in Index often have two codes

Example:

- Diabetic iritis 250.5X for diabetes (etiology)
- [364.42] for iritis (manifestation)

5th digit indicates type of diabetes

> 0 type II or unspecified type, not stated as uncontrolled
>
> > Fifth-digit 0 is for use for type II patients, even if the patient requires insulin
>
> 1 type I [juvenile type], not stated as uncontrolled
>
> 2 type II or unspecified type, uncontrolled
>
> > Fifth-digit 2 is for use for type II diabetic patients, even if the patient requires insulin
>
> 3 type I [juvenile type], uncontrolled

V58.67 used in addition to diabetes code to show long-term use if insulin

> If type is not indicated, code type II diabetes
>
> > Patient with type II diabetes can receive insulin for periods when diabetes is uncontrolled
>
> > Type I diabetic is one who is insulin-dependent

Other Metabolic and Immunity Disorders Section

Disorders such as gout and dehydration

Disorders often have many names

> *Example:* 242.0X Toxic diffuse goiter, also known as

- Basedow's disease
- Graves' disease
- Primary thyroid hyperplasia

ICD-9-CM, CHAPTER 4, DISEASES OF BLOOD AND BLOOD-FORMING ORGANS

Short chapter with 10 sections

Includes anemia, blood disorders, coagulation defects

Often used code, anemia

Many different types of anemia

- Hereditary hemolytic (282)
- Iron deficiency (280)

- Acquired hemolytic (283)
- Aplastic (284)
- Other and Unspecified (285)

Multiple coding often necessary

Identify underlying disease condition

ICD-9-CM, CHAPTER 5, MENTAL DISORDERS

Includes codes for

- Personality disorders
- Stress disorders
- Neuroses
- Psychoses
- Sexual deviation/dysfunction, etc.

5th digit = status of episode

Example: 304.2, cocaine dependence, is assigned the following 5th digits:

- 0 unspecified (episode)
- 1 continuous
- 2 episodic
- 3 in remission

ICD-9-CM, CHAPTER 6, DISEASES OF NERVOUS SYSTEM AND SENSE ORGANS

Central Nervous System

Peripheral Nervous System

Disorders of Eye

Diseases of Ear

Pain—Category 338

Acute or chronic pain not elsewhere classified due to:

- Trama
- Neoplasm
- Postoperative
- Psychosocial dysfunction

Principal/Primary diagnosis

- When definitive diagnosis not established
- Pain management is reason for encounter/admission

ICD-9-CM, CHAPTER 7, DISEASES OF CIRCULATORY SYSTEM

Three types of hypertension

1. Malignant accelerated, severe, poor prognosis
2. Benign continuous, mild (BP elevated) controllable
3. Unspecified NOT indicated as either malignant or benign

Hypertension (401-405)

Hypertension table located in Index of ICD-9-CM

- Under "H," Hypertension
- Codes divided based on type (malignant, benign, unspecified)

Hypertension, Essential, or NOS

Assign hypertension (arterial, essential, primary, systemic, NOS) to 401

4th digit indicates type

- 0 Malignant
- 1 Benign
- 9 Unspecified

Hypertension with Heart Disease

402 Category

Certain heart conditions when stated "due to hypertension" or implied ("hypertensive")

Add 4th digit for type

Use additional code to specify type of heart failure (428)

Hypertensive Chronic Kidney Disease

Cause-and-effect relationship assumed in chronic kidney disease (CKD) with hypertension

Category 403, Hypertensive chronic kidney disease, used when following present:

- Chronic kidney disease (585.X)
- Kidney failure, unspecified (586)
- Kidney sclerosis, unspecified (587)

5th digit assignment required for stage of CKD

- 0 CKD stage I through IV
- 1 CKD stage V or end stage

Hypertensive Heart and Chronic Kidney Disease

Assign 404 when both hypertensive chronic kidney disease and hypertensive heart disease stated

Assume cause-and-effect relationship

Assign 5th digit for mention kidney stage of chronic disease and/or heart failure

- Use additional code to specify type of heart failure (428)

Hypertensive Cerebrovascular Disease

Code

- Cerebrovascular disease (430-438)
- Type of hypertension (401-405)

Hypertensive Retinopathy

Code

- Hypertensive retinopathy (362.11)
- Type of hypertension (401-405)

Hypertension, Secondary

Hypertension caused by an underlying condition

- Code
  - Underlying condition
  - Type of hypertension (405)

Hypertension, Transient

Transient hypertension: Temporary elevated BP

Do NOT assign 401-405, Hypertensive Disease

- Hypertension dx is NOT established
- Use
  - 796.2, Elevated blood pressure or
  - 642.3X, Transient hypertension of pregnancy

Hypertension, Controlled

Hypertension controlled by therapy

- Assign code from 401-405

Hypertension, Uncontrolled

Untreated or uncontrolled hypertension

- Assign code from 401-405

Documentation must state malignant hypertension to use 404

Elevated Blood Pressure

Elevated blood pressure coded 796.2

- Elevated BP reading without hypertension is dx
- Hypertension NOT stated, NOT coded to 401

ICD-9-CM, CHAPTER 8, DISEASES OF RESPIRATORY SYSTEM

Watch for "Use additional code to identify infectious organism"

Some codes indicate specific organism and do not need an additional code

Respiratory failure sequencing

If the respiratory failure is due to an acute condition (such as MI [myocardial infarction]) or acute exacerbation of a chronic condition (such as COPD [chronic obstructive pulmonary disease]), sequence the acute condition first

Example: MI (acute condition) and respiratory failure

- Sequence MI first and respiratory failure second

If the respiratory failure (acute condition) is due to a chronic nonrespiratory condition (such as myasthenia gravis), sequence the respiratory failure first

Example: Acute respiratory failure (acute) and myasthenia gravis (chronic)

- Sequence acute respiratory failure first and myasthenia gravis second

Acute Respiratory Infection Section

Frequently used codes, such as

- Common cold (460, acute nasopharyngitis)
- Sore throat (462, acute pharyngitis)
- Acute tonsillitis (463)
- Bronchitis (490-491)
- Acute upper respiratory infection (465, URI)
- Influenza (487, flu)

ICD-9-CM, CHAPTER 9, DISEASES OF DIGESTIVE SYSTEM

Mouth to anus + accessory organs

Extensive subcategories

- 574 Cholelithiasis (10 subcategories)
- Each has 5th digit subclassification

Commonly used codes

- Ulcers (531-534)
  - Gastric (531)
  - Duodenal (532)
  - Peptic (533)
  - Gastrojejunal (534)
- Hernias (550-553)

ICD-9-CM, CHAPTER 10, DISEASES OF GENITOURINARY SYSTEM

Commonly used codes

- Urinary tract infection (599.0)

- Inflammation of prostate (601.X)
- Disorders of menstruation (625-627)

Stages of chronic kidney disease

- Stage I: Blood flow through kidney increases, kidney enlarges (585.1)
- Stage II: (mild) Small amounts of blood protein (albumin) leak into urine (microalbuminuria) (585.2)
- Stage III: (moderate) Albumin and other protein losses increase. Patient may develop high blood pressure and kidney loses ability to filter waste (585.3)
- Stage IV: (severe) Large amounts of urine pass through kidney, blood pressure increases (585.4)
- Stage V: Ability to filter waste nearly stops (585.5)
- End-stage renal failure (585.6)

    When documentation indicates chronic renal disease (CKD) and ESRD, report ESRD

- Unspecified 585.9

Status post kidney transplant, assign V42.0

- Patient may still have CKD

ICD-9-CM, CHAPTER 11, COMPLICATIONS OF PREGNANCY, CHILDBIRTH, AND PUERPERIUM

Extensive multiple coding with many 5th digit assignments and notes

Admission for pregnancy, complication

- Obstetric complication = primary dx

Chapter 11 ICD-9-CM codes take precedence over codes from other chapters

Codes 640-676.9 share same 5th digit subclassification

- Denotes current episode of care
- 0 Unspecified as to episode of care or not applicable
- 1 Delivered, with or without mention of antepartum condition
- 2 Delivered, with mention of postpartum complication
- 3 Antepartum condition or complication
- 4 Postpartum condition or complication

General Rules

Not all encounters are pregnancy-related

Example: Pregnant woman, broken ankle (medial malleolus, open)

- Broken ankle (824.1)
- V22.2 Pregnant state incidental; must be documented in medical record that condition being treated not affecting pregnancy

Complications of Pregnancy, Childbirth, and Puerperium

Chapter 11 codes (630-677)

Used only on mother's medical record

Not on newborn medical record

Selection of Primary Diagnosis

Routine prenatal visits, no complications:

- V22.0, Supervision, normal **first** pregnancy or
- V22.1, Supervision, **other** normal pregnancy

Prenatal outpatient visits for high-risk pregnancies:

- V23, Supervision of high-risk pregnancy

Fifth Digit

All categories EXCEPT 650 (Normal delivery)

Requires 5th digit for

- Antepartum
- Postpartum
- If delivery has occurred

Appropriate 5th digit listed under each code

Example: 640.0, Threatened abortion

- 0 unspecified episode
- 1 delivered with or without complication
- 3 antepartum condition or complication

Note that NOT all 5th digits are applicable (640.0, cannot assign 2 or 4)

Postpartum Period

After delivery +6 weeks

Abortions

Codes 634-637 require 5th digits

- 0 unspecified
- 1 incomplete; POC (product of conception) NOT expelled
- 2 complete; all POC expelled prior to care

Abortions with Liveborn Fetus
Attempted abortion results in liveborn fetus

- 644.21 (Early onset of delivery)
- Use V27.X (Outcome of delivery)
- Attempted abortion code also assigned

ICD-9-CM, CHAPTER 12, DISEASES OF SKIN AND SUBCUTANEOUS TISSUE

Skin

Epidermis

Dermis

Subcutaneous tissue

Infectious skin/subcutaneous tissue

Scar tissue

Accessory Organs

Sweat glands

Sebaceous glands

Nails

Hair and hair follicles

Other

Multiple Codes Often Necessary

Example: Cellulitis due to *Staphylococcus,* report

- Cellulitis 682.X
- Staph 041.X

ICD-9-CM, CHAPTER 13, DISEASES OF MUSCULOSKELETAL SYSTEM AND CONNECTIVE TISSUE

Bone

Bursa

Cartilage

Fascia

Ligaments

Muscle

Synovia

Tendons

Chapter 13 Sections

Extensive notes and 5th digits

- Arthropathies (joint disease) and related disorders
- Dorsopathies (curvature of spine)
- Rheumatism, Excluding Back
- Osteopathies, Chondropathies, and Acquired Musculoskeletal Deformities

ICD-9-CM, CHAPTERS 14 AND 15, CONGENITAL ANOMALIES AND CONDITIONS ORIGINATING IN PERINATAL PERIOD

Congenital Anomalies (abnormalities at birth), 740-759

Conditions Originating in Perinatal Period

- Perinatal period through 28th day following birth
- Codes can be used after 28th day if documented that condition originated during perinatal period

Chapter 17 codes are only for the newborn record; never on the maternal record

Assign V30-V39 as first listed according to type of birth

ICD-9-CM, CHAPTER 16, SYMPTOMS, SIGNS, AND ILL-DEFINED CONDITIONS

Do NOT code a sign or symptom if

- Definitive dx made (symptoms are part of disease)

Used only if no specific dx made

ICD-9-CM, CHAPTER 17, INJURY AND POISONING

Section Examples

Fractures

Dislocations

Sprains and Strains

Intracranial Injury

Internal Injury

Crushing Injury

Foreign Body

Burns

Late Effects

Poisoning

Acute fracture care vs. aftercare

Use aftercare codes after completion of active treatment

- Cast change/removal (V53.7)
- Removal of external/internal devices (V54.0X)
- Medication adjustments
- Follow-up visits following fracture treatment

E Codes

Provide supplemental information

Never principal diagnosis

Index and Tabular
E code Index located in Section III

    Directly before the Tabular

    Not in the Index to Disease, Volume 2

E codes are located after the V codes in the Tabular

Identify

- Cause of an injury or poisoning
- Intent (unintentional or intentional)
- Place it occurred

General E Code Guidelines
Use with any code in Volume 1

Initial encounter

- Use E code

Subsequent encounter

- Use late effects E codes, if appropriate

Intent
Unknown, Undetermined (E980-E989)

Unspecified, Undetermined (E980-E989)

Questionable, Undetermined (E980-E989)

Table of Drugs and Chemicals
Alphabetic listing with codes (see Figure 3-15)

Do NOT code directly from Table

Always reference Tabular

Two or more substances involved
If two or more substances involved

- Code each unless combination code exists
- Code substance more closely related to principal dx
- Include one code from each category (cause, intent, place)

Interaction of drug(s) and alcohol

- Use poisoning and E codes for both

Unknown or suspected intent
Unknown

Unspecified

Questionable

Undetermined cause
Intent known, cause unknown, use

- E928.9, Unspecified accident

- E958.9, Suicide and self-inflicted injury by unspecified means
- E968.9, Assault by unspecified means

Late effects of external cause
Should be used with late effect of a previous injury/poisoning

Should NOT be used with related current injury code

Coding of Burns
Multiple injuries and burns
Sequence most severe injury first (physician determined)

Current burns
Sequence highest-degree burn first

Current burns (940-948) classified by

- Depth (severity)
- Extent (% body surface)
- Agent (if necessary)

Depth of burn
1st degree: Erythema

2nd degree: Blistering

3rd degree: Full-thickness involvement

Burns classified
- According to extent of body surface involved

Category 948
- 4th digits = % body surface involved
- 5th digits = % body surface involved in 3rd-degree burns
- Rule of Nines applies

Burn Example: 3rd-degree burn of abdomen (10%) and 2nd-degree burn of thigh (5%) by hot water
- 942.33 Burn, abdomen, 3rd degree
- 945.26 Burn, thigh, 2nd degree
- 948.11 15% total burn area and 10% 3rd degree
- E924.0 Burn by hot liquid

Coding for multiple injuries
Separate code for each injury

Sequence most serious injury first

Vessel and nerve damage
Code primary injury first

- Use additional code if minor nerve damage

Primary injury = nerve damage
- Code nerve damage first

Multiple fractures

Same coding principles as multiple injuries

Code multiple fractures by site

Sequenced by severity

Fractures

Not indicated as closed or open = closed

Same bone fractured AND dislocated:

- Code fracture ONLY (highest level of injury)

UNIT IV

Coding Challenge

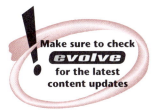

UNIT IV   Coding Challenge

EXAMINATIONS

> **DISCLAIMER:** Every effort has been made to ensure that the content of the practice exams in Unit IV and on the companion CD resemble the format and content of the current CPC certification examination. However, the Academy may revise the examinations at any time and it is your responsibility to review all certification information published by the American Academy of Professional Coders as they are the definitive source for information regarding the CPC certification examination.

You have three opportunities to practice taking an examination:

- Pre-Examination (before study)
- Post-Examination (after study)
- Final Examination (at the end of your complete program of study)

You should have a current edition of the following texts:

- ICD-9-CM (*International Classification of Diseases,* 9th Edition, Clinical Modification), Volumes 1 and 2
- HCPCS (Healthcare Common Procedure Coding System)
- CPT *(Current Procedural Terminology)*

No other reference material is allowed for any of the examinations.

- For the Pre-Examination and Post-Examination, you will need a computer that can use a CD-ROM and the three coding references listed above (ICD-9-CM [Vols. 1 and 2], HCPCS, CPT).
- For the Final Examination, you will need paper, pencils, and an eraser, along with the three coding references.
- Each organization's certification examination has different scoring requirements, but as you take the examinations with this text, you should strive for 80% to 90% on the Post-Examination and 70% as a minimum on the Final Examination.

> **NOTE:** To enable the learner to calculate an examination score, minimums have been identified as "passing" within this text; however, this may or may not be the percentage identified by the American Academy of Professional Coders as a "passing" grade. It is your responsibility to review all certification information published by the American Academy of Professional Coders as they are the definitive source for information regarding the CPC certification examination.

> **NOTE:** It is expected that the examine is able to assign key components when reporting evaluation and management services. See updated E/M questions for examples of the new format. All categories of codes (I, II, and III) are potentially on the examination.

PRE-EXAMINATION AND POST-EXAMINATION

The Pre-Examination contains 150 questions and is located on the CD-ROM. The purpose of the Pre-Examination is only to assess your beginning level of knowledge and skill—your starting place. Based on your scores, you can tailor your study to target your weakest areas and increase your scores. Take the Pre-Examination before you begin your studies.

Your score will automatically be calculated for you on each of the three sections. A passing score for the examinations in this text requires the following:

Section 1   **63%** or 27 of the 43 questions correct

Section 2   **73%** or 44 of the 60 questions correct

Section 3   **60%** or 28 of the 47 questions correct

The software will calculate and retain your scoring information.

Immediately on completion of your study, you should complete the Post-Examination on the CD-ROM. After you are finished, the CD-ROM will automatically compare your Pre-Examination scores with your Post-Examination scores and will store your results. By comparing the results of the Pre-Examination and the Post-Examination (the same examination will be taken twice), the software illustrates the improvements you have achieved or the areas that you will need to practice more on before taking the Final Examination.

Rationales for each question are available for review after you complete the Post-Examination. Study the questions for which you did not choose the right response. Did you misread the question, did you not know the material well enough to answer correctly, or did you run out of time? Knowing why you missed a question is an important step toward improving your skill level.

Ideally, you should complete each examination in one sitting ($5\frac{1}{2}$ hours, or 330 minutes); if time does not allow, spread the examination times over several periods. There are no time extensions during an actual examination setting, and learning how to judge the amount of time you to spend on each question is an important part of this learning experience to prepare you for the real certification examination.

FINAL EXAMINATION

If you scored well on all areas of the Post-Examination (80% to 90%), you are ready to move on to the Final Examination, located in Unit 4 of the text.

There is an answer sheet on which to place your answers; it is located directly before the examination. Remove your answer sheet from this text, and enter your answer for each of the 150 questions using paper and pencil.

NOTE: The real certification examination is currently paper and pencil.

Once you have completed the Final Examination, go to the CD-ROM to enter your answers on the electronic score sheet. The software will then provide you with the answers and compare your scores to illustrate your improvement.

A passing score for the Final Examination is the same as listed for the Pre/Post Examination.

If you did not attain a minimum score on each section, you should develop a plan to restudy those particular areas where the examination indicates you are having difficulties. There are rationales for each question in the Final Examination, and you should review that information as well as material in the text. You can take any of the practice examinations again after your additional study.

FINAL EXAMINATION ANSWER SHEET

SECTION 1

Medical terminology
1. A B C D
2. A B C D
3. A B C D
4. A B C D
5. A B C D
6. A B C D
7. A B C D
8. A B C D
9. A B C D
10. A B C D
11. A B C D
12. A B C D
13. A B C D

Anatomy
14. A B C D
15. A B C D
16. A B C D
17. A B C D
18. A B C D
19. A B C D
20. A B C D
21. A B C D
22. A B C D

ICD-9-CM
23. A B C D
24. A B C D
25. A B C D
26. A B C D
27. A B C D
28. A B C D
29. A B C D
30. A B C D
31. A B C D
32. A B C D
33. A B C D

HCPCS
34. A B C D
35. A B C D
36. A B C D
37. A B C D
38. A B C D

Practice management
39. A B C D
40. A B C D
41. A B C D
42. A B C D
43. A B C D

SECTION 2

10000
44. A B C D
45. A B C D
46. A B C D
47. A B C D
48. A B C D
49. A B C D
50. A B C D
51. A B C D
52. A B C D
53. A B C D

20000
54. A B C D
55. A B C D
56. A B C D
57. A B C D
58. A B C D
59. A B C D
60. A B C D
61. A B C D
62. A B C D
63. A B C D

30000
64. A B C D
65. A B C D
66. A B C D
67. A B C D
68. A B C D
69. A B C D
70. A B C D
71. A B C D
72. A B C D
73. A B C D

40000
74. A B C D
75. A B C D
76. A B C D
77. A B C D
78. A B C D
79. A B C D
80. A B C D
81. A B C D
82. A B C D
83. A B C D

50000
84. A B C D
85. A B C D
86. A B C D
87. A B C D
88. A B C D
89. A B C D
90. A B C D
91. A B C D
92. A B C D
93. A B C D

60000
94. A B C D
95. A B C D
96. A B C D
97. A B C D
98. A B C D
99. A B C D
100. A B C D
101. A B C D
102. A B C D
103. A B C D

SECTION 3

E/M
104. A B C D
105. A B C D
106. A B C D
107. A B C D
108. A B C D
109. A B C D
110. A B C D
111. A B C D
112. A B C D
113. A B C D
114. A B C D
115. A B C D

Anesthesia
116. A B C D
117. A B C D
118. A B C D
119. A B C D
120. A B C D
121. A B C D

70000
122. A B C D
123. A B C D
124. A B C D
125. A B C D
126. A B C D
127. A B C D
128. A B C D
129. A B C D
130. A B C D

80000
131. A B C D
132. A B C D
133. A B C D
134. A B C D
135. A B C D
136. A B C D
137. A B C D
138. A B C D
139. A B C D
140. A B C D

90000
141. A B C D
142. A B C D
143. A B C D
144. A B C D
145. A B C D
146. A B C D
147. A B C D
148. A B C D
149. A B C D
150. A B C D

FINAL EXAMINATION
SECTION 1

QUESTIONS 1-43

Medical Terminology

1. This term means the surgical removal of the fallopian tube:
   A. ligation
   B. hysterectomy
   C. salpingostomy
   D. salpingectomy

2. This combining form means thirst:
   A. dips/o
   B. acr/o
   C. cortic/o
   D. somat/o

3. This term is also known as a homograft:
   A. autograft
   B. allograft
   C. xenograft
   D. zenograft

4. Which of the following terms does NOT describe a receptor of the body?
   A. mechanoreceptor
   B. proprioceptor
   C. thermoreceptor
   D. endoreceptor

5. Which of the following terms means taste?
   A. Meissner
   B. pacinian
   C. gustatory
   D. astrocytes

6. This suffix means removal:
   A. -penia
   B. -ectomy
   C. -itis
   D. -pexy

7. This term means abnormal thickening of the skin:
   A. ductus
   B. dermatofibroma
   C. dermatitis
   D. pachyderma

8. The term that defines the relaxation phase of the heartbeat is:
   A. systole
   B. sinoatrial
   C. diastole
   D. septa

UNIT IV Coding Challenge

9. This abbreviation refers to a resection of the prostate that is accomplished by means of a scope passed through the urethra.
   A. TURP
   B. TURBT
   C. BPH
   D. UPJ

10. What does EGD stand for?
    A. esophagogastroduodenoscopy
    B. esophagogastric junction
    C. endoscopic retrograde cholangiopancreatography
    D. enterocolostomy

11. This term means the use of electric current to destroy tissue:
    A. eventration
    B. enterolysis
    C. evisceration
    D. fulguration

12. This gland secretes a factor that causes T-cells to mature; it is larger in infants, then shrinks with age.
    A. spleen
    B. lymph
    C. thymus
    D. adrenal

13. This suffix means to act upon:
    A. -in
    B. -ine
    C. -tropin
    D. -agon

Anatomy

14. This is the first portion of the small intestine:
    A. jejunum
    B. ileum
    C. duodenum
    D. cecum

15. This is a part of the inner ear:
    A. vestibule
    B. malleus
    C. incus
    D. stapes

16. This is the area behind the cornea:
    A. anterior chamber
    B. choroid layer
    C. ciliary body
    D. fundus

17. This is the collarbone:
    A. patella
    B. tibia
    C. scapula
    D. clavicle

18. The act of turning upward, such as the hand turned palm upward:
    A. supination
    B. adduction
    C. pronation
    D. circumduction

19. The middle layer of the skin, also known as the corium or true skin, is the:
    A. epidermis.
    B. stratum corneum.
    C. dermis.
    D. subcutaneous.

20. The shaft of a long bone:
    A. diaphysis
    B. epiphysis
    C. metaphysis
    D. periosteum

21. Which of the following is NOT a covering of the chamber walls of the heart?
    A. endocardium
    B. myocardium
    C. pericardium
    D. epicardium

22. The name of the entire motor nervous system:
    A. autonomic nervous system
    B. parasympathetic system
    C. peripheral nervous system
    D. sympathetic system

ICD-9-CM

23. Three-week-old female with obstructive apnea.
    A. 770.8
    B. 770.82
    C. 769
    D. 770.83

24. Congenital hypothyroidism with mild retardation.
    A. 243, 317
    B. 244.8, 317
    C. 243, 318.0
    D. 317, 243

UNIT IV Coding Challenge

25. Glomerulonephritis due to infectious hepatitis.
    A. 580.9, 070
    B. 070, 580.9
    C. 580.81, 070.9
    D. 070.9, 580.81

26. Bloody stool.
    A. 772.4
    B. 792.1
    C. 578.1
    D. 578.0

27. A lethargic patient with vomiting and severe cramping ingested five tablets of Tylenol with codeine and half a bottle of whiskey.
    A. 965.01, 965.4, 980.0, 780.79, 787.03, 789.00, E980.0, E980
    B. 965.09, 965.61, 980.0, 780.79, 787.03, 789.00, E980.0
    C. 966.09, 965.4, 980.0, 780.71, 787.03, 789.00, E980.4, E980.9
    D. 965.09, 965.4, 980.0, 780.79, 787.03, 789.00, E980.0, E980.9

28. Admission for hemodialysis because of acute renal failure.
    A. V56.31, 584.9
    B. V56, 584
    C. V56.0, 584.9
    D. 584.9, V56.0

29. Sarcoidosis with cardiomyopathy.
    A. 135, 517.8
    B. 135, 425.8
    C. 425.8, 135
    D. 135, 425.8, V71.7

30. Open wound of left hand.
    A. 882.0
    B. 883.0
    C. 887.2
    D. 882.2

31. Fracture of the right patella with abrasion.
    A. 822.0, 916.0
    B. 822.0
    C. 916.0, 822.1
    D. 823.00

32. Mr. Hallberger is 62 and has multiple problems. I am examining him in the intensive critical care unit. I understand he has fluid overload with acute renal failure and was started on ultrafiltration by the nephrologist on duty. He has an abnormal chest x-ray. He has preexisting type II diabetes mellitus and sepsis. We are left with a patient now who is still sedated and on a ventilator because of respiratory failure. Code the diagnoses only.
    A. 782.3, 585.9, 792, 250.40, 039.9, 518.81
    B. 789.59, 584.7, 793.1, 250.4, 039.9, 518.81
    C. 276.50, 587, 793.1, 250.00, 038.9, 518.81, 99223
    D. 276.6, 038.9, 995.91, 584.9, 518.81, 250.00, 793.1

33. Susan Oster, 45, was admitted to the hospital with septicemia and SIRS. Her temperature was 38.5° C, heart rate 102 beats/min, respiration 20/min, WBC 12,500. Her respiratory and acute hepatic failure are due to septicemia.
   A. 038.9, 995.92
   B. 038.9, 518.81, 570
   C. 995.92, 038.9
   D. 038.9, 995.92, 518.81, 570

HCPCS

34. A patient is issued a 22-inch seat cushion for his wheelchair.
   A. E2601
   B. E0950
   C. E0190
   D. E2602

35. A patient with chronic lumbar pain previously purchased a TENS and now needs replacement batteries.
   A. E1592
   B. A5082
   C. A4772
   D. A4630

36. Which HCPCS modifier indicates the great toe of the right foot?
   A. T1
   B. T3
   C. T4
   D. T5

37. A patient with chronic obstructive pulmonary disease is issued a medically necessary nebulizer with a compressor and humidifier for extensive use with oxygen delivery.
   A. E0570, E0550
   B. E0555, E0571
   C. E0580, E0550
   D. E0575, E0550

38. A patient presents for trimming of 10 dystrophic toenails.
   A. G0127 × 2, 703.8
   B. G0127, G0127 × 9, 703.0
   C. G0127, 703.8
   D. G0127 × 5, G0127 × 5, 703.9

Practice Management

39. Specific coding guidelines in the CPT manual are located in:
   A. the index.
   B. the introduction.
   C. the beginning of each section.
   D. Appendix A.

UNIT IV Coding Challenge

40. Which punctuation mark between codes in the index of the CPT manual indicates a range of codes is available?
    A. period
    B. comma
    C. semicolon
    D. hyphen

41. The term that indicates this is the type of code for which the full code description can be known only if the common part of the code (the description preceding the semicolon) of a preceding entry is referenced:
    A. stand-alone
    B. indented
    C. independent
    D. add-on

42. The symbol that indicates an add-on code is:
    A. ▲
    B. ●
    C. +
    D. ▶◀

43. When you see the symbol "⊘" next to a code in the CPT manual, you know that:
    A. the code is a new code.
    B. the code contains new or revised text
    C. the code is a modifier -51 exempt code.
    D. FDA approval is pending.

SECTION 2

QUESTIONS 44-103

10000 Intmentary System

44. **OPERATIVE REPORT**

    OPERATIVE PROCEDURE: Excision of back lesion.

    INDICATIONS FOR SURGERY: The patient has an enlarging lesion on the upper midback.

    FINDINGS AT SURGERY: There was a 5-cm, upper midback lesion.

    OPERATIVE PROCEDURE: With the patient prone, the back was prepped and draped in the usual sterile fashion. The skin and underlying tissues were anesthetized with 30 mL of 1% lidocaine with epinephrine.
    Through a 5-cm transverse skin incision, the lesion was excised. Hemostasis was ensured. The incision was closed using 3-0 Vicryl for the deep layers and running 3-0 Prolene subcuticular stitch with Steri-Strips for the skin.
    The patient was returned to the same-day surgery center in stable postoperative condition. All sponge, needle, and instrument counts were correct. Estimated blood loss is 0 mL.

PATHOLOGY REPORT LATER INDICATED: Dermatofibroma, skin of back. Assign code(s) for the physician service only.
A. 11406, 12002, 216.5
B. 11424, 215.7
C. 11406, 12032, 216.5
D. 11606, 232.5

45. **EMERGENCY DEPARTMENT REPORT CHIEF COMPLAINT:** Nasal bridge laceration.

    SUBJECTIVE: The patient is a 74-year-old male who presents to the emergency department with a laceration to the bridge of his nose. He fell in the bathroom tonight. He recalls the incident. He just sort of lost his balance. He denies any vertigo. He denies any chest pain or shortness of breath. He denies any head pain or neck pain. There was no loss of consciousness. He slipped on a wet floor in the bathroom and lost his balance; that is how it happened. He has not had any blood from the nose or mouth.

    PAST MEDICAL HISTORY:
    1. Parkinson's
    2. Back pain
    3. Constipation

    MEDICATIONS: See the patient record for a complete list of medications.

    ALLERGIES: NKDA.

    REVIEW OF SYSTEMS: Per HPI. Otherwise, negative.

    PHYSICAL EXAMINATION: The exam showed a 74-year-old male in no acute distress. Examination of the HEAD showed no obvious trauma other than the bridge of the nose, where there is approximately a 1.5- to 2-cm laceration. He had no bony tenderness under this. Pupils were equal, round, and reactive. EARS and NOSE: OROPHARYNX was unremarkable. NECK was soft and supple. HEART was regular. LUNGS were clear but slightly diminished in the bases.

    PROCEDURE: The wound was draped in a sterile fashion and anesthetized with 1% Xylocaine with sodium bicarbonate. It was cleansed with sterile saline and then repaired using interrupted 6-0 Ethilon sutures (Dr. Barney Teller, first-year resident, assisted with the suturing).

    ASSESSMENT: Nasal bridge laceration, status post fall.

    PLAN: Keep clean. Sutures out in 5 to 7 days. Watch for signs of infection.
    A. 12051, 873.20, E885.9
    B. 12011, 873.20, E885.9
    C. 12011, 873.32, E888.8
    D. 12011, 11000, 873.32, E929.9

UNIT IV Coding Challenge

46. **SAME-DAY SURGERY**

    DIAGNOSIS: Inverted nipple with mammary duct ectasia, left.

    OPERATION: Excision of mass deep to left nipple.

    With the patient under general anesthesia, a circumareolar incision was made with sharp dissection and carried down into the breast tissue. The nipple complex was raised up using a small retractor. We gently dissected underneath to free up the nipple entirely. Once this was done, we had the nipple fully unfolded, and there was some evident mammary duct ectasis. An area 3 × 4 cm was excised using electrocautery. Hemostasis was maintained with the electrocautery, and then the breast tissue deep to the nipple was reconstructed using sutures of 3-0 chromic. Subcutaneous tissue was closed using 3-0 chromic, and then the skin was closed using 4-0 Vicryl. Steri-Strips were applied. The patient tolerated the procedure well and was returned to the recovery area in stable condition. At the end of the procedure, all sponges and instruments were accounted for.
    A. 19120-RT, 610.4
    B. 11404-LT, 611.1
    C. 19112, 610.4
    D. 19120-LT, 610.4

47. This patient returns today for palliative care to her feet. Her toenails have become elongated and thickened, and she is unable to trim them on her own. She states that she has had no problems and no acute signs of any infection or otherwise to her feet. She returns today strictly for nail debridement to her feet.

    EXAMINATION: Her pedal pulses are palpable bilaterally. The nails are mycotic, 1 through 4 on the left, and 1 through 3 on the right.

    ASSESSMENT: Onychomycosis, 1 through 4 on the left and 1 through 3 on the right.

    PLAN: Mild debridement of mycotic nails × 7. This patient is to return to the clinic in 3 to 4 months for follow-up palliative care.
    A. 11721 × 7, 117.9
    B. 99212, 11721, 110.1
    C. 11719, 110.1
    D. 11721, 110.1

48. **OPERATIVE REPORT**
    With the patient having had a wire localization performed by radiology, she was taken to the operating room and, under local anesthesia of the left breast, was prepped and draped in a sterile manner. A breast line incision was made through the entry point of the wire, and a core of tissue surrounding the wire (approximately 1 × 2 cm) was removed using electrocautery for hemostasis. The specimen, including the wire, was then submitted to radiology, and the presence of the lesion within the specimen was confirmed. The wound was checked for hemostasis, and this was maintained with electrocautery. The breast tissue was reapproximated using 2-0 and 3-0 chromic. The skin was closed using 4-0 Vicryl in a subcuticular manner. Steri-Strips were applied. The patient tolerated the procedure well

and was discharged from the operating room in stable condition. At the end of the procedure, all sponges and instruments were accounted for.

Pathology report later indicated: Benign lesion.

A. 11602-LT, 238.3
B. 11400-LT, 174.9
C. 19125-LT, 217
D. 19125-LT, 239.3

49. What CPT code(s) would be used to code a split-thickness skin graft, both thighs to the abdomen, measuring 45 × 21 cm? The patient has third-degree burns of the abdomen. Documentation stated 2-% of the body surface was burned with 9% third degree. The patient also sustained second-degree burns of the back.

A. 15100 × 2, 949.3, 949.2, 948.00
B. 15100, 15101 × 9, 942.33, 942.24, 948.20
C. 15100, 15101 × 9-51, 946.3, 949.2, 948.02
D. 15100, 15101 × 8, 948.01, 942.29

50. What CPT code would be used to report a massive debridement of an open anterior abdominal wound, including subcutaneous tissue and muscle? The patient fell while speed walking and landed on a sharp rock.

A. 11000, 879.2, E880.1, E920.8
B. 11010, 879.6, E880.1
C. 11042, 879.2
D. 11043, 879.3, E888.0, E920.8

51. The patient is brought to surgery for repair of an accidentally inflicted open wound of the left thigh, the total extent measuring approximately 40 × 35 cm.

DESCRIPTION OF PROCEDURE: The legs were prepped with Betadine scrub and solution and then draped in a routine sterile fashion. Split-thickness skin grafts measuring about a 10,000th inch thick were taken from both thighs, meshed with a 3:1 ratio mesher, and stapled to the wounds. The donor sites were dressed with scarlet red, and the recipient sites were dressed with Xeroform, Kerlix fluffs, and Kerlix roll, and a few ABD pads were used for absorption. Estimated blood loss was negligible. The patient tolerated the procedure well and left surgery in good condition.

A. 15120, 15121 × 12, 891.0, E929.9
B. 15100, 15101, 11010, 891.0, E928.9
C. 15220, 15221 × 13, 890.0, E928.9
D. 15100, 15101 × 13, 890.0, E928.9

52. What CPT code would be used to code the destruction of a malignant lesion on the genitalia measuring 1.6 cm using cryosurgery?

A. 17272, 184.4
B. 11602, 199.0
C. 11420, 198.82
D. 11622, 184.4

UNIT IV   Coding Challenge

53. What code(s) is used by the radiologist when performing preoperative placement of a needle localization wire of a single lesion of the breast? The patient was diagnosed with adenocarcinoma of the upper outer quadrant of the right breast, primary site.
    A. 19290, 19125, 174.5
    B. 19125, 174.4
    C. 19290, 174.4
    D. 19295, 174.5

20000 Musculoskeletal System

54. Carl Ostrick, a 21-year-old male, slipped on a patch of ice on his sidewalk while shoveling snow. When he fell, his left hand was wedged under his body and his carpometacarpal joint was dislocated. After manipulating the joint back into normal alignment, the surgeon fixed the dislocation by placing a wire percutaneously through the carpometacarpal joint to maintain alignment.
    A. 26608-F1, 833.01, E886.0
    B. 26650-FA, 833.14, E888.9
    C. 26706-LT, 833.00, E885.9
    D. 26676-LT, 833.04, E885.9

55. John, an 84-year-old male, tripped while on his morning walk. He stated he was thinking about something else when he inadvertently tripped over the sidewalk curb and fell to his knees. X-ray indicated a fracture of his right patella. With the patient under general anesthesia, the area was opened and extensively irrigated. The left aspect of the patella was severely fragmented, and a portion of the patella was subsequently removed. The remaining patella fractures were wired. The surrounding tissue was repaired, thoroughly irrigated, and closed in the usual manner.
    A. 27524-RT, 822.0, E880.1
    B. 27520-RT, 822.0, E880.1
    C. 27524-RT, 822.1, E888.9
    D. 27524-RT, 822.0, E888.9

56. Maryann received a blow to her right tibial shaft while moving a large stuffed chair up a flight of stairs when the person in front of the chair slipped and released his hold on the chair. The full weight of the chair was pushed against her; when she was unable to hold the chair in place, both she and the chair fell to the landing a dozen steps below. The chair tipped on its side and landed on her tibia. On x-ray, the right tibia shaft was fractured in three places. Percutaneous screws and pins were placed to secure the fracture sites.
    A. 27750-RT, 823.80, E880.9
    B. 27756-RT, 823.80, E888.9
    C. 27756-RT, 823.20, E880.9
    D. 27750-RT, 823.20, E880.9

57. Darin was a passenger in an automobile rollover accident and was not wearing a seat belt at the time. He was thrown from the automobile and was pinned under the rear of the overturned vehicle. He sustained craniofacial separation, Le Forte III fracture, that required complicated internal and external fixation using an open approach to repair the extensive damage. A halo device was used to hold the head immobile.
    A. 21435, 20661
    B. 21435
    C. 21432
    D. 21436, 20661

58. Libby was thrown from a horse while riding in the ditch; a truck that honked the horn as it passed her startled her horse. The horse reared up, and Libby was thrown to the ground. Her left tibia was fractured and required insertion of multiple pins to stabilize the defect area. A unilateral multiplane external fixation system was then attached to the pins. Code the placement of the fixation device and diagnosis only.
    A. 20661-LT, 823.82, E828.9
    B. 20692-LT, 823.80, E828.2
    C. 20692-LT, 823.82, E828.2
    D. 20690-LT, 823.80, E828.2

59. A small incision was made over the left proximal tibia, and a traction pin was inserted through the bone to the opposite side. Weights were then affixed to the pins to stabilize the closed tibial fracture temporarily until fracture repair could be performed. Assign codes for the physician service.
    A. 20650-LT, 823.80
    B. 20663-LT, 823.90
    C. 20690-LT, 823.40
    D. 20692-LT, 823.90

60. Mary tells her physician that she has been having pain in her left wrist for several weeks. The physician examines the area and palpates a ganglion cyst of the tendon sheath. He marks the injection sites, sterilizes the area, and injects corticosteroid into two areas.
    A. 20550-LT × 2, 727.42
    B. 20551-LT, 727.41
    C. 20551-LT × 2, 727.43
    D. 20612-LT, 20612-59-LT, 727.42

61. The physician applies a Minerva-type fiberglass body cast from the hips to the shoulders and to the head. Before application, a stockinette is stretched over the patient's torso, and further padding of the bony areas with felt padding was done. The patient was diagnosed with Morquio-Brailsford kyphosis. Assign codes for the physician service only.
    A. 29040, 277.5, 737.41
    B. 29590, 737.41
    C. 29025, 737.41, 277.5
    D. 29000, 737.10, 277.5

62. OPERATIVE REPORT

PREOPERATIVE DIAGNOSIS: Open fracture, left humerus, with possible loss of left radial pulse.

PROCEDURE PERFORMED: Open reduction internal fixation, left open humerus fracture.

PROCEDURE: While under a general anesthetic, the patient's left arm was prepped with Betadine and draped in sterile fashion. We then created a longitudinal incision over the anterolateral aspect of his left arm and carried the dissection through the subcutaneous tissue. We attempted to identify the lateral intermuscular septum and progressed to the fracture site, which was actually fairly easy to do because there was some significant tearing and rupturing of the biceps and brachialis muscles. These were partial ruptures, but the bone was relatively easy to expose through this. We then identified the fracture site and thoroughly irrigated it with several liters of saline. We also noted that the radial nerve was easily visible, crossing along the posterolateral aspect of the fracture site. It was intact. We carefully detected it throughout the remainder of the procedure. We then were able to strip the periosteum away from the lateral side of the shaft of the humerus both proximally and distally from the fracture site. We did this just enough to apply a 6-hole plate, which we eventually held in place with six cortical screws. We did attempt to compress the fracture site. Due to some comminution, the fracture was not quite anatomically aligned, but certainly it was felt to be very acceptable.

Once we had applied the plate, we then checked the radial pulse with a Doppler. We found that the radial pulse was present using the Doppler, but not with palpation. We then applied Xeroform dressings to the wounds and the incision. After padding the arm thoroughly, we applied a long-arm splint with the elbow flexed about 75 degrees. He tolerated the procedure well, and the radial pulse was again present on Doppler examination at the end of the procedure.

A. 24515-RT, 812.30, E887
B. 24500-LT, 812.20, E888.9
C. 24515-LT, 812.31, E887
D. 24505-LT, 812.20, E888.9

63. OPERATIVE REPORT

PREOPERATIVE DIAGNOSIS: Left thigh abscess.

PROCEDURE PERFORMED: Incision and drainage of left thigh abscess.

OPERATIVE NOTE: With the patient under general anesthesia, he was placed in the lithotomy position. The area around the anus was carefully inspected, and we saw no evidence of communication with the perirectal space. This appears to have risen in the crease at the top of the leg, extending from the posterior buttocks region up toward the side of the base of the penis. In any event, the area was prepped and draped in a sterile manner. Then we incised the area in fluctuation. We obtained a lot of very foul-smelling, almost stool-like material (it was not stool, but it was brown and very foul-smelling material). This was not the typical pus one sees with a *Staphylococcus aureus*–type infection. The incision was widened to allow us to probe the cavity fully. Again, I could see no evidence of communication to the rectum, but there was extension down the thigh and extension up into the groin crease. The fascia was darkened from the purulent material. I

opened some of the fascia to make sure the underlying muscle was viable. This appeared viable. No gas was present. There was nothing to suggest a necrotizing fasciitis. The patient did have a very extensive inflammation within this abscess cavity. The abscess cavity was irrigated with peroxide and saline and packed with gauze vaginal packing. The patient tolerated the procedure well and was discharged from the operating room in stable condition.
A. 26990-LT, 682.6
B. 27301-LT, 682.6
C. 27301-LT, 682.60
D. 27025-LT, 682.6

30000 Respiratory System and Cardiovascular System

64. **OPERATIVE REPORT**
    Code only the operative procedure and diagnosis(es).

    PREOPERATIVE DIAGNOSIS:
    1. Hypoxia
    2. Pneumothorax

    POSTOPERATIVE DIAGNOSIS:
    1. Hypoxia
    2. Pneumothorax

    PROCEDURE: Chest tube placement

    DESCRIPTION OF PROCEDURE: The patient was previously sedated with Versed and paralyzed with Nimbex. Lidocaine was used to numb the incision area in the midlateral left chest at about nipple level. After the lidocaine, an incision was made, and we bluntly dissected to the area of the pleural space, making sure we were superior to the rib. On entrance to the pleural space, there was immediate release of air noted. An 18-gauge chest tube was subsequently placed and sutured to the skin. There were no complications for the procedure, and blood loss was minimal.

    DISPOSITION: Follow-up, single-view, chest x-ray showed significant resolution of the pneumothorax except for a small apical pneumothorax that was noted.
    A. 32422, 799.02, 512.8
    B. 32551, 71010, 799.00, 512.8
    C. 32551, 512.8, 799.02
    D. 32422, 799.00, 512.0

65. **OPERATIVE PROCEDURE**

    PREOPERATIVE DIAGNOSIS: 68-year-old male in a coma.

    POSTOPERATIVE DIAGNOSIS: 68-year-old male in a coma.

    PROCEDURE PERFORMED: Placement of a triple lumen central line in right subclavian vein.

    With the usual Betadine scrub to the right subclavian vein area and with a second attempt, the subclavian vein was cannulated and the wire was threaded. The first time the wire did not thread right, and so the attempt was aborted to make sure we had good identification of structures. Once the wire was in place, the needle was removed and a tissue dilator was pushed into position over the wire. Once that was removed, then the

central lumen catheter was pushed into position at 17 cm and the wire removed. All three ports were flushed. The catheter was sewn into position, and a dressing applied.
A. 36011, 780.09
B. 36011, 780.01
C. 36556, 780.09
D. 36556, 780.01

66. **OPERATIVE REPORT:** The patient is in for a bone marrow biopsy. The patient was sterilized by standard procedure. Bone marrow core biopsies were obtained from the left posterior iliac crest with minimal discomfort. At the end of the procedure, the patient denied discomfort, without evidence of complications. The patient has diffuse, malignant lymphoma. Assign codes for the physician service only.
A. 20225, 229.0
B. 38221, 202.80
C. 38230, 200.10
D. 38220, 202.80

67. What CPT code would you use to report the percutaneous insertion of a dual-chamber pacemaker by means of the subclavian vein? The patient has sick sinus syndrome, tachy-brady.
A. 33249, 427.0, 427.81
B. 33217, 427.81
C. 33208, 427.81
D. 33240, 426.12, 427.0

68. Patient is a 40-year-old male who was involved in a motor vehicle crash. He is having some pulmonary insufficiency.

PROCEDURE: Bronchoscope was inserted through the accessory point on the end of the ET tube and was then advanced through the ET tube. The ET tube came pretty close down to the carina. We selectively intubated the right mainstem bronchus with the bronchoscope. There were some secretions here, and these were aspirated. We then advanced this selectively into first the lower and then the middle and upper lobes. Secretions were present, more so in the middle and lower lobes. No mucous plug was identified. We then went into the left mainstem and looked at the upper and lower lobes. There was really not much in the way of secretions present. We did inject some saline and aspirated this out. We then removed the bronchoscope and put the patient back on the supplemental O2. We waited a few minutes. The oxygen level actually stayed pretty good during this time. We then reinserted the bronchoscope and went down to the right side again. We aspirated out all secretions and made sure everything was clear. We then removed the bronchoscope and pulled back on the ET tube about 1.5 cm. We then again placed the patient on supplemental oxygenation.

FINDINGS: No mucous plug was identified. Secretions were found mainly in the right lung and were aspirated. The left side looked pretty clear.
A. 31646, 518.5, E819.9
B. 32654, 518.82, E812
C. 31645-50, 518.5, E819.9
D. 31645-RT, 31622-51-LT, 518.5, E988.5

69. This 52-year-old male has undergone several attempts at extubation, all of which failed. He also has morbid obesity and significant subcutaneous fat in his neck. The patient is now in for a flap tracheostomy and cervical lipectomy. The cervical lipectomy is necessary for adequate exposure and access to the trachea and also to secure tracheotomy tube placement. Assign code(s) for the physician service only.
    A. 31610, 15839-51
    B. 31610
    C. 31610, 15838
    D. 31603, 15839-51

70. This patient returns to the operating room for placement of an additional chest tube for an anterior pneumothorax due to a contusion lung injury. The same physician had just placed a chest tube 4 days earlier.
    A. 32551, 860.0
    B. 32420, 861.21
    C. 32551-58, 861.21
    D. 32551, 861.3

71. **OPERATIVE REPORT**

    PREOPERATIVE DIAGNOSIS: Atelectasis of the left lower lobe.

    PROCEDURE PERFORMED: Fiberoptic bronchoscopy with brushings and cell washings.

    PROCEDURE: The patient was already sedated, on a ventilator, and intubated; so his bronchoscopy was done through the ET tube. It was passed easily down to the carina. About 2 to 2.5 cm above the carina, we could see the trachea, which appeared good, as was the carina. In the right lung, all segments were patent and entered, and no masses were seen. The left lung, however, had petechial ecchymotic areas scattered throughout the airways. The tissue was friable and swollen, but no mucous plugs were noted, and all the airways were open, just somewhat swollen. No abnormal secretions were noted at all. Brushings were taken as well as washings, including some with Mucomyst to see whether we could get some distal mucous plug, but nothing really significant was returned. The specimens were sent to appropriate cytological and bacteriological studies. The patient tolerated the procedure fairly well.
    A. 31622, 31623-51, 518.0
    B. 31623, 770.4
    C. 31622-RT, 31623-51-LT, 518.0
    D. 31624, 770.4

72. **OPERATIVE REPORT**

    PREOPERATIVE DIAGNOSIS: Atherosclerotic heart disease.

    POSTOPERATIVE DIAGNOSIS: Atherosclerotic heart disease.

    OPERATIVE PROCEDURE: Coronary bypass grafts × 2 with a single graft from the aorta to the distal left anterior descending and from the aorta to the distal right coronary artery.

    PROCEDURE: The patient was brought to the operating room and placed in a supine position. Under general intubation anesthesia, the anterior chest and legs were prepped and draped in the usual manner. A segment of greater saphenous vein was harvested from the left thigh, utilizing the endoscopic vein harvesting technique, and prepared for grafting. The sternum was opened in the usual fashion, and the left internal mammary artery was taken down and prepared for grafting. The flow through the internal mammary artery was very poor. The patient did have a 25-mm difference in arterial pressure between the right and left arms, the right arm being higher. The left internal mammary artery was therefore not used. The pericardium was incised sharply and a pericardial well created. The patient was systemically heparinized and placed on bicaval to aortic cardiopulmonary bypass with the sump in the main pulmonary artery for cardiac decompression. The patient was cooled to 26°C, and on fibrillation an aortic cross-clamp was applied and potassium-rich cold crystalline cardioplegic solution was administered through the aortic root with satisfactory cardiac arrest. Subsequent doses were given down the vein grafts as the anastomoses were completed and via the coronary sinus in a retrograde fashion. Attention was directed to the right coronary artery. The end of the greater saphenous vein was then anastomosed thereto with 7-0 continuous Prolene distally. The remaining graft material was then grafted to the left anterior descending at the junction of the middle and distal third. The aortic cross-clamp was removed after 149 minutes with spontaneous cardioversion. The usual maneuvers to remove air from the left heart were then carried out using transesophageal echocardiographic technique. After all the air was removed and the patient had returned to a satisfactory temperature, he was weaned from cardiopulmonary bypass after 213 minutes utilizing 5 g per kilogram per minute of dopamine. The chest was closed in the usual fashion. A sterile compression dressing was applied, and the patient returned to the surgical intensive care unit in satisfactory condition.

A. 33511, 33517, 440.9
B. 33511, 33508, 414.01
C. 33534, 33508, 414.00
D. 33511, 33517, 414.01

73. Connie was brought to the operating room for a sliding hiatal hernia, and transthoracic repair was performed.
A. 39520, 553.3
B. 39503, 756.6
C. 39530, 553.3
D. 39540, 756.6

40000 Digestive System

74. What CPT code would you use if the physician performs a pyloroplasty and vagotomy in the same surgical session?
A. 43865
B. 50400
C. 43635
D. 43640

75. **OPERATIVE REPORT**

    PREOPERATIVE DIAGNOSIS: Leaking from intestinal anastomosis.

    POSTOPERATIVE DIAGNOSIS: Leaking from intestinal anastomosis.

    PROCEDURE PERFORMED: Proximal ileostomy for diversion of colon. Oversew of right colonic fistula.

Final Examination

OPERATIVE NOTE: This patient was taken back to the operating room from the intensive care unit. She was having acute signs of leakage from an anastomosis I performed 3 days previously. We took down some of the sutures holding the wound together. We basically exposed all of this patient's intestine. It was evident that she was leaking from the small bowel as well as from the right colon. I thought the only thing we could do would be to repair the right colon. This was done in two layers, and then we freed up enough bowel to try to make an ileostomy proximal to the area of leakage. We were able to do this with great difficulty, and there was only a small amount of bowel to be brought out. We brought this out as an ileostomy stoma, realizing that it was of questionable viability and that it should be watched closely. With that accomplished, we then packed the wound and returned the patient to the intensive care unit.
A. 44310, 998.31
B. 44310-78, 997.4, E878.2
C. 45136, 996.5, E878.2
D. 45136-78, 998.32, E879.1

76. This patient is taken to the operating room from the intensive care unit (ICU). The area of the stoma appears to be necrotic, and on this basis the surgeon indicates that the patient has been taken back to the operating room. The surgeon performing the revision is not the same surgeon that originally placed the stoma, nor is the stoma being revised during the postoperative period of any previous procedure.

    PROCEDURE PERFORMED: Revision ileostomy stoma.

    OPERATIVE NOTE: With the patient moved onto the operating table, the abdomen was prepped and draped. The segment of bowel that was serving as the ileostomy was freed up. Going in through this large open wound, we were able to identify which segment of bowel this was. We resected the end of the bowel that was necrotic and freed up enough of the distal small bowel so that we could bring it out through a new stoma that was placed lateral to the original stoma. The stoma was created, the bowel was brought out, and the mucosa was sewn onto the skin. With this accomplished, we appeared to have a viable stoma. The patient tolerated this procedure and was returned to the ICU in stable condition.
    A. 44310, 560.1, E878.1
    B. 45136, 009.0, E878.0
    C. 44312, 569.69, 557.0, E878.3
    D. 44314, 557.0

77. This patient is brought back to the operating room during the postoperative period by the same physician to repair an esophagogastrostomy leak, transthoracic approach, done 2 days ago. The patient is status post esophagectomy for cancer. Code the procedure and the diagnosis for the complication.
    A. 43320-78, 530.10
    B. 43340-78, 578.9
    C. 43341, 997.4, E878.2
    D. 43415-78, 997.4, E878.2

UNIT IV Coding Challenge

78. The physician is using an abdominal approach to perform a proctopexy combined with a sigmoid resection, the patient was diagnosed with colon cancer, primary site sigmoid flexure of the colon:
    A. 45540, 153.3
    B. 45541, 153.7
    C. 45550, 153.3
    D. 45345, 154.0

79. **OPERATIVE REPORT**

    PREOPERATIVE DIAGNOSIS: Melena.

    POSTOPERATIVE DIAGNOSIS: Normal endoscopy.

    PROCEDURE: The video therapeutic endoscope was passed without difficulty into the oropharynx. The gastroesophageal junction was seen at 40 cm. Inspection of the esophagus revealed no erythema, ulceration, varices, or other mucosal abnormalities. The stomach was entered and the endoscope advanced to the second duodenum. Inspection of the second duodenum, first duodenum, duodenal bulb, and pylorus revealed no abnormalities. Retroflexion revealed no lesions along the curvature. Inspection of the antrum, body, and fundus of the stomach revealed no abnormalities. The patient tolerated the procedure well. The patient complained of abdominal pain and weight loss.
    A. 45378, 789.00, 783.21
    B. 43235, 789.00, 783.21
    C. 49320, 783.0, 789.00
    D. 43255, 278.01, 789.01

80. This 70-year-old male is brought to the operating room for a biopsy of the pancreas. A wedge biopsy is taken and sent to pathology. The report comes back immediately indicating that primary malignant cells were present in the specimen. The decision was made to perform a total pancreatectomy. Code the operative procedure(s) and diagnosis only.
    A. 48100, 197.8
    B. 48155, 157.8
    C. 48155, 48100-51, 157.9
    D. 48155, 48100-51, 88309, 157.9

81. The patient was taken to the operating room for a repair of a recurrent strangulated inguinal hernia.
    A. 49521, 550.91
    B. 49520, 550.10
    C. 49492, 550.90
    D. 49521-78, 550.93

82. This 43-year-old female comes in with a peritonsillar abscess. The patient is brought to same-day surgery and given general anesthetic. On examination of the peritonsillar abscess, an incision was made and fluid was drained. The area was examined again, saline was applied, and then the area was packed with gauze. The patient tolerated the procedure well.
    A. 42825, 475
    B. 42700, 475
    C. 42825, 463
    D. 42700, 474.0

83. What code would you use to report a rigid proctosigmoidoscopy with removal of two nonadenomatous polyps of the rectum by snare technique?
    A. 45320, 569.0
    B. 45383, 211.3
    C. 45309 × 2, M8210/0
    D. 45315, 569.0

50000 Urinary System, Male Genital System, Female Genital System, and Maternity Care and Delivery

84. **OPERATIVE REPORT**

    PREOPERATIVE DIAGNOSIS: Missed abortion with fetal demise, 11 weeks.

    POSTOPERATIVE DIAGNOSIS: Missed abortion with fetal demise, 11 weeks.

    PROCEDURE: Suction D&C.

    The patient was prepped and draped in a lithotomy position under general mask anesthesia, and the bladder was straight catheterized; a weighted speculum was placed in the vagina. The anterior lip of the cervix was grasped with a single-tooth tenaculum. The uterus was then sounded to a depth of 8 cm. The cervical os was then serially dilated to allow passage of a size 10 curved suction curette. A size 10 curved suction curette was then used to evacuate the intrauterine contents. Sharp curette was used to gently palpate the uterine wall with negative return of tissue, and the suction curette was again used with negative return of tissue. The tenaculum was removed from the cervix. The speculum was removed from the vagina. All sponges and needles were accounted for at completion of the procedure. The patient left the operating room in apparent good condition having tolerated the procedure well.
    A. 59812, 634.92
    B. 59812, 638.90
    C. 59820, 632
    D. 59856, 632

85. **OPERATIVE REPORT**

    PREOPERATIVE DIAGNOSIS: Right ureteral stricture.

    POSTOPERATIVE DIAGNOSIS: Right ureteral stricture.

    PROCEDURE PERFORMED: Cystoscopy, right ureteral stent change.

    PROCEDURE NOTE: The patient was placed in the lithotomy position after receiving IV sedation. He was prepped and draped in the lithotomy position. The 21-French cystoscope was passed into the bladder, and urine was collected for culture. Inspection of the bladder demonstrated findings consistent with radiation cystitis, which has been previously diagnosed. There is no frank neoplasia. The right ureteral stent was grasped and removed through the urethral meatus; under fluoroscopic control, a guide wire was advanced up the stent, and the stent was exchanged for a 7-French 26-cm stent under fluoroscopic control in the usual fashion. The patient tolerated the procedure well.

A. 51702-LT, 593.3
B. 52005-RT, 595.9
C. 52332-RT, 595.9
D. 52332-RT, 593.3

86. This patient is a 42-year-old female who has been having prolonged and heavy bleeding.

    SURGICAL FINDINGS: On pelvic exam under anesthesia, the uterus was normal size and firm. The examination revealed no masses. She had a few small endometrial polyps in the lower uterine segment.

    DESCRIPTION OF PROCEDURE: After induction of general anesthesia, the patient was placed in the dorsolithotomy position, after which the perineum and vagina were prepped, the bladder straight catheterized, and the patient draped. After bimanual exam was performed, a weighted speculum was placed in the vagina and the anterior lip of the cervix was grasped with a single toothed tenaculum. An endocervical curettage was then done with a Kevorkian curet. The uterus was then sounded to 8.5 cm. The endocervical canal was dilated to 7 mm with Hegar dilators. A 5.5-mm Olympus hysteroscope was introduced using a distention medium. The cavity was systematically inspected, and the preceding findings noted. The hysteroscope was withdrawn and the cervix further dilated to 10 mm. Polyp forceps was introduced, and a few small polyps were removed. These were sent separately. Sharp endometrial curettage was then done. The hysteroscope was then reinserted, and the polyps had essentially been removed. The patient tolerated the procedure well and returned to the recovery room in stable condition. Pathology confirmed benign endometrial polyps.
    A. 58558, 57460-51, 626.2, 621.0
    B. 58558, 626.2, 621.0
    C. 58558, 57558-51, 626.2, 621.0
    D. 58558, 626.6, 239.5

87. This patient is 35 years old at 36 weeks' gestation. She presented in spontaneous labor. Because of her prior cesarean section, she is taken to the operating room to have a repeat lower-segment transverse cesarean section performed. The patient also desires sterilization, and so a bilateral tubal ligation will also be performed. A single, liveborn infant was the outcome of the delivery.
    A. 59510, 58600-51, V25.2
    B. 59620, 58615-51, 644.21, V27.0
    C. 59514, 58605-51, V27.0, 644.21
    D. 59514, 58611, 654.21, 644.21, V27.0, V25.2

88. **OPERATIVE REPORT**

    PREOPERATIVE DIAGNOSIS: Possible recurrent transitional cell carcinoma of the bladder.

    POSTOPERATIVE DIAGNOSIS: No evidence of recurrence.

PROCEDURE PERFORMED: Cystoscopy with multiple bladder biopsies.

PROCEDURE NOTE: The patient was given a general mask anesthetic, prepped, and draped in the lithotomy position. The 21-French cystoscope was passed into the bladder. There was a hyperemic area on the posterior wall of the bladder, and a biopsy was taken. Random biopsies of the bladder were also performed. This area was fulgurated. A total of 7 sq cm of bladder was fulgurated. A catheter was left at the end of the procedure. The patient tolerated the procedure well and was transferred to the recovery room in good condition. The pathology report indicated no evidence of recurrence.
A. 52224, V10.51
B. 51020, 52204, V16.52
C. 52234, V10.51
D. 52224 × 4, 236.7

89. This 41-year-old female presented with a right labial lesion. A biopsy was taken, and the results were reported as VIN III, cannot rule out invasion. The decision was therefore made to proceed with wide local excision of the right vulva.

    PROCEDURE: The patient was taken to the operating room, and general anesthesia was administered. The patient was then prepped and draped in the usual manner in lithotomy position, and the bladder was emptied with a straight catheter. The vulva was then inspected. On the right labium minora at approximately the 11 o'clock position, there was a multifocal lesion. A marking pen was then used to mark out an elliptical incision, leaving a 1-cm border on all sides. The skin ellipse was then excised using a knife. Bleeders were cauterized with electrocautery. A running locked suture of 2-0 Vicryl was then placed in the deeper tissue. The skin was finally reapproximated with 4-0 Vicryl in an interrupted fashion. Good hemostasis was thereby achieved. The patient tolerated this procedure well. There were no complications.
    A. 56605, 184.4
    B. 56625, 233.32
    C. 56620, 233.32
    D. 11620, 184.4

90. This 1-year-old boy has a midshaft hypospadias with a very mild degree of chordee. He also has a persistent right hydrocele. The surgeon brought the boy to surgery to perform a right hydrocele repair and one-stage repair of hypospadias with preputial onlay flap.
    A. 54322, 55040, 752.61, 752.63
    B. 54322, 55041-51, 752.61, 752.63, 603.9
    C. 54324, 55060-51, 752.61, 752.63, 603.9
    D. 54324, 55060, 752.63, 603.9

91. The pediatric physician takes this newborn male to the nursery to perform a clamp circumcision.
    A. 54160, V50.2
    B. 54150, V50.21
    C. 54160, V50.21
    D. 54150, V50.2

UNIT IV Coding Challenge

92. This gentleman has worsening bilateral hydronephrosis. He did not have much of a post void residual on bladder scan. He is taken to the operating room to have a bilateral cystoscopy and retrograde pyelogram. The results come back as gross prostatic hyperplasia.
    A. 52005, 600.3
    B. 52000, 591, 600.9
    C. 52005-50, 600.91, 591
    D. 52000-50, 591, 600.9

93. This 32-year-old female presents with an ectopic pregnancy. The physician performs a laparoscopic salpingectomy.
    A. 59120, 633.90
    B. 59151, 633.90
    C. 58943, 633.10
    D. 59120, 633.80

60000 Endocrine System, Hemic and Lymphatic Systems, Nervous System, Eye and Ocular Adnexa, Auditory System

94. Left frontal ventricular puncture for implanting catheter, layered repair of 8-cm scalp laceration, and repair of multiple facial and eyelid lacerations with an approximate total length of 12 cm. Assign code(s) for the physician service only.
    A. 61020, 12015-51
    B. 61107, 12034-51, 12015-51
    C. 61215, 12015-51
    D. 61107, 12034-51

95. Marginal laceration involving the left lower eyelid and laceration of the left upper eyelid involving the tarsus. Both required full-thickness repair. Also, there were multiple stellate lacerations above the left eye, totaling 24.2 cm and requiring full-thickness layered repair. Assign code(s) for the physician service only.
    A. 67935-E2, 12017
    B. 67930-E2, 13152-51, 13153
    C. 67935-E2, 67935-E1-51, 12056-51
    D. 67935-E2, 12017-51

96. **OPERATIVE REPORT**

    PREOPERATIVE DIAGNOSIS: Fever.

    PROCEDURE PERFORMED: Lumbar puncture.

    DESCRIPTION OF PROCEDURE: The patient was placed in the lateral decubitus position with the left side up. The legs and hips were flexed into the fetal position. The lumbosacral area was sterilely prepped. It was then numbed with 1% Xylocaine. I then placed a 22-gauge spinal needle on the first pass into the intrathecal space between the L4 and L5 spinous processes. The fluid was minimally xanthochromic. I sent the fluid for cell count for differential, protein, glucose, Gram stain, and culture. The patient tolerated the procedure well without apparent complication. The needle was removed at the end of the procedure. The area was cleansed, and a Band-Aid was placed.
    A. 62272, 780.91
    B. 62268, 780.60
    C. 62272, 782.3, 780.60
    D. 62270, 780.60

97. **OPERATIVE REPORT**

    PREOPERATIVE DIAGNOSIS: Herniated disk L4-5 on the left.

    PROCEDURE PERFORMED: Laminotomy, foraminotomy, removal of herniated disk L4-5 on the left.

    PROCEDURE: Under general anesthesia, the patient was placed in the prone position and the back was prepped and draped in the usual manner. An incision was made in the skin extending through subcutaneous tissue. Lumbodorsal fascia was divided. The erector spinae muscles were bluntly dissected from the lamina of L4-5 on the left. The interspace was localized. I then performed a generous laminotomy and foraminotomy here, and retracted on the nerve root. It was obvious there was a herniated disk. I removed it, entered the space, and removed degenerating material, satisfied that I had decompressed the root well. There were free fragments lying around beneath the nerve root. We removed all of these. I was able to pass a hockey stick down the foramen across the midline, satisfied I had taken out the large fragments from the interspace at L4-5, and decompressed it well. I irrigated the wound well, put a Hemovac drain in the wound, and then closed the wound in layers using double-knotted 0 chromic on the lumbodorsal fascia with Vicryl, 2-0 plain in the subcutaneous tissue, and surgical staples on the skin. A dressing was applied. The patient was discharged to the recovery room.
    A. 63030-LT, 722.10
    B. 63012-LT, 722.32
    C. 63047-LT, 722.92
    D. 63047-LT, 63048-LT, 722.10

98. **OPERATIVE REPORT**

    PREOPERATIVE DIAGNOSIS: Brain tumor versus abscess.

    PROCEDURE: Craniotomy.

    DESCRIPTION OF PROCEDURE: Under general anesthesia, the patient's head was prepped and draped in the usual manner. It was placed in Mayfield pins. We then proceeded with a craniotomy. An inverted U-shaped incision was made over the posterior right occipital area. The flap was turned down. Three burr holes were made. Having done this, I then localized the tumor through the burr holes and dura. We then made an incision in the dura in an inverted U-shaped fashion. The cortex looked a little swollen but normal. We then used the localizer to locate the cavity. I separated the gyrus and got right into the cavity and saw pus, which was removed. Cultures were taken and sent for pathology report, which came back later describing the presence of clusters of gram-positive cocci, confirming that this was an abscess. We cleaned out the abscessed cavity using irrigation and suction. The bed of the abscessed cavity was cauterized. Then a small piece of Gelfoam was used for hemostasis. Satisfied that it was dry, I closed the dura. I approximated the scalp. A dressing was applied. The patient was discharged to the recovery room.
    A. 61154, 324.0
    B. 61154, 239.6
    C. 61320, 324.0
    D. 61150, 239.6

UNIT IV   Coding Challenge

99. This patient came in with an obstructed ventriculoperitoneal shunt. The procedure performed was to be a revision of shunt. After inspecting the shunt system, the entire cerebrospinal fluid shunt system was removed and a similar replacement shunt system was placed. Patient has normal pressure hydrocephalus (NPH).
    A. 62180, 996.1, 331.3
    B. 62258, 996.2, 331.5
    C. 62256, 996.2, 331.4
    D. 62190, 996.2, 331.5

100. This patient is in for a recurrent herniated disk at L5-S1 on the left. The procedure performed is a repeat laminotomy and foraminotomy at the L5-S1 interspace.
    A. 63030-LT, 722.10
    B. 63030-LT, 722.11
    C. 63042-LT, 722.11
    D. 63042-LT, 722.10

101. What CPT code would you assign to report a left partial thyroid lobectomy, with isthmusectomy? The diagnosis was benign growth of the thyroid.
    A. 60210, 226
    B. 60220, 237.4
    C. 60212, 239.7
    D. 60225, 226, 239.7

102. **OPERATIVE REPORT**

    PREOPERATIVE DIAGNOSIS: Paralytic ectropion, left eye.

    PROCEDURE PERFORMED: Medial tarsorrhaphy, left eye.

    In the operating room, after intravenous sedation, the patient was given a total of about 0.5 mL of local infiltrative anesthetic. The skin surfaces on the medial area of the lid, medial to the punctum, were denuded. A bolster had been prepared and double 5-0 silk suture was passed through the bolster, which was passed through the inferior skin and raw lid margin, then through the superior margin, and out through the skin. A superior bolster was then applied. The puncta were probed with wire instrument and found not to be obstructed. The suture was then fully tied and trimmed. Bacitracin ointment was placed on the surface of the skin. The patient left the operating room in stable condition, without complications, having tolerated the procedure well.
    A. 67875-LT, 374.12
    B. 67710-LT, 374.11
    C. 67882-LT, 374.10
    D. 67880-LT, 374.12

103. This 66-year-old male has been diagnosed with a senile cataract of the posterior subcapsular and is scheduled for a cataract extraction by phacoemulsification of the right eye. The physician has taken the patient to the operating room to perform a posterior subcapsular cataract extraction with IOL placement, diffuse of the right eye.
    A. 66982-RT, 366.09
    B. 66984-RT, 366.14
    C. 66983-RT, 366.12
    D. 66830-RT, 366.14

SECTION 3

QUESTIONS 104-150

Evaluation and Management (E/M)

104. Bill, a retired U.S. Air Force pilot, was on observation status 12 hours to assess the outcome of a fall from the back of a parked pickup truck into a gravel pit.

    History of Present Illness: The patient is a 42-year-old gentleman who works at the local garden shop. He explained that yesterday he fell from his pickup truck as he was loading gravel for a landscaping project. He lost his footing when attempting to climb from the pickup bed and fell approximately four feet and landed on a rock that was protruding from the ground 4 inches striking his head on the rock. He did not lose consciousness, but was dizzy. He subsequently developed a throbbing headache (8/10) and swelling at the point of impact. The duration of the dizziness was approximately 10 minutes; but, the headache still persists 26 hours after the fall. He did take ibuprofen without significant improvement in the pain level. Review of Systems: Constitutional, eyes, ears, nose, throat, lungs, cardiovascular, gastrointestinal, skin, neurologic, lymphatic, and immunologic negative except for HPI statements. PFSH: He is married and has 2 children. He has been working at the garden shop for four years. He currently smokes one pack of cigarettes a day and has smoked for 10 years. His father died of heart disease when he was 52. He has one brother with ankylosing spondylitis and one sister who is healthy as far as he knows. His mother died when he was 14 years old. He is currently on no prescribed medications. A comprehensive exam is documented and rendered. The medical decision making is low complexity.

    The physician discharged Bill from observation that same day after 10 hours, after determining that no further monitoring of his condition was necessary. The physician provided a detailed examination and indicated that the medical decision making was of a low complexity.
    A. 99218, V71.9, E888.8
    B. 99234, V71.4, E884.9
    C. 99217, V71.4, E888.8
    D. 99234, 99217, V71.4, E884.9

105. Dr. Martin admits a 65-year-old female patient to the hospital to rule out acute pericarditis following a severe viral infection. The patient has complained of retrosternal, sharp, intermittent pain of 2 days' duration that is reduced by sitting up and leaning forward, accompanied by tachypnea. ROS: She does not currently have chest pain but is complaining of shortness of breath. She states that her legs and feet have been swollen of late. She reports no change in her vision or her hearing, and she has not had a rash. No dyspnea stated. PFSH: She states that she has had and echocardiogram in the past when she complained of chest tightness and her family physician gave her some medication, but she is not certain what it was. She has three adult children, all healthy. Her husband is deceased. She does not smoke or consume alcohol. Her father died at age 69 from congestive heart failure and her mother died of influenza at 70. Refer to the

UNIT IV   Coding Challenge

admission form for a list of current medications. The examination was detailed. The medical decision making was high complexity.
A. 99236, 786.51, 786.06
B. 99223, 420.91, 411.1, 442.9, 415.19, 530.9
C. 99245, 420.91, 411.1, 442.9, 415.19, 530.9
D. 99221, 786.51, 786.06

106. A gynecologist admits an established patient, a 35-year-old female with dysfunctional uterine bleeding, after seeing her in the clinic that day. During the course of the history, the physician notes that the patient has a history of infrequent periods of heavy flow. She has had irregular heavy periods and intermittent spotting for 4 years. The patient has been on a 3-month course of oral contraceptives for symptoms with no relief. The patient states that she has occasional headaches. A complete ROS was performed, consisting of constitutional factors, ophthalmologic, otolaryngologic, cardiovascular, respiratory, gastrointestinal, genitourinary, musculoskeletal, integumentary, neurologic, psychiatric, endocrine, hematologic, lymphatic, allergic, and immunologic which were all negative, except for the symptoms described above. The family history is positive for endometrial cancer, with mother, two aunts, and two sisters who had endometrial cancer. The patient has a personal history of cervical and endometrial polyp removal 3 years prior to admission. The patients states that she does not smoke and only drinks socially. As a part of the comprehensive examination, the physician notes the patient has a large amount of blood in the vault and an enlarged uterus. The prolonged hemorrhaging has resulted in a very thin and friable endometrial lining. The physician orders the patient to be started on intravenous Premarin and orders a full laboratory workup. The medical decision making is of moderate complexity.
A. 99215, 99222, V13.29, V16.49
B. 99222, 626.8, V13.29, V16.49
C. 99215, 99222, 623.8, V13.29, V16.4
D. 99222, 626.1, V16.49

107. Dr. Black admits a patient with an 8-day history of a low-grade fever, tachycardia, tachypnea, and radiologic evidence of basal consolidation of the lung and limited pleural effusion on the left side, per patient as seen at outside clinic several days prior. The patient has also been experiencing swelling of the extremities. The pulse is rapid and thready, as checked by patient on her own during the past couple days. A complete ROS of constitutional factors, ophthalmologic, otolaryngologic, cardiovascular, respiratory, gastrointestinal, genitourinary, musculoskeletal, integumentary, neurologic, psychiatric, endocrine, hematologic, lymphatic, allergic, and immunologic was performed and negative except for the symptoms described above. Past history includes tachycardia and pneumonia. Family history includes heart disease, hypertension and high cholesterol in both parents. The patient drinks only occasionally and quit smoking four years ago. The comprehensive examination was performed and diminished bowel sounds were noted. The physician orders laboratory tests and radiographic studies, including a follow-up chest x-ray as he considers the extensive diagnostic options and the medical decision making complexity is high for this patient.
A. 99233, 780.6, 785.0, 786.06, 511.9, 787.5
B. 99233, 780.6, 427.0, 786.06, 486, 511.9
C. 99223, 780.6, 785.0, 786.06
D. 99223, 780.6, 785.0, 786.06, 511.9, 787.5

108. Dr. Stephanopolis makes subsequent hospital visits to Salanda Ortez, who has been in the hospital for primary viral pneumonia. She was experiencing severe dyspnea, rales, fever, and chest pain for over a week. The patient states that this morning she had nausea and her heart was racing while she was experiencing some dyspnea and SOB. The chest radiography showed patchy bilateral infiltrates and basilar streaking. Sputum microbiology was positive for a secondary bacterial pneumonia. An expanded problem-focused physical examination was performed. The medical decision making was moderate. The patient was given intravenous antibiotic as treatment for the bacterial pneumonia.
    A. 99233, 786.09, 786.7, 780.6, 729.1, 786.50, 793.1, 795.39
    B. 99232, 482.9, 480.9
    C. 99221, 786.09, 786.7, 780.6, 729.1, 786.50, 793.1, 795.39
    D. 99234, 482.89

109. A 57-year-old male was sent by his family physician to a urologist for an office consultation due to hematuria. The patient has had bright red blood in his urine sporadically for the past 3 weeks. His family physician gave him a dose of antibiotic therapy for urinary tract infection; however, the symptom still persists. The patient states that he does experience some lower back discomfort when urinating, with no fever, chills or nausea. The patient is currently taking Lotrel 10/20 for his hypertension which is stable at this time and has allergies to Sulfa. The urologist performs a detailed history and physical examination. The urologist recommends a cystoscopy to be scheduled for the following day and discusses the procedure and risks with the patient. The urologist also contacted the family physician with the recommendations and is requested to proceed with the cystoscopy and any further follow-up required. The medical decision making is of moderate complexity. A report was sent to attending physician. Report only the office service.
    A. 99243, 599.7 724.2
    B. 99244-57, 52000, 599.0, 724.2
    C. 99253, 599.9, 724.2
    D. 99221, 599.7, 724.2

110. A neurological consultation in the emergency department of the local hospital is requested for a 25-year-old male with suspected closed head trauma by the ED physician. The neurologist saw the patient in the ED. The patient had a loss of consciousness this morning after receiving a blow to the head in a basketball game. He presents to the emergency department with a headache, dizziness, and confusion. During the course of the history, the patient relates that he has been very irritable, confused and has had a bit of nausea since the incident. All other systems reviewed and are negative: Constitutional, ophthalmologic, otolaryngologic, cardiovascular, respiratory, genitourinary, musculoskeletal, integumentary, psychiatric, endocrine, hematologic, lymphatic, allergic, and immunologic. The patients states that he does have a history of headaches and that both parents have hypertension, also a grandfather with heart disease. He also states that he does drink beer on the weekends and does not smoke. Physical examination reveals the patient to be unsteady and exhibiting difficulty in concentration when stating months in reverse. The pupils dilate unequally. The physician continues with a complete comprehensive examination involving an extensive review of neurological function. The neurologist orders a stat CT and MRI. The physician suspects a subdural hematoma or an epidural hematoma and the medical decision-making complexity is

high. The neurologist admits the patient to the hospital. Assign only the physician services.
A. 99285, 780.09, 780.4, 784.0
B. 99253, 784.0, 780.09, 780.4
C. 99255, 784.0, 298.9, 780.4
D. 99245, 784.0, 780.09, 780.4

111. An obstetrician is requested to provide an office consultation to a 23-year-old female with first-trimester bleeding from Dr A. The patient presents with a history of brownish discharge and occasional pinkish discharge. During the history, the patient relates that she has had suprapubic pain in the past week and cramping. She states her pain is 8/10. She has felt nausea and has vomited on three occasions. On one occasion, the nausea was accompanied by dizziness and vertigo, all other systems are negative at this time and included: Constitutional factors, ophthalmologic, otolaryngologic, cardiovascular, respiratory, musculoskeletal, integumentary, neurologic, psychiatric, endocrine, hematologic, lymphatic, allergic, and immunologic. The PFSH included patient history of tonsillectomy with family history of breast cancer on her mother's side. The patient does not smoke or drink. The physician conducts a comprehensive examination focused on the chief complaint and related systems. The uterus is found to be soft and involuted. There is cervical motion tenderness and significant abdominal tenderness on palpation. A left pelvic mass is palpated in the left quadrant. The physician orders a pelvic ultrasound, a complete CBC, and differential. Considering the range of possible diagnoses, the medical decision-making complexity is high.
A. 99255, 634.91, 719.65
B. 99242, 634.90, 719.65
C. 99245, 640.93, 789.3
D. 99245, 649.53, 789.3

112. A 56-year-old established male patient presents to his family physician for a preventive checkup at the local outpatient clinic. The physician conducts a multi-system history and physical examination, and the checkup takes 45 minutes.
A. 99214, V70.4
B. 99403, V70.7
C. 99386, V70.0
D. 99396, V70.0

113. Karra Hendricks, a 37-year-old female, is an established patient who presents to the office with right lower quadrant abdominal pain with fever. The patient states she has had the pain for 3 days. She has taken Tylenol for her fever with some relief. The patient does have occasional diarrhea and headaches. She smokes approximately 5-10 cigarettes a day and drinks socially. The physician performs a problem focused examination. The medical decision making is noted to be of a moderate complexity.
A. 99203, 789.03
B. 99213, 789.04, 780.6
C. 99214, 789.03, 780.6
D. 99221, 789.05, 780.6

114. Sam, a 4-year-old male, was brought to the emergency department by his mother, where Dr. Black, the emergency department physician, examined the child. Dr. Black has not provided service to this child in the past. During the history, the mother stated that the child has had a temperature of 101° F for the past 24 hours, has been very, very, fussy and crying, and has been pulling on his left ear. Child states "it hurts". The physician examined the child during an expanded problem-focused examination, ear, NMT, and diagnosed acute suppurative otitis media, for which he prescribed a 10-day course of amoxicillin. MDM was low complexity.
    A. 99283, 382.9, 780.95
    B. 99212, 282.41, 780.95
    C. 99241, 382.01, 780.95
    D. 99282, 382.00, 780.95

115. Dr. Robertson provided the first month of care planning oversight for a home health agency's home care of a 64-year-old male patient with advanced pancreatic cancer. The physician developed a plan that included home oxygen, intravenous diuretics, pain control management by means of intravenous morphine, review of records and lab studies, and communication with the agency. The time spent in oversight for the month was 45 minutes.
    A. 99378
    B. 99340
    C. 99375
    D. 99380

Anesthesia

116. If the anesthesia service were provided to a patient who had severe systemic disease, what would the physical status modifier be?
    A. P1
    B. P2
    C. P3
    D. P4

117. What qualifying circumstances code would be used to identify the administration of anesthesia that is complicated by an emergency condition?
    A. 99100
    B. 99116
    C. 99135
    D. 99140

118. Anesthesia service includes the following care:
    A. Preoperative, intraoperative
    B. Preoperative, intraoperative, postoperative
    C. Intraoperative, postoperative
    D. Preoperative, postoperative

119. The following is the anesthesia formula:
    A. BTC
    B. TBC
    C. BTQ
    D. BTM

UNIT IV Coding Challenge

120. Which HCPCS modifier indicates an anesthesia service in which the anesthesiologist medically directs one CRNA?
    A. QX
    B. QY
    C. QZ
    D. QK

121. Anesthesia service for a pneumocentesis for lung aspiration, 32420.
    A. 00522
    B. 00500
    C. 00520
    D. 00524

70000 Radiology

Direction: Report only the professional component unless specifically directed to do otherwise within the question.

122. This 69-year-old female is in for a magnetic resonance examination of the brain because of new seizure activity. After imaging without contrast, contrast was administered and further sequences were performed. Examination results indicated no apparent neoplasm or vascular malformation.
    A. 70543-26, 780.31
    B. 70543-26, 780.39
    C. 70553-26, 780.39
    D. 70553, 345.90

123. This patient undergoes a gallbladder sonogram due to epigastric pain. The report indicates that the visualized portions of the liver are normal. No free fluid noted within Morison's pouch. The gallbladder is identified and is empty. No evidence of wall thickening or surrounding fluid is seen. There is no ductal dilatation. The common hepatic duct and common bile duct measure 0.4 and 0.8 cm, respectively. The common bile duct measurement is at the upper limits of normal.
    A. 76700-26, 789.07
    B. 76705-26, 789.06
    C. 76775-26, 789.05
    D. 76705, 789.07

124. **EXAMINATION OF:** Chest.

    CLINICAL SYMPTOMS: Pneumonia.

    PA AND LATERAL CHEST X-RAY WITH FLUOROSCOPY.

    CONCLUSION: Ventilation within the lung fields has improved compared with previous study.
    A. 71020-26, 482.89
    B. 71034, 482.83
    C. 71023-26, 486
    D. 71023, 486

125. **EXAMINATION OF:** Abdomen and pelvis.

    CLINICAL SYMPTOMS: Ascites.

    CT OF ABDOMEN AND PELVIS: Technique: CT of the abdomen and pelvis was performed without oral or IV contrast material per physician request. No previous CT scans for comparison.

    FINDINGS: No ascites. Moderate-sized pleural effusion on the right.
    A. 74160-26, 789.59
    B. 74150-26, 511.9
    C. 74150, 511.9
    D. 74160, 789.59

126. **EXAMINATION OF:** Brain.

    CLINICAL FINDING: Headache.

    COMPUTED TOMOGRAPHY OF THE BRAIN was performed without contrast material.

    FINDINGS: There is blood within the third ventricle. The lateral ventricles show mild dilatation with small amounts of blood.

    IMPRESSION: Acute subarachnoid hemorrhage.
    A. 70460-26, 784.0
    B. 70250, 784.0
    C. 70450-26, 430
    D. 70450-26, 784.0

127. Report both the technical and professional components of the following service: This 68-year-old male is seen in Radiation Oncology Department for prostate cancer. The oncologist performs a complex clinical treatment planning, dosimetry calculation, complex isodose plan; treatment devices include blocks, special shields, wedges, and treatment management. The patient had 5 days of radiation treatments for 2 weeks, a total of 10 days of treatment.
    A. 77263, 77300, 77315, 77334, 185
    B. 77300, 77315, 77334, 77427 × 2, 185
    C. 77263, 77300, 77315, 77334, 77427 × 2, 185
    D. 77263, 77427 × 2, 185

128. **EXAMINATION OF:** Right hip.

    DIAGNOSIS: Osteoarthritis right hip.

    ONE-VIEW RIGHT HIP: A single frontal view is obtained of the right hip. No previous studies are available for comparison. Right hip arthroplasty is seen. Alignment appears grossly unremarkable on this single view. There are skin staples present. Air is seen in the soft tissues, likely due to recent surgery. There appear to be two drains present. The tip of one overlies the soft tissues superolateral to the greater trochanter. The second one is more inferior. The tip overlies the right proximal femoral prosthesis.

    IMPRESSION: Single view of the right hip with findings consistent with recent right total hip arthroplasty.
    A. 72100, 719
    B. 73500-RT, 715.95
    C. 72100-26, 715.9
    D. 73500-26-RT, 715.95, V43.64

129. **EXAMINATION OF:** Cervical spine.

    CLINICAL SYMPTOMS: Herniated disk.

    FINDINGS: A single spot fluoroscopic film from the operating room is submitted for interpretation. The cervical spine is not well demonstrated above the level of the inferior aspect of C6. There is a metallic surgical plate seen anterior to the cervical spine. The cephalic portion of the plate is at the level of C6 at its superior endplate. That extends in an inferior direction, presumably anterior to C7; however, there is not adequate visualization of C7 to confirm location. Density overlies the C6-7 intervertebral disk space, suggesting the presence of a bone plug in this area; however, again visualization is not adequate in this area. Further evaluation with plain radiographs is recommended.
    A. 72100-26, 722.10
    B. 72020-26, 722.0
    C. 72100-52-26, 722.0
    D. 72020-52-26, 722.11

130. This patient is suffering from primary lung cancer and is in for a follow-up CT scan of the thorax with contrast material. Code the physician component only.
    A. 71250-26, 197.0
    B. 71260, 162.9
    C. 71260-26, 162.9
    D. 71270-26, 239.1

80000 Pathology and Laboratory

Direction: Report only the professional component of the service unless directed to do so otherwise.

131. **CLINICAL HISTORY:** Boil, left groin.

    SPECIMEN RECEIVED: Necrotic fascia left groin and leg (anterior and posterior).

    GROSS DESCRIPTION: The specimen is labeled with the patient's name and "fascia left groin and leg" and consists of multiple segments of skin and soft tissue measuring up to 30 cm in greatest dimension. The skin is unremarkable, with the soft tissue being hemorrhagic and friable and foul smelling.

    MICROSCOPIC DESCRIPTION: Sections of skin and soft tissue show coagulative necrosis with neutrophilic exudates.

    DIAGNOSIS: Skin and soft tissue, left groin and leg, anterior and posterior showing coagulative necrosis and acute inflammation.
    A. 88304, 680.9
    B. 88305-26, 709.8
    C. 88304-26, 709.8, 686.9
    D. 88305, 680.2

132. **Report the global service.**

    CLINICAL HISTORY: Mass, left atrium.

    SPECIMEN RECEIVED: Left atrium.

    GROSS DESCRIPTION: The specimen is labeled with patient's name and "left atrial myxoma" and consists of a 4 × 4 × 2-cm ovoid mass with a partially calcified hemorrhagic white-tan tissue.

    INTRAOPERATIVE FROZEN SECTION DIAGNOSIS: Myxoma

    MICROSCOPIC DESCRIPTION: Sections show a well-circumscribed mass consisting of fibromyxoid tissue showing numerous vascular channels. Areas of superficial ulceration and chronic inflammatory infiltrate are noted. Areas of calcification are also present.

    DIAGNOSIS: Myxoma, benign, left atrium.
    A. 88305, 239.8
    B. 88307, 88331, 212.7
    C. 88307, 88331-26, 212.7
    D. 88305, 212.7

133. This patient is in for a kidney biopsy (50200) because a mass was identified by ultrasound. The specimen is sent to pathology for gross and microscopic examination. Report the technical and professional components for this service. The results were inconclusive.
    A. 88305-26, 593.9
    B. 88307-26, 593.89
    C. 88307, 593.9
    D. 88305, 593.9

134. This 69-year-old female presents to the laboratory after her physician ordered troponin, quantitative, and troponin, qualitative assays, to assist in the diagnosis of her chief complaint of acute onset of chest pain.
    A. 84484, 80299, 786.51
    B. 84512, 84484, 80299, 786.59
    C. 84484, 84512, 786.50
    D. 84484, 84512, 786.59

135. **CLINICAL HISTORY:** Necrotic soleus muscle, right leg.

    SPECIMEN RECEIVED: Soleus muscle, right leg.

    GROSS DESCRIPTION: Submitted in formalin, labeled with the patient's name and "soleus muscle right leg," are multiple irregular fragments of tan, gray, brown soft tissue measuring 8 × 8 × 2.5 cm in aggregate. Multiple representative fragments are submitted in four cassettes.

    MICROSCOPIC DESCRIPTION: The slides show multiple sections of skeletal muscle showing severe coagulative and liquefactive necrosis. Patchy neutrophilic infiltrates are present within the necrotic tissue.

    DIAGNOSIS: Soft tissue, soleus muscle, right leg debridement; necrosis and patchy acute inflammation, skeletal muscle—infective myositis.
    A. 88305-26, 728.2
    B. 88304-26, 728.0
    C. 88307-26, 785.4
    D. 88304-26, 728.2

UNIT IV   Coding Challenge

136. This 34-year-old established female patient is in for her yearly physical and lab. The physician orders a comprehensive metabolic panel, hemogram automated and manual differential WBC count (CBC), and a thyroid-stimulating hormone. Code the lab only.
   A. 99395, 80050
   B. 80050-52
   C. 80069, 80050
   D. 80050

137. This is a patient with atrial fibrillation who comes to the clinic laboratory routinely for a quantitative digoxin level.
   A. 80101, 80102, 428.0
   B. 81001, V58.83, V58.69, 427.41
   C. 80162, V58.83, V58.69, 427.31
   D. 80162, 785.0

138. This patient presented to the laboratory yesterday for a creatine measurement. The results came back at higher than normal levels; therefore, the patient was asked to return to the laboratory today for a repeat creatine test before the nephrologist is consulted. Report the second day of test only.
   A. 82540 × 2, 790.6
   B. 82550, 790.6
   C. 82550, 790.91
   D. 82540, 790.6

139. Code a pregnancy test, urine.
   A. 84702
   B. 84703
   C. 81025
   D. 84702 × 2

140. What CPT code would you use to code a bilirubin, total (transcutaneous)?
   A. 82252
   B. 82247
   C. 82248
   D. 88720

90000 Medicine

141. **DIALYSIS INPATIENT NOTE:** This 24-year-old male patient is on continuous ambulatory peritoneal dialysis (CAPD) using 1.5%. He drains more than 600 mL. He is tolerating dialysis well. He continues to have some abdominal pain, but his abdomen is not distended. He has some diarrhea. His abdomen does not look like acute abdomen. His vitals, other than blood pressure in the 190s over 100s, are fine. He is afebrile.
   At this time, I will continue with 1.5% dialysate. I gave him labetalol IV for blood pressure. Because of diarrhea, I am going to check stool for white cells, culture. Next we will see what the primary physician says today. His HIDA scan was normal. The patient suffers from ESRD and has had 6 encounters this month. Code the month of service.
   A. 90947, 90960, 585.6, 787.91, V45.11
   B. 90945, 585.6, 787.91, V45.11
   C. 90960, 585.6, V45.11
   D. 90945, 585.6

142. **INDICATION:** Pulmonary hypertension with newly diagnosed acute myocardial infarction.

PROCEDURE PERFORMED: Insertion of Swan-Ganz catheter.

DESCRIPTION OF PROCEDURE: The right internal jugular and subclavian area was prepped with antiseptic solution. Sterile drapes were applied. Under usual sterile precautions, the right internal jugular vein was cannulated. A 9-French introducer was inserted, and a 7-French Swan-Ganz catheter was inserted without difficulty. Right atrial pressures were 2 to 3, right ventricular pressures 24/0, and pulmonary artery 26/9 with a wedge pressure of 5. This is a Trendelenburg position. The patient tolerated the procedure well.
A. 93501, 93503-51, 410.91
B. 93508, 416.8
C. 93503, 93539, 401.9, 410.91
D. 93503, 410.91, 416.8

143. **DIAGNOSIS:** Atrial flutter.

PROCEDURE PERFORMED: Electrical cardioversion.

DESCRIPTION OF PROCEDURE: The patient was sedated with Versed and morphine. She was given a total of 5 mg of Versed. She was cardioverted with 50 joules into sinus tachycardia.

The patient was given a 20-mg Cardizem IV push. Her heart rate went down to the 110s, and she was definitely in sinus tachycardia.

CONCLUSION: Successful electrical cardioversion of atrial flutter into sinus tachycardia.
A. 92961, 427.61
B. 92960, 427.32
C. 92960, 92973, 427.32
D. 92960, 427.89

144. A patient presents for a pleural cavity chemotherapy session with 10 mg doxorubicin HCl that requires a thoracentesis to be performed.
A. 96445, J9000
B. 96440, 32421, J9000
C. 96440, J9000
D. 96445, 32421, J9000

145. What CPT code would be used to report a home visit for a respiratory patient to care for the mechanical ventilation?
A. 99503
B. 99504
C. 99505
D. 99509

146. What CPT code would be used to code the technical aspect of an evaluation of swallowing by video recording using a flexible fiberoptic endoscope?
A. 92611
B. 92612
C. 92610
D. 92613

UNIT IV Coding Challenge

147. Which code would be used to report an EEG (electroencephalogram) provided during carotid surgery?
    A. 95816
    B. 95819
    C. 95822
    D. 95955

148. This 40-year-old patient who is a type II diabetic is seen in an inpatient setting for psychotherapy. The doctor spends 50 minutes face to face with the patient. The patient is seen for depression.
    A. 90818, 311, 250.90
    B. 90817, 311, 250.90
    C. 90818, 311
    D. 90817, 311

149. How would you report a screening hearing test?
    A. 92551, V80.3
    B. 92555, V72.19
    C. 92553, V72.19
    D. 92620, V80.3

150. The patient presented for a spontaneous nystagmus test that included gaze, fixation, and recording and used vertical electrodes. Assign code(s) for the physician service only.
    A. 92541
    B. 92547
    C. 92541, 92544, 92547
    D. 92541, 92547

Appendix A

ICD-9-CM Official Guidelines for Coding and Reporting

Reprinted as released by the Centers for Medicare and Medicaid Services and the National Center for Health Statistics. See http://www.cdc.gov/nchs/datawh/ftpserv/ftpicd9/ftpicd9.htm#guidelines. **You can also check the Evolve website for the latest updates at http://evolve.elsevier.com/Buck/cpc.**

**Effective October 1, 2007
Narrative changes appear in bold text
Items underlined have been moved within the guidelines since November 15, 2006
The guidelines include the updated V Code Table**

The Centers for Medicare and Medicaid Services (CMS) and the National Center for Health Statistics (NCHS), two departments within the U.S. Federal Government's Department of Health and Human Services (DHHS) provide the following guidelines for coding and reporting using the International Classification of Diseases, 9th Revision, Clinical Modification (ICD-9-CM). These guidelines should be used as a companion document to the official version of the ICD-9-CM as published on CD-ROM by the U.S. Government Printing Office (GPO).

These guidelines have been approved by the four organizations that make up the Cooperating Parties for the ICD-9-CM: the American Hospital Association (AHA), the American Health Information Management Association (AHIMA), CMS, and NCHS. These guidelines are included on the official government version of the ICD-9-CM, and also appear in *"Coding Clinic for ICD-9-CM"* published by the AHA.

These guidelines are a set of rules that have been developed to accompany and complement the official conventions and instructions provided within the ICD-9-CM itself. These guidelines are based on the coding and sequencing instructions in Volumes I, II and III of ICD-9-CM, but provide additional instruction. Adherence to these guidelines when assigning ICD-9-CM diagnosis and procedure codes is required under the Health Insurance Portability and Accountability Act (HIPAA). The diagnosis codes (Volumes 1-2) have been adopted under HIPAA for all healthcare settings. Volume 3 procedure codes have been adopted for inpatient procedures reported by hospitals. A joint effort between the healthcare provider and the coder is essential to achieve complete and accurate documentation, code assignment, and reporting of diagnoses and procedures. These guidelines have been developed to assist both the healthcare provider and the coder in identifying those diagnoses and procedures that are to be reported. The importance of consistent, complete documentation in the medical record cannot be overemphasized. Without such documentation accurate coding cannot be achieved. The entire record should be reviewed to determine the specific reason for the encounter and the conditions treated.

Appendix A   ICD-9-CM Official Guidelines for Coding and Reporting

The term encounter is used for all settings, including hospital admissions. In the context of these guidelines, the term provider is used throughout the guidelines to mean physician or any qualified health care practitioner who is legally accountable for establishing the patient's diagnosis. Only this set of guidelines, approved by the Cooperating Parties, is official.

The guidelines are organized into sections. Section I includes the structure and conventions of the classification and general guidelines that apply to the entire classification, and chapter-specific guidelines that correspond to the chapters as they are arranged in the classification. Section II includes guidelines for selection of principal diagnosis for non-outpatient settings. Section III includes guidelines for reporting additional diagnoses in non-outpatient settings. Section IV is for outpatient coding and reporting.

ICD-9-CM Official Guidelines for Coding and Reporting

Section I.   Conventions, general coding guidelines and chapter specific guidelines

   A. Conventions for the ICD-9-CM
      1. Format:
      2. Abbreviations
         a. Index abbreviations
         b. Tabular abbreviations
      3. Punctuation
      4. Includes and Excludes Notes and Inclusion terms
      5. Other and Unspecified codes
         a. "Other" codes
         b. "Unspecified" codes
      6. Etiology/manifestation convention ("code first", "use additional code" and "in diseases classified elsewhere" notes)
      7. "And"
      8. "With"
      9. "See" and "See Also"
   B. General Coding Guidelines
      1. Use of Both Alphabetic Index and Tabular List
      2. Locate each term in the Alphabetic Index
      3. Level of Detail in Coding
      4. Code or codes from 001.0 through V84.8
      5. Selection of codes 001.0 through 999.9
      6. Signs and symptoms
      7. Conditions that are an integral part of a disease process
      8. Conditions that are not an integral part of a disease process
      9. Multiple coding for a single condition
      10. Acute and Chronic Conditions

11. Combination Code
12. Late Effects
13. Impending or Threatened Condition
14. **Reporting Same Diagnosis Code More Than Once**
15. **Admissions/Encounters for Rehabilitation**
16. **Documenting for BMI and Pressure Ulcer Stages**

C. Chapter-Specific Coding Guidelines
1. Chapter 1: Infectious and Parasitic Diseases (001-139)
   a. Human Immunodeficiency Virus (HIV) Infections
   b. Septicemia, Systemic Inflammatory Response Syndrome (SIRS), Sepsis, Severe Sepsis, and Septic Shock
   c. **Methicillin Resistant Staphylococcus aureus (MRSA) Conditions**
2. Chapter 2: Neoplasms (140-239)
   a. Treatment directed at the malignancy
   b. Treatment of secondary site
   c. Coding and sequencing of complications
   d. Primary malignancy previously excised
   e. Admissions/Encounters involving chemotherapy, immunotherapy and radiation therapy
   f. Admission/encounter to determine extent of malignancy
   g. Symptoms, signs, and ill-defined conditions listed in Chapter 16 associated with neoplasms
   h. Admission/encounter for pain control/management
   i. **Malignant neoplasm associated with transplanted organ**
3. Chapter 3: Endocrine, Nutritional, and Metabolic Diseases and Immunity Disorders (240-279)
   a. Diabetes mellitus
4. Chapter 4: Diseases of Blood and Blood Forming Organs (280-289)
   a. Anemia of chronic disease
5. Chapter 5: Mental Disorders (290-319)

   Reserved for future guideline expansion
6. Chapter 6: Diseases of Nervous System and Sense Organs (320-389)
   a. Pain – Category
7. Chapter 7: Diseases of Circulatory System (390-459)
   a. Hypertension
   b. Cerebral infarction/stroke/cerebrovascular accident (CVA)

c. Postoperative cerebrovascular accident

d. Late Effects of Cerebrovascular Disease

e. Acute myocardial infarction (AMI)

8. Chapter 8: Diseases of Respiratory System (460-519)

    a. Chronic Obstructive Pulmonary Disease [COPD] and Asthma

    b. Chronic Obstructive Pulmonary Disease [COPD] and Bronchitis

    c. Acute Respiratory Failure

    d. Influenza due to identified avian influenza virus (avian influenza)

9. Chapter 9: Diseases of Digestive System (520-579)

    Reserved for future guideline expansion

10. Chapter 10: Diseases of Genitourinary System (580-629)

    a. Chronic kidney disease

11. Chapter 11: Complications of Pregnancy, Childbirth, and the Puerperium (630-679)

    a. General Rules for Obstetric Cases

    b. Selection of OB Principal or First-listed Diagnosis

    c. Fetal Conditions Affecting the Management of the Mother

    d. HIV Infection in Pregnancy, Childbirth and the Puerperium

    e. Current Conditions Complicating Pregnancy

    f. Diabetes mellitus in pregnancy

    g. Gestational diabetes

    h. Normal Delivery, Code 650

    i. The Postpartum and Peripartum Periods

    j. Code 677, Late effect of complication of pregnancy

    k. Abortions

12. Chapter 12: Diseases Skin and Subcutaneous Tissue (680-709)

    a. Pressure ulcer stage codes

13. Chapter 13: Diseases of Musculoskeletal and Connective Tissue (710-739)

    a. Coding of Pathologic Fractures

14. Chapter 14: Congenital Anomalies (740-759)

    a. Codes in categories 740-759, Congenital Anomalies

15. Chapter 15: Newborn (Perinatal) Guidelines (760-779)

    a. General Perinatal Rules

    b. Use of codes V30-V39

c. Newborn transfers

d. Use of category V29

e. Use of other V codes on perinatal records

f. Maternal Causes of Perinatal Morbidity

g. Congenital Anomalies in Newborns

h. Coding Additional Perinatal Diagnoses

i. Prematurity and Fetal Growth Retardation

j. Newborn sepsis

16. Chapter 16: Signs, Symptoms and Ill-Defined Conditions (780-799)

    Reserved for future guideline expansion

17. Chapter 17: Injury and Poisoning (800-999)

    a. Coding of Injuries

    b. Coding of Traumatic Fractures

    c. Coding of Burns

    d. Coding of Debridement of Wound, Infection, or Burn

    e. Adverse Effects, Poisoning and Toxic Effects

    f. Complications of care

    g. SIRS due to Non-infectious Process

18. Classification of Factors Influencing Health Status and Contact with Health Service (Supplemental V01-V89)

    a. Introduction

    b. V codes use in any healthcare setting

    c. V Codes indicate a reason for an encounter

    d. Categories of V Codes

    e. V Code Table

19. Supplemental Classification of External Causes of Injury and Poisoning (E-codes, E800-E999)

    a. General E Code Coding Guidelines

    b. Place of Occurrence Guideline

    c. Adverse Effects of Drugs, Medicinal and Biological Substances Guidelines

    d. Multiple Cause E Code Coding Guidelines

    e. Child and Adult Abuse Guideline

    f. Unknown or Suspected Intent Guideline

    g. Undetermined Cause

    h. Late Effects of External Cause Guidelines

    i. Misadventures and Complications of Care Guidelines

    j. Terrorism Guidelines

Appendix A ICD-9-CM Official Guidelines for Coding and Reporting

Section II. Selection of Principal Diagnosis
- A. Codes for symptoms, signs, and ill-defined conditions
- B. Two or more interrelated conditions, each potentially meeting the definition for principal diagnosis
- C. Two or more diagnoses that equally meet the definition for principal diagnosis
- D. Two or more comparative or contrasting conditions
- E. A symptom(s) followed by contrasting/comparative diagnoses
- F. Original treatment plan not carried out
- G. Complications of surgery and other medical care
- H. Uncertain Diagnosis
- I. Admission from Observation Unit
    1. Admission Following Medical Observation
    2. Admission Following Post-Operative Observation
- J. Admission from Outpatient Surgery

Section III. Reporting Additional Diagnoses
- A. Previous conditions
- B. Abnormal findings
- C. Uncertain Diagnosis

Section IV. Diagnostic Coding and Reporting Guidelines for Outpatient Services
- A. Selection of first-listed condition
    1. Outpatient Surgery
    2. Observation Stay
- B. Codes from 001.0 through **V89.09**
- C. Accurate reporting of ICD-9-CM diagnosis codes
- D. Selection of codes 001.0 through 999.9
- E. Codes that describe symptoms and signs
- F. Encounters for circumstances other than a disease or injury
- G. Level of Detail in Coding
    1. ICD-9-CM codes with 3, 4, or 5 digits
    2. Use of full number of digits required for a code
- H. ICD-9-CM code for the diagnosis, condition, problem, or other reason for encounter/visit
- I. Uncertain diagnosis
- J. Chronic diseases
- K. Code all documented conditions that coexist
- L. Patients receiving diagnostic services only

Appendix A ICD-9-CM Official Guidelines for Coding and Reporting

    M. Patients receiving therapeutic services only

    N. Patients receiving preoperative evaluations only

    O. Ambulatory surgery

    P. Routine outpatient prenatal visits

Appendix I: Present on Admission Reporting Guidelines

SECTION I. CONVENTIONS, GENERAL CODING GUIDELINES AND CHAPTER SPECIFIC GUIDELINES

The conventions, general guidelines and chapter-specific guidelines are applicable to all health care settings unless otherwise indicated.

A. Conventions for the ICD-9-CM

The conventions for the ICD-9-CM are the general rules for use of the classification independent of the guidelines. These conventions are incorporated within the index and tabular of the ICD-9-CM as instructional notes. The conventions are as follows:

1. Format:

The ICD-9-CM uses an indented format for ease in reference

2. Abbreviations

  a. Index abbreviations

    NEC "Not elsewhere classifiable" This abbreviation in the index represents "other specified" when a specific code is not available for a condition the index directs the coder to the "other specified" code in the tabular.

  b. Tabular abbreviations

    NEC "Not elsewhere classifiable" This abbreviation in the tabular represents "other specified". When a specific code is not available for a condition the tabular includes an NEC entry under a code to identify the code as the "other specified" code.

    (See Section I.A.5.a. "Other" codes").

    NOS "Not otherwise specified" This abbreviation is the equivalent of unspecified.

    (See Section I.A.5.b., "Unspecified" codes)

3. Punctuation

  [ ] Brackets are used in the tabular list to enclose synonyms, alternative wording or explanatory phrases. Brackets are used in the index to identify manifestation codes.

  (See Section I.A.6. "Etiology/manifestations")

  ( ) Parentheses are used in both the index and tabular to enclose supplementary words that may be present or absent in the statement of a disease or procedure without affecting the code number to which it is assigned. The terms within the parentheses are referred to as nonessential modifiers.

: Colons are used in the Tabular list after an incomplete term which needs one or more of the modifiers following the colon to make it assignable to a given category.

4. Includes and Excludes Notes and Inclusion terms

Includes: This note appears immediately under a three-digit code title to further define, or give examples of, the content of the category.

Excludes: An excludes note under a code indicates that the terms excluded from the code are to be coded elsewhere. In some cases the codes for the excluded terms should not be used in conjunction with the code from which it is excluded. An example of this is a congenital condition excluded from an acquired form of the same condition. The congenital and acquired codes should not be used together. In other cases, the excluded terms may be used together with an excluded code. An example of this is when fractures of different bones are coded to different codes. Both codes may be used together if both types of fractures are present.

Inclusion terms: List of terms is included under certain four and five digit codes. These terms are the conditions for which that code number is to be used. The terms may be synonyms of the code title, or, in the case of "other specified" codes, the terms are a list of the various conditions assigned to that code. The inclusion terms are not necessarily exhaustive. Additional terms found only in the index may also be assigned to a code.

5. Other and Unspecified codes

a. "Other" codes

Codes titled "other" or "other specified" (usually a code with a 4th digit 8 or fifth-digit 9 for diagnosis codes) are for use when the information in the medical record provides detail for which a specific code does not exist. Index entries with NEC in the line designate "other" codes in the tabular. These index entries represent specific disease entities for which no specific code exists so the term is included within an "other" code.

b. "Unspecified" codes

Codes (usually a code with a 4th digit 9 or 5th digit 0 for diagnosis codes) titled "unspecified" are for use when the information in the medical record is insufficient to assign a more specific code.

6. Etiology/manifestation convention ("code first", "use additional code" and "in diseases classified elsewhere" notes)

Certain conditions have both an underlying etiology and multiple body system manifestations due to the underlying etiology. For such conditions, the ICD-9-CM has a coding convention that requires the underlying condition be sequenced first followed by the manifestation. Wherever such a combination exists, there is a "use additional code" note at the etiology code, and a "code first" note at the manifestation code. These instructional notes indicate the proper sequencing order of the codes, etiology followed by manifestation.

In most cases the manifestation codes will have in the code title, "in diseases classified elsewhere." Codes with this title are a component of the etiology/manifestation convention. The code title indicates that it is a manifestation code. "In diseases classified elsewhere" codes are never permitted to be used as first listed or principal diagnosis codes. They must be used in conjunction with an underlying condition code and they must be listed following the underlying condition.

There are manifestation codes that do not have "in diseases classified elsewhere" in the title. For such codes a "use additional code" note will still be present and the rules for sequencing apply.

In addition to the notes in the tabular, these conditions also have a specific index entry structure. In the index both conditions are listed together with the etiology code first followed by the manifestation codes in brackets. The code in brackets is always to be sequenced second.

The most commonly used etiology/manifestation combinations are the codes for Diabetes mellitus, category 250. For each code under category 250 there is a use additional code note for the manifestation that is specific for that particular diabetic manifestation. Should a patient have more than one manifestation of diabetes, more than one code from category 250 may be used with as many manifestation codes as are needed to fully describe the patient's complete diabetic condition. The category 250 diabetes codes should be sequenced first, followed by the manifestation codes.

"Code first" and "Use additional code" notes are also used as sequencing rules in the classification for certain codes that are not part of an etiology/manifestation combination.

See – Section I.B.9. "Multiple coding for a single condition".

7. "And"

The word "and" should be interpreted to mean either "and" or "or" when it appears in a title.

8. "With"

The word "with" in the alphabetic index is sequenced immediately following the main term, not in alphabetical order.

9. "See" and "See Also"

The "see" instruction following a main term in the index indicates that another term should be referenced. It is necessary to go to the main term referenced with the "see" note to locate the correct code.

A "see also" instruction following a main term in the index instructs that there is another main term that may also be referenced that may provide additional index entries that may be useful. It is not necessary to follow the "see also" note when the original main term provides the necessary code.

B. General Coding Guidelines

1. Use of Both Alphabetic Index and Tabular List

Use both the Alphabetic Index and the Tabular List when locating and assigning a code. Reliance on only the Alphabetic Index or the Tabular List leads to errors in code assignments and less specificity in code selection.

2. Locate each term in the Alphabetic Index

Locate each term in the Alphabetic Index and verify the code selected in the Tabular List. Read and be guided by instructional notations that appear in both the Alphabetic Index and the Tabular List.

3. Level of Detail in Coding

Diagnosis and procedure codes are to be used at their highest number of digits available.

ICD-9-CM diagnosis codes are composed of codes with 3, 4, or 5 digits. Codes with three digits are included in ICD-9-CM as the heading of a category of codes that may be further subdivided by the use of fourth and/or fifth digits, which provide greater detail.

A three-digit code is to be used only if it is not further subdivided. Where fourth-digit subcategories and/or fifth-digit subclassifications are provided, they must be assigned. A code is invalid if it has not been coded to the full number of digits required for that code. For example, Acute myocardial infarction, code 410, has fourth digits that describe the location of the infarction (e.g., 410.2, Of inferolateral wall), and fifth digits that identify the episode of care. It would be incorrect to report a code in category 410 without a fourth and fifth digit.

ICD-9-CM Volume 3 procedure codes are composed of codes with either 3 or 4 digits. Codes with two digits are included in ICD-9-CM as the heading of a category of codes that may be further subdivided by the use of third and/or fourth digits, which provide greater detail.

4. Code or codes from 001.0 through V89.09

The appropriate code or codes from 001.0 through **V89.09** must be used to identify diagnoses, symptoms, conditions, problems, complaints or other reason(s) for the encounter/visit.

5. Selection of codes 001.0 through 999.9

The selection of codes 001.0 through 999.9 will frequently be used to describe the reason for the admission/encounter. These codes are from the section of ICD-9-CM for the classification of diseases and injuries (e.g., infectious and parasitic diseases; neoplasms; symptoms, signs, and ill-defined conditions, etc.).

6. Signs and symptoms

Codes that describe symptoms and signs, as opposed to diagnoses, are acceptable for reporting purposes when a related definitive diagnosis has not been established (confirmed) by the provider. Chapter 16 of ICD-9-CM, Symptoms, Signs, and Ill-defined conditions (codes 780.0-799.9) contain many, but not all codes for symptoms.

7. Conditions that are an integral part of a disease process

Signs and symptoms that are **associated routinely with a** disease process should not be assigned as additional codes, unless otherwise instructed by the classification.

8. Conditions that are not an integral part of a disease process

Additional signs and symptoms that may not be associated routinely with a disease process should be coded when present.

9. Multiple coding for a single condition

In addition to the etiology/manifestation convention that requires two codes to fully describe a single condition that affects multiple body systems, there are other single conditions that also require more than one code. "Use additional code" notes are found in the tabular at codes that are not part of an etiology/manifestation pair where a secondary code is useful to fully describe a condition. The sequencing rule is the same as the etiology/manifestation pair – , "use additional code" indicates that a secondary code should be added.

For example, for infections that are not included in chapter 1, a secondary code from category 041, Bacterial infection in conditions classified elsewhere and of unspecified site, may be required to identify the bacterial organism causing the infection. A "use additional code" note will normally be found at the infectious disease code, indicating a need for the organism code to be added as a secondary code.

"Code first" notes are also under certain codes that are not specifically manifestation codes but may be due to an underlying cause. When a "code first" note is present and an underlying condition is present the underlying condition should be sequenced first.

"Code, if applicable, any causal condition first", notes indicate that this code may be assigned as a principal diagnosis when the causal condition is unknown or not applicable. If a causal condition is known, then the code for that condition should be sequenced as the principal or first-listed diagnosis.

Multiple codes may be needed for late effects, complication codes and obstetric codes to more fully describe a condition. See the specific guidelines for these conditions for further instruction.

10. Acute and Chronic Conditions

If the same condition is described as both acute (subacute) and chronic, and separate subentries exist in the Alphabetic Index at the same indentation level, code both and sequence the acute (subacute) code first.

11. Combination Code

A combination code is a single code used to classify:

Two diagnoses, or

A diagnosis with an associated secondary process (manifestation)

A diagnosis with an associated complication

Combination codes are identified by referring to subterm entries in the Alphabetic Index and by reading the inclusion and exclusion notes in the Tabular List.

Assign only the combination code when that code fully identifies the diagnostic conditions involved or when the Alphabetic Index so directs. Multiple coding should not be used when the classification provides a combination code that clearly identifies all of the elements documented in the diagnosis. When the combination code lacks necessary specificity in describing the manifestation or complication, an additional code should be used as a secondary code.

12. Late Effects

A late effect is the residual effect (condition produced) after the acute phase of an illness or injury has terminated. There is no time limit on when a late effect code can be used. The residual may be apparent early, such as in cerebrovascular accident cases, or it may occur months or years later, such as that due to a previous injury. Coding of late effects generally requires two codes sequenced in the following order: The condition or nature of the late effect is sequenced first. The late effect code is sequenced second.

An exception to the above guidelines are those instances where the code for late effect is followed by a manifestation code identified in the Tabular List and title, or the late effect code has been expanded (at the fourth and fifth-digit levels) to include the manifestation(s). The code for the acute phase of an illness or injury that led to the late effect is never used with a code for the late effect.

13. Impending or Threatened Condition

Code any condition described at the time of discharge as "impending" or "threatened" as follows:

If it did occur, code as confirmed diagnosis.

If it did not occur, reference the Alphabetic Index to determine if the condition has a subentry term for "impending" or "threatened" and also reference main term entries for "Impending" and for "Threatened."

If the subterms are listed, assign the given code.

If the subterms are not listed, code the existing underlying condition(s) and not the condition described as impending or threatened.

14. Reporting Same Diagnosis Code More than Once

Each unique ICD-9-CM diagnosis code may be reported only once for an encounter. This applies to bilateral conditions or two different conditions classified to the same ICD-9-CM diagnosis code.

15. Admissions/Encounters for Rehabilitation

When the purpose for the admission/encounter is rehabilitation, sequence the appropriate V code from category V57, Care involving use of rehabilitation procedures, as the principal/first-listed diagnosis. The code for the condition for which the service is being performed should be reported as an additional diagnosis.

Only one code from category V57 is required. Code V57.89, Other specified rehabilitation procedures, should be assigned if more than one type of rehabilitation is performed during a single encounter. A procedure code should be reported to identify each type of rehabilitation therapy actually performed.

16. Documentation for BMI and Pressure Ulcer Stages

For the Body Mass Index (BMI) and pressure ulcer stage codes, code assignment may be based on medical record documentation from clinicians who are not the patient's provider (i.e., physician or other qualified healthcare

practitioner legally accountable for establishing the patient's diagnosis), since this information is typically documented by other clinicians involved in the care of the patient (e.g., a dietitian often documents the BMI and nurses often documents the pressure ulcer stages). However, the associated diagnosis (such as overweight, obesity, or pressure ulcer) must be documented by the patient's provider. If there is conflicting medical record documentation, either from the same clinician or different clinicians, the patient's attending provider should be queried for clarification.

The BMI and pressure ulcer stage codes should only be reported as secondary diagnoses. As with all other secondary diagnosis codes, the BMI and pressure ulcer stage codes should only be assigned when they meet the definition of a reportable additional diagnosis (see Section III, Reporting Additional Diagnoses).

C. Chapter-Specific Coding Guidelines

In addition to general coding guidelines, there are guidelines for specific diagnoses and/or conditions in the classification. Unless otherwise indicated, these guidelines apply to all health care settings. Please refer to Section II for guidelines on the selection of principal diagnosis.

1. **Chapter 1: Infectious and Parasitic Diseases (001-139)**

    a. **Human Immunodeficiency Virus (HIV) Infections**

    1) **Code only confirmed cases**

        Code only confirmed cases of HIV infection/illness. This is an exception to the hospital inpatient guideline Section II, H.

        In this context, "confirmation" does not require documentation of positive serology or culture for HIV; the provider's diagnostic statement that the patient is HIV positive, or has an HIV-related illness is sufficient.

    2) **Selection and sequencing of HIV codes**

        (a) **Patient admitted for HIV-related condition**

            If a patient is admitted for an HIV-related condition, the principal diagnosis should be 042, followed by additional diagnosis codes for all reported HIV-related conditions.

        (b) **Patient with HIV disease admitted for unrelated condition**

            If a patient with HIV disease is admitted for an unrelated condition (such as a traumatic injury), the code for the unrelated condition (e.g., the nature of injury code) should be the principal diagnosis. Other diagnoses would be 042 followed by additional diagnosis codes for all reported HIV-related conditions.

        (c) **Whether the patient is newly diagnosed**

            Whether the patient is newly diagnosed or has had previous admissions/encounters for HIV conditions is irrelevant to the sequencing decision.

(d) Asymptomatic human immunodeficiency virus

V08 Asymptomatic human immunodeficiency virus [HIV] infection, is to be applied when the patient without any documentation of symptoms is listed as being "HIV positive," "known HIV," "HIV test positive," or similar terminology. Do not use this code if the term "AIDS" is used or if the patient is treated for any HIV-related illness or is described as having any condition(s) resulting from his/her HIV positive status; use 042 in these cases.

(e) Patients with inconclusive HIV serology

Patients with inconclusive HIV serology, but no definitive diagnosis or manifestations of the illness, may be assigned code 795.71, Inconclusive serologic test for Human Immunodeficiency Virus [HIV].

(f) Previously diagnosed HIV-related illness

Patients with any known prior diagnosis of an HIV-related illness should be coded to 042. Once a patient has developed an HIV-related illness, the patient should always be assigned code 042 on every subsequent admission/encounter. Patients previously diagnosed with any HIV illness (042) should never be assigned to 795.71 or V08.

(g) HIV Infection in Pregnancy, Childbirth and the Puerperium

During pregnancy, childbirth or the puerperium, a patient admitted (or presenting for a health care encounter) because of an HIV-related illness should receive a principal diagnosis code of 647.6X, Other specified infectious and parasitic diseases in the mother classifiable elsewhere, but complicating the pregnancy, childbirth or the puerperium, followed by 042 and the code(s) for the HIV-related illness(es). Codes from Chapter 15 always take sequencing priority.

Patients with asymptomatic HIV infection status admitted (or presenting for a health care encounter) during pregnancy, childbirth, or the puerperium should receive codes of 647.6X and V08.

(h) Encounters for testing for HIV

If a patient is being seen to determine his/her HIV status, use code V73.89, Screening for other specified viral disease. Use code V69.8, Other problems related to lifestyle, as a secondary code if an asymptomatic patient is in a known high risk group for HIV. Should a patient with signs or symptoms or illness, or a confirmed HIV related diagnosis be tested for HIV, code the signs and symptoms or the diagnosis. An additional counseling code V65.44 may be used if counseling is provided during the encounter for the test.

When a patient returns to be informed of his/her HIV test results use code V65.44, HIV counseling, if the results of the test are negative.

If the results are positive but the patient is asymptomatic use code V08, Asymptomatic HIV infection. If the results are positive and the patient is symptomatic use code 042, HIV infection, with codes for the HIV related symptoms or diagnosis. The HIV counseling code may also be used if counseling is provided for patients with positive test results.

b. Septicemia, Systemic Inflammatory Response Syndrome (SIRS), Sepsis, Severe Sepsis, and Septic Shock

  1) SIRS, Septicemia, and Sepsis

  (a) The terms septicemia and sepsis are often used interchangeably by providers, however they are not considered synonymous terms. The following descriptions are provided for reference but do not preclude querying the provider for clarification about terms used in the documentation:

  (i) Septicemia generally refers to a systemic disease associated with the presence of pathological microorganisms or toxins in the blood, which can include bacteria, viruses, fungi or other organisms.

  (ii) Systemic inflammatory response syndrome (SIRS) generally refers to the systemic response to infection, trauma/burns, or other insult (such as cancer) with symptoms including fever, tachycardia, tachypnea, and leukocytosis.

  (iii) Sepsis generally refers to SIRS due to infection.

  (iv) Severe sepsis generally refers to sepsis with associated acute organ dysfunction.

  (b) The Coding of SIRS, sepsis, and severe sepsis

  The coding of SIRS, sepsis and severe sepsis requires a minimum of 2 codes: a code for the underlying cause (such as infection or trauma) and a code from subcategory 995.9 Systemic inflammatory response syndrome (SIRS).

  (i) The code for the underlying cause (such as infection or trauma) must be sequenced before the code from subcategory 995.9 Systemic inflammatory response syndrome (SIRS).

  (ii) Sepsis and severe sepsis require a code for the systemic infection (038.xx, 112.5, etc.) and either code 995.91, Sepsis, or 995.92, Severe sepsis. If the causal organism is not documented, assign code 038.9, Unspecified septicemia.

  (iii) Severe sepsis requires additional code(s) for the associated acute organ dysfunction(s).

  (iv) If a patient has sepsis with multiple organ dysfunctions, follow the instructions for coding severe sepsis.

  (v) Either the term sepsis or SIRS must be documented to assign a code from subcategory 995.9.

  (vi) See Section I.C.17.g), Injury and poisoning, for information regarding systemic inflammatory response syndrome (SIRS) due to trauma/burns and other non-infectious processes.

(c) Due to the complex nature of sepsis and severe sepsis, some cases may require querying the provider prior to assignment of the codes.

2) Sequencing sepsis and severe sepsis

(a) Sepsis and severe sepsis as principal diagnosis

If sepsis or severe sepsis is present on admission, and meets the definition of principal diagnosis, the systemic infection code (e.g., 038.xx, 112.5, etc) should be assigned as the principal diagnosis, followed by code 995.91, Sepsis, or 995.92, Severe sepsis, as required by the sequencing rules in the Tabular List. Codes from subcategory 995.9 can never be assigned as a principal diagnosis. A code should also be assigned for any localized infection, if present.

If the sepsis or severe sepsis is due to a postprocedural infection, see Section **I.C.1.6.10** for guidelines related to sepsis due to postprocedural infection.

(b) Sepsis and severe sepsis as secondary diagnoses

When sepsis or severe sepsis develops during the encounter (it was not present on admission), the systemic infection code and code 995.91 or 995.92 should be assigned as secondary diagnoses.

(c) Documentation unclear as to whether sepsis or severe sepsis is present on admission

Sepsis or severe sepsis may be present on admission but the diagnosis may not be confirmed until sometime after admission. If the documentation is not clear whether the sepsis or severe sepsis was present on admission, the provider should be queried.

3) Sepsis/SIRS with Localized Infection

If the reason for admission is both sepsis, severe sepsis, or SIRS and a localized infection, such as pneumonia or cellulitis, a code for the systemic infection (038.xx, 112.5, etc) should be assigned first, then code 995.91 or 995.92, followed by the code for the localized infection. If the patient is admitted with a localized infection, such as pneumonia, and sepsis/SIRS doesn't develop until after admission, see guideline I.C.1.b2.b).

If the localized infection is postprocedural, *see Section* **I.C.1.6.10** *for guidelines related to sepsis due to postprocedural infection.*

Note: The term urosepsis is a nonspecific term. If that is the only term documented then only code 599.0 should be assigned based on the default for the term in the ICD-9-CM index, in addition to the code for the causal organism if known.

4) Bacterial Sepsis and Septicemia

In most cases, it will be a code from category 038, Septicemia, that will be used in conjunction with a code from subcategory 995.9 such as the following:

(a) Streptococcal sepsis

If the documentation in the record states streptococcal sepsis, codes 038.0, Streptococcal septicemia, and code 995.91 should be used, in that sequence.

(b) Streptococcal septicemia

If the documentation states streptococcal septicemia, only code 038.0 should be assigned, however, the provider should be queried whether the patient has sepsis, an infection with SIRS.

5) Acute organ dysfunction that is not clearly associated with the sepsis

If a patient has sepsis and an acute organ dysfunction, but the medical record documentation indicates that the acute organ dysfunction is related to a medical condition other than the sepsis, do not assign code 995.92, Severe sepsis. An acute organ dysfunction must be associated with the sepsis in order to assign the severe sepsis code. If the documentation is not clear as to whether an acute organ dysfunction is related to the sepsis or another medical condition, query the provider.

6) Septic shock

(a) Sequencing of septic shock

Septic shock generally refers to circulatory failure associated with severe sepsis, and, therefore, it represents a type of acute organ dysfunction.

For all cases of septic shock, the code for the systemic infection should be sequenced first, followed by codes 995.92 and 785.52. Any additional codes for other acute organ dysfunctions should also be assigned. As noted in the sequencing instructions in the Tabular List, the code for septic shock cannot be assigned as a principal diagnosis.

(b) Septic Shock without documentation of severe sepsis

Septic shock indicates the presence of severe sepsis.

Code 995.92, Severe sepsis, must be assigned with code 785.52, Septic shock, even if the term severe sepsis is not documented in the record. The "use additional code" note and the "code first" note in the tabular support this guideline.

7) Sepsis and septic shock complicating abortion and pregnancy

Sepsis and septic shock **complicating** abortion, ectopic pregnancy, and molar pregnancy are classified to category codes in Chapter 11 (630-639).

See section I.C.11.

Appendix A   ICD-9-CM Official Guidelines for Coding and Reporting

8) Negative or inconclusive blood cultures

Negative or inconclusive blood cultures do not preclude a diagnosis of septicemia or sepsis in patients with clinical evidence of the condition, however, the provider should be queried.

9) Newborn sepsis

See Section I.C.15.j for information on the coding of newborn sepsis.

10) Sepsis due to a Postprocedural Infection

(a) Documentation of causal relationship

As with all postprocedural complications, code assignment is based on the provider's documentation of the relationship between the infection and the procedure.

(b) Sepsis due to postprocedural infection

In cases of postprocedural sepsis, the complication code, such as code 998.59, Other postoperative infection, or 674.3x, Other complications of obstetrical surgical wounds, should be coded first followed by the appropriate sepsis codes (systemic infection code and either code 995.91 or 995.92). An additional code(s) for any acute organ dysfunction should also be assigned for cases of severe sepsis.

11) External cause of injury codes with SIRS

Refer to Section I.C.19.a.7 for instruction on the use of external cause of injury codes with codes for SIRS resulting from trauma.

12) Sepsis and Severe Sepsis Associated with Non-infectious Process

In some cases, a non-infectious process, such as trauma, may lead to an infection which can result in sepsis or severe sepsis. If sepsis or severe sepsis is documented as associated with a non-infectious condition, such as a burn or serious injury, and this condition meets the definition for principal diagnosis, the code for the non-infectious condition should be sequenced first, followed by the code for the systemic infection and either code 995.91, Sepsis, or 995.92, Severe sepsis. Additional codes for any associated acute organ dysfunction(s) should also be assigned for cases of severe sepsis. If the sepsis or severe sepsis meets the definition of principal diagnosis, the systemic infection and sepsis codes should be sequenced before the non-infectious condition. When both the associated non-infectious condition and the sepsis or severe sepsis meet the definition of principal diagnosis, either may be assigned as principal diagnosis.

See Section I.C.1.b.2)(a) for guidelines pertaining to sepsis or severe sepsis as the principal diagnosis.

(b) **Only one SIRS (subcategory 995.9) code should be assigned**

Only one code from subcategory 995.9 should be assigned. Therefore, when a non-infectious condition leads to an infection resulting in sepsis or severe sepsis, assign either code 995.91 or 995.92. Do

not additionally assign code 995.93, Systemic inflammatory response syndrome due to non-infectious process without acute organ dysfunction, or 995.94, Systemic inflammatory response syndrome with acute organ dysfunction.

See Section I.C.17.g for information on the coding of SIRS due to trauma/burns or other non-infectious disease processes.

c. **Methicillin Resistant *Staphylococcus aureus* (MRSA) Conditions**

   1) **Selection and sequencing of MRSA codes**

      (a) **Combination codes for MRSA infection**

      When a patient is diagnosed with an infection that is due to methicillin resistant *Staphylococcus aureus* (MRSA), and that infection has a combination code that includes the causal organism (e.g., septicemia, pneumonia) assign the appropriate code for the condition (e.g., code 038.12, Methicillin resistant Staphylococcus aureus septicemia or code 482.42, Methicillin resistant pneumonia due to Staphylococcus aureus). Do not assign code 041.12, Methicillin resistant Staphylococcus aureus, as an additional code because the code includes the type of infection and the MRSA organism. Do not assign a code from subcategory V09.0, Infection with microorganisms resistant to penicillins, as an additional diagnosis.

      See Section C.1.b.1 for instructions on coding and sequencing of septicemia.

      (b) **Other codes for MRSA infection**

      When there is documentation of a current infection (e.g., wound infection, stitch abscess, urinary tract infection) due to MRSA, and that infection does not have a combination code that includes the causal organism, select the appropriate code to identify the condition along with code 041.12, Methicillin resistant Staphylococcus aureus, for the MRSA infection. Do not assign a code from subcategory V09.0, Infection with microorganisms resistant to penicillins.

      (c) **Methicillin susceptible Staphylococcus aureus (MSSA) and MRSA colonization**

      The condition or state of being colonized or carrying MSSA or MRSA is called colonization or carriage, while an individual person is described as being colonized or being a carrier. Colonization means that MSSA or MSRA is present on or in the body without necessarily causing illness. A positive MRSA colonization test might be documented by the provider as "MRSA screen positive" or "MRSA nasal swab positive".

Assign code V02.54, Carrier or suspected carrier, Methicillin resistant Staphylococcus aureus, for patients documented as having MRSA colonization. Assign code V02.53, Carrier or suspected carrier, Methicillin susceptible Staphylococcus aureus, for patient documented as having MSSA colonization. Colonization is not necessarily indicative of a disease process or as the cause of a specific condition the patient may have unless documented as such by the provider.

Code V02.59, Other specified bacterial diseases, should be assigned for other types of staphylococcal colonization (e.g., *S. epidermidis*, *S. saprophyticus*). Code V02.59 should not be assigned for colonization with any type of *Staphylococcus aureus* (MRSA, MSSA).

(d) **MRSA colonization and infection**

If a patient is documented as having both MRSA colonization and infection during a hospital admission, code V02.54, Carrier or suspected carrier, Methicillin resistant *Staphylococcus aureus*, and a code for the MRSA infection may both be assigned.

2. **Chapter 2: Neoplasms (140-239)**

<u>General guidelines</u>

Chapter 2 of the ICD-9-CM contains the codes for most benign and all malignant neoplasms. Certain benign neoplasms, such as prostatic adenomas, may be found in the specific body system chapters. To properly code a neoplasm it is necessary to determine from the record if the neoplasm is benign, in-situ, malignant, or of uncertain histologic behavior. If malignant, any secondary (metastatic) sites should also be determined.

The neoplasm table in the Alphabetic Index should be referenced first. However, if the histological term is documented, that term should be referenced first, rather than going immediately to the Neoplasm Table, in order to determine which column in the Neoplasm Table is appropriate. For example, if the documentation indicates "adenoma," refer to the term in the Alphabetic Index to review the entries under this term and the instructional note to "see also neoplasm, by site, benign." The table provides the proper code based on the type of neoplasm and the site. It is important to select the proper column in the table that corresponds to the type of neoplasm. The tabular should then be referenced to verify that the correct code has been selected from the table and that a more specific site code does not exist.

See Section I. C. 18.d.4. for information regarding V codes for genetic susceptibility to cancer.

a. **Treatment directed at the malignancy**

If the treatment is directed at the malignancy, designate the malignancy as the principal diagnosis.

The only exception to this guideline is if a patient admission/encounter is solely for the administration of chemotherapy, immunotherapy or radiation therapy, assign the appropriate V58.x code as the first-listed or principal

diagnosis, and the diagnosis or problem for which the service is being performed as a secondary diagnosis.

b. Treatment of secondary site

When a patient is admitted because of a primary neoplasm with metastasis and treatment is directed toward the secondary site only, the secondary neoplasm is designated as the principal diagnosis even though the primary malignancy is still present.

c. Coding and sequencing of complications

Coding and sequencing of complications associated with the malignancies or with the therapy thereof are subject to the following guidelines:

1) **Anemia associated with malignancy**

   When admission/encounter is for management of an anemia associated with the malignancy, and the treatment is only for anemia, the appropriate anemia code (such as code 285.22, Anemia in neoplastic disease) is designated as the principal diagnosis and is followed by the appropriate code(s) for the malignancy.

   Code 285.22 may also be used as a secondary code if the patient suffers from anemia and is being treated for the malignancy.

2) **Anemia associated with chemotherapy, immunotherapy and radiation therapy**

   When the admission/encounter is for management of an anemia associated with chemotherapy, immunotherapy or radiotherapy and the only treatment is for the anemia, the anemia is sequenced first followed by code E933.1. The appropriate neoplasm code should be assigned as an additional code.

3) **Management of dehydration due to the malignancy**

   When the admission/encounter is for management of dehydration due to the malignancy or the therapy, or a combination of both, and only the dehydration is being treated (intravenous rehydration), the dehydration is sequenced first, followed by the code(s) for the malignancy.

4) **Treatment of a complication resulting from a surgical procedure**

   When the admission/encounter is for treatment of a complication resulting from a surgical procedure, designate the complication as the principal or first-listed diagnosis if treatment is directed at resolving the complication.

d. Primary malignancy previously excised

When a primary malignancy has been previously excised or eradicated from its site and there is no further treatment directed to that site and there is no evidence of any existing primary malignancy, a code from category V10, Personal history of malignant neoplasm, should be used to indicate the former site of the malignancy. Any mention of extension, invasion, or metastasis to another site is coded as a secondary malignant neoplasm to that site.

The secondary site may be the principal or first-listed with the V10 code used as a secondary code.

e. **Admissions/Encounters involving chemotherapy, immunotherapy and radiation therapy**

   1) **Episode of care involves surgical removal of neoplasm**

   When an episode of care involves the surgical removal of a neoplasm, primary or secondary site, followed by adjunct chemotherapy or radiation treatment during the same episode of care, the neoplasm code should be assigned as principal or first-listed diagnosis, using codes in the 140-198 series or where appropriate in the 200-203 series.

   2) **Patient admission/encounter solely for administration of chemotherapy, immunotherapy and radiation therapy**

   If a patient admission/encounter is solely for the administration of chemotherapy, immunotherapy or radiation therapy assign code V58.0, Encounter for radiation therapy, or V58.11, Encounter for antineoplastic chemotherapy, or V58.12, Encounter for antineoplastic immunotherapy as the first-listed or principal diagnosis. If a patient receives more than one of these therapies during the same admission more than one of these codes may be assigned, in any sequence.

   The malignancy for which the therapy is being administered should be assigned as a secondary diagnosis.

   3) **Patient admitted for radiotherapy/chemotherapy and immunotherapy and develops complications**

   When a patient is admitted for the purpose of radiotherapy, immunotherapy or chemotherapy and develops complications such as uncontrolled nausea and vomiting or dehydration, the principal or first-listed diagnosis is V58.0, Encounter for radiotherapy, or V58.11, Encounter for antineoplastic chemotherapy, or V58.12, Encounter for antineoplastic immunotherapy followed by any codes for the complications.

f. **Admission/encounter to determine extent of malignancy**

When the reason for admission/encounter is to determine the extent of the malignancy, or for a procedure such as paracentesis or thoracentesis, the primary malignancy or appropriate metastatic site is designated as the principal or first-listed diagnosis, even though chemotherapy or radiotherapy is administered.

g. **Symptoms, signs, and ill-defined conditions listed in Chapter 16 associated with neoplasms**

Symptoms, signs, and ill-defined conditions listed in Chapter 16 characteristic of, or associated with, an existing primary or secondary site malignancy cannot be used to replace the malignancy as principal or first-listed diagnosis, regardless of the number of admissions or encounters for treatment and care of the neoplasm.

See section I.C.18.d.14, Encounter for prophylactic organ removal.

h. Admission/encounter for pain control/management

See Section I.C.6.a.5 for information on coding admission/encounter for pain control/management.

i. Malignant neoplasm associated with transplanted organ

A malignant neoplasm of a transplanted organ should be coded as a transplant complication. Assign first the appropriate code from subcategory 996.8, Complications of transplanted organ, followed by code 199.2, Malignant neoplasm associated with transplanted organ. Use an additional code for the specific malignancy.

3. Chapter 3: Endocrine, Nutritional, and Metabolic Diseases and Immunity Disorders (240-279)

a. Diabetes mellitus

Codes under category 250, Diabetes mellitus, identify complications/manifestations associated with diabetes mellitus. A fifth-digit is required for all category 250 codes to identify the type of diabetes mellitus and whether the diabetes is controlled or uncontrolled.

See I.C.3.a.7 for secondary diabetes.

1) Fifth-digits for category 250:

The following are the fifth-digits for the codes under category 250:

0   type II or unspecified type, not stated as uncontrolled

1   type I, [juvenile type], not stated as uncontrolled

2   type II or unspecified type, uncontrolled

3   type I, [juvenile type], uncontrolled

The age of a patient is not the sole determining factor, though most type I diabetics develop the condition before reaching puberty. For this reason type I diabetes mellitus is also referred to as juvenile diabetes.

2) Type of diabetes mellitus not documented

If the type of diabetes mellitus is not documented in the medical record the default is type II.

3) Diabetes mellitus and the use of insulin

All type I diabetics must use insulin to replace what their bodies do not produce. However, the use of insulin does not mean that a patient is a type I diabetic. Some patients with type II diabetes mellitus are unable to control their blood sugar through diet and oral medication alone and do require insulin. If the documentation in a medical record does not indicate the type of diabetes but does indicate that the patient uses insulin, the appropriate fifth-digit for type II must be used. For type II patients who routinely use insulin, code V58.67, Long-term (current) use of insulin, should also be assigned to indicate that the patient uses insulin. Code V58.67 should not be assigned if insulin is given temporarily to bring a type II patient's blood sugar under control during an encounter.

4) **Assigning and sequencing diabetes codes and associated conditions**

When assigning codes for diabetes and its associated conditions, the code(s) from category 250 must be sequenced before the codes for the associated conditions. The diabetes codes and the secondary codes that correspond to them are paired codes that follow the etiology/manifestation convention of the classification *(See Section I.A.6., Etiology/manifestation convention).* Assign as many codes from category 250 as needed to identify all of the associated conditions that the patient has. The corresponding secondary codes are listed under each of the diabetes codes.

(a) **Diabetic retinopathy/diabetic macular edema**

Diabetic macular edema, code 362.07, is only present with diabetic retinopathy. Another code from subcategory 362.0, Diabetic retinopathy, must be used with code 362.07. Codes under subcategory 362.0 are diabetes manifestation codes, so they must be used following the appropriate diabetes code.

5) **Diabetes mellitus in pregnancy and gestational diabetes**

(a) For diabetes mellitus complicating pregnancy, see Section I.C.11.f., Diabetes mellitus in pregnancy.

(b) For gestational diabetes, see Section I.C.11, g., Gestational diabetes.

6) **Insulin pump malfunction**

(a) **Underdose of insulin due insulin pump failure**

An underdose of insulin due to an insulin pump failure should be assigned 996.57, Mechanical complication due to insulin pump, as the principal or first listed code, followed by the appropriate diabetes mellitus code based on documentation.

(b) **Overdose of insulin due to insulin pump failure**

The principal or first listed code for an encounter due to an insulin pump malfunction resulting in an overdose of insulin, should also be 996.57, Mechanical complication due to insulin pump, followed by code 962.3, Poisoning by insulins and antidiabetic agents, and the appropriate diabetes mellitus code based on documentation.

7) **Secondary Diabetes Mellitus**

Codes under category 249, Secondary diabetes mellitus, identify complications/manifestations associated with secondary diabetes mellitus. Secondary diabetes is always caused by another condition or event (e.g., cystic fibrosis, malignant neoplasm of pancreas, pancreatectomy, adverse effect of drug, or poisoning).

(a) **Fifth-digits for category 249:**

A fifth-digit is required for all category 249 codes to identify whether the diabetes is controlled or uncontrolled.

(b) **Secondary diabetes mellitus and the use of insulin**

For patients who routinely use insulin, code V58.67, Long-term (current) use of insulin, should also be assigned. Code V58.67 should not be assigned if insulin is given temporarily to bring a patient's blood sugar under control during an encounter.

(c) **Assigning and sequencing secondary diabetes codes and associated conditions**

When assigning codes for secondary diabetes and its associated conditions (e.g. renal manifestations), the code(s) from category 249 must be sequenced before the codes for the associated conditions. The secondary diabetes codes and the diabetic manifestation codes that correspond to them are paired codes that follow the etiology/manifestation convention of the classification. Assign as many codes from category 249 as needed to identify all of the associated conditions that the patient has. The corresponding codes for the associated conditions are listed under each of the secondary diabetes codes. For example, secondary diabetes with diabetic nephrosis is assigned to code 249.40, followed by 581.81.

(d) **Assigning and sequencing secondary diabetes codes and its causes**

The sequencing of the secondary diabetes codes in relationship to codes for the cause of the diabetes is based on the reason for the encounter, applicable ICD-9-CM sequencing conventions, and chapter-specific guidelines.

If a patient is seen for treatment of the secondary diabetes or one of its associated conditions, a code from category 249 is sequenced as the principal or first-listed diagnosis, with the cause of the secondary diabetes (e.g. cystic fibrosis) sequenced as an additional diagnosis.

If, however, the patient is seen for the treatment of the condition causing the secondary diabetes (e.g., malignant neoplasm of pancreas), the code for the cause of the secondary diabetes should be sequenced as the principal or first-listed diagnosis followed by a code from category 249.

(i) Secondary diabetes mellitus due to pancreatectomy

For postpancreatectomy diabetes mellitus (lack of insulin due to the surgical removal of all or part of the pancreas), assign code 251.3, Postsurgical hypoinsulinemia. A code from subcategory 249 should not be assigned for secondary diabetes mellitus due to pancreatectomy. Code also any diabetic manifestations (e.g. diabetic nephrosis 581.81).

(ii) **Secondary diabetes due to drugs**

Secondary diabetes may be caused by an adverse effect of correctly administered medications, poisoning or late effect of poisoning.

See section I.C.17.e for coding of adverse effects and poisoning, and section I.C.19 for E code reporting.

4. **Chapter 4: Diseases of Blood and Blood Forming Organs (280-289)**

   a. **Anemia of chronic disease**

   Subcategory 285.2, Anemia in chronic illness, has codes for anemia in chronic kidney disease, code 285.21; anemia in neoplastic disease, code 285.22; and anemia in other chronic illness, code 285.29. These codes can be used as the principal/first listed code if the reason for the encounter is to treat the anemia. They may also be used as secondary codes if treatment of the anemia is a component of an encounter, but not the primary reason for the encounter. When using a code from subcategory 285 it is also necessary to use the code for the chronic condition causing the anemia.

   1) **Anemia in chronic kidney disease**

   When assigning code 285.21, Anemia in chronic kidney disease, it is also necessary to assign a code from category 585, Chronic kidney disease, to indicate the stage of chronic kidney disease.

   See I.C.10.a. Chronic kidney disease (CKD).

   2) **Anemia in neoplastic disease**

   When assigning code 285.22, Anemia in neoplastic disease, it is also necessary to assign the neoplasm code that is responsible for the anemia. Code 285.22 is for use for anemia that is due to the malignancy, not for anemia due to antineoplastic chemotherapy drugs, which is an adverse effect.

   See I.C.2.c.1 Anemia associated with malignancy.

   See I.C.2.c.2 Anemia associated with chemotherapy, immunotherapy and radiation therapy.

   See I.C.17.e.1. Adverse effects.

5. **Chapter 5: Mental Disorders (290-319)**

   Reserved for future guideline expansion

6. **Chapter 6: Diseases of Nervous System and Sense Organs (320-389)**

   a. **Pain – Category 338**

   1) **General coding information**

   Codes in category 338 may be used in conjunction with codes from other categories and chapters to provide more detail about acute or chronic pain and neoplasm-related pain, unless otherwise indicated below.

If the pain is not specified as acute or chronic, do not assign codes from category 338, except for post-thoracotomy pain, postoperative pain or neoplasm related pain, or central pain syndrome.

A code from subcategories 338.1 and 338.2 should not be assigned if the underlying (definitive) diagnosis is known, unless the reason for the encounter is pain control/management and not management of the underlying condition.

(a) **Category 338 Codes as Principal or First-Listed Diagnosis**

   Category 338 codes are acceptable as principal diagnosis or the first-listed code:

   - When pain control or pain management is the reason for the admission/encounter (e.g., a patient with displaced intervertebral disc, nerve impingement and severe back pain presents for injection of steroid into the spinal canal). The underlying cause of the pain should be reported as an additional diagnosis, if known.

   - When an admission or encounter is for a procedure aimed at treating the underlying condition (e.g., spinal fusion, kyphoplasty), a code for the underlying condition (e.g., vertebral fracture, spinal stenosis) should be assigned as the principal diagnosis. No code from category 338 should be assigned.

   - When a patient is admitted for the insertion of a neurostimulator for pain control, assign the appropriate pain code as the principal of first listed diagnosis. When an admission or encounter is for a procedure aimed at treating the underlying condition and a neurostimulator is inserted for pain control during the same admission/encounter, a code for the underlying condition should be assigned as the principal diagnosis and the appropriate pain code should be assigned as a secondary diagnosis.

(b) **Use of Category 338 Codes in Conjunction with Site Specific Pain Codes**

   (i) **Assigning Category 338 Codes and Site-Specific Pain Codes**

   Codes from category 338 may be used in conjunction with codes that identify the site of pain (including codes from chapter 16) if the category 338 code provides additional information. For example, if the code describes the site of the pain, but does not fully describe whether the pain is acute or chronic, then both codes should be assigned.

   (ii) **Sequencing of Category 338 Codes with Site-Specific Pain Codes**

   The sequencing of category 338 codes with site-specific pain codes (including chapter 16 codes), is dependent on the circumstances of the encounter/admission as follows:

- If the encounter is for pain control or pain management, assign the code from category 338 followed by the code identifying the specific site of pain (e.g., encounter for pain management for acute neck pain from trauma is assigned code 338.11, Acute pain due to trauma, followed by code 723.1, Cervicalgia, to identify the site of pain).

- If the encounter is for any other reason except pain control or pain management, and a related definitive diagnosis has not been established (confirmed) by the provider, assign the code for the specific site of pain first, followed by the appropriate code from category 338.

2) **Pain due to devices, implants and grafts**

   Pain associated with devices, implants or grafts left in a surgical site (for example painful hip prothesis) is assigned to the appropriate code(s) found in Chapter 17, Injury and Poisoning. Use additional code(s) from category 338 to identify acute or chronic pain due to presence of the device, implant or graft (338.18-338.19 or 338.28-338.29).

3) **Postoperative Pain**

   Post-thoracotomy pain and other postoperative pain are classified to subcategories 338.1 and 338.2, depending on whether the pain is acute or chronic. The default for post-thoracotomy and other postoperative pain not specified as acute or chronic is the code for the acute form.

   Routine or expected postoperative pain immediately after surgery should not be coded.

   (a) **Postoperative pain not associated with specific postoperative complication**

   Postoperative pain not associated with a specific postoperative complication is assigned to the appropriate postoperative pain code in category 338.

   (b) **Postoperative pain associated with specific postoperative complication**

   Postoperative pain associated with a specific postoperative complication (such as painful suture wires) is assigned to the appropriate code(s) found in Chapter 17, Injury and Poisoning. If appropriate, use additional code(s) from category 338 to identify acute or chronic pain (338.18 or 338.28). If pain control/management is the reason for the encounter, a code from category 338 should be assigned as the principal or first-listed diagnosis in accordance with *Section I.C.6.a.1.a above.*

   (c) **Postoperative pain as principal or first-listed diagnosis**

   Postoperative pain may be reported as the principal or first-listed diagnosis when the stated reason for the admission/encounter is documented as postoperative pain control/management.

(d) Postoperative pain as secondary diagnosis

Postoperative pain may be reported as a secondary diagnosis code when a patient presents for outpatient surgery and develops an unusual or inordinate amount of postoperative pain.

Routine or expected postoperative pain immediately after surgery should not be coded.

The provider's documentation should be used to guide the coding of postoperative pain, as well as *Section III. Reporting Additional Diagnoses* and *Section IV. Diagnostic Coding and Reporting in the Outpatient Setting.*

See Section II.I.2 for information on sequencing of diagnoses for patients admitted to hospital inpatient care following postoperative observation.

See Section II.J for information on sequencing of diagnoses for patients admitted to hospital inpatient care from outpatient surgery.

See Section IV.A.2 for information on sequencing of diagnoses for patients admitted for observation.

4) Chronic pain

Chronic pain is classified to subcategory 338.2. There is no time frame defining when pain becomes chronic pain. The provider's documentation should be used to guide use of these codes.

5) Neoplasm Related Pain

Code 338.3 is assigned to pain documented as being related, associated or due to cancer, primary or secondary malignancy, or tumor. This code is assigned regardless of whether the pain is acute or chronic.

This code may be assigned as the principal or first-listed code when the stated reason for the admission/encounter is documented as pain control/pain management. The underlying neoplasm should be reported as an additional diagnosis.

When the reason for the admission/encounter is management of the neoplasm and the pain associated with the neoplasm is also documented, code 338.3 may be assigned as an additional diagnosis.

See Section I.C.2 for instructions on the sequencing of neoplasms for all other stated reasons for the admission/encounter (except for pain control/pain management).

6) Chronic pain syndrome

This condition is different than the term "chronic pain," and therefore this code should only be used when the provider has specifically documented this condition.

7. Chapter 7: Diseases of Circulatory System (390-459)

a. Hypertension

Hypertension Table

The Hypertension Table, found under the main term, "Hypertension", in the Alphabetic Index, contains a complete listing of all conditions due to or associated with hypertension and classifies them according to malignant, benign, and unspecified.

1) **Hypertension, Essential, or NOS**

   Assign hypertension (arterial) (essential) (primary) (systemic) (NOS) to category code 401 with the appropriate fourth digit to indicate malignant (.0), benign (.1), or unspecified (.9). Do not use either .0 malignant or .1 benign unless medical record documentation supports such a designation.

2) **Hypertension with Heart Disease**

   Heart conditions (425.8, 429.0-429.3, 429.8, 429.9) are assigned to a code from category 402 when a causal relationship is stated (due to hypertension) or implied (hypertensive). Use an additional code from category 428 to identify the type of heart failure in those patients with heart failure. More than one code from category 428 may be assigned if the patient has systolic or diastolic failure and congestive heart failure.

   The same heart conditions (425.8, 429.0-429.3, 429.8, 429.9) with hypertension, but without a stated causal relationship, are coded separately. Sequence according to the circumstances of the admission/encounter.

3) **Hypertensive Chronic Kidney Disease**

   Assign codes from category 403, Hypertensive chronic kidney disease, when conditions classified to **category** 585 are present. Unlike hypertension with heart disease, ICD-9-CM presumes a cause-and-effect relationship and classifies chronic kidney disease (CKD) with hypertension as hypertensive chronic kidney disease.

   Fifth digits for category 403 should be assigned as follows:

   - 0 with CKD stage I through stage IV, or unspecified.
   - 1 with CKD stage V or end stage renal disease. The appropriate code from category 585, Chronic kidney disease, should be used as a secondary code with a code from category 403 to identify the stage of chronic kidney disease.

   See Section I.C.10.a for information on the coding of chronic kidney disease.

4) **Hypertensive Heart and Chronic Kidney Disease**

   Assign codes from combination category 404, Hypertensive heart and chronic kidney disease, when both hypertensive kidney disease and hypertensive heart disease are stated in the diagnosis. Assume a relationship between the hypertension and the chronic kidney disease, whether or not the condition is so designated. Assign an additional code from category 428, to identify the type of heart failure. More than one code from category 428 may be assigned if the patient has systolic or diastolic failure and congestive heart failure.

Fifth digits for category 404 should be assigned as follows:

- 0 without heart failure and with chronic kidney disease (CKD) stage I through stage IV, or unspecified
- 1 with heart failure and with CKD stage I through stage IV, or unspecified
- 2 without heart failure and with CKD stage V or end stage renal disease
- 3 with heart failure and with CKD stage V or end stage renal disease

The appropriate code from category 585, Chronic kidney disease, should be used as a secondary code with a code from category 404 to identify the stage of kidney disease.

See Section I.C.10.a for information on the coding of chronic kidney disease.

5) Hypertensive Cerebrovascular Disease

First assign codes from 430-438, Cerebrovascular disease, then the appropriate hypertension code from categories 401-405.

6) Hypertensive Retinopathy

Two codes are necessary to identify the condition. First assign the code from subcategory 362.11, Hypertensive retinopathy, then the appropriate code from categories 401-405 to indicate the type of hypertension.

7) Hypertension, Secondary

Two codes are required: one to identify the underlying etiology and one from category 405 to identify the hypertension.

Sequencing of codes is determined by the reason for dmission/encounter.

8) Hypertension, Transient

Assign code 796.2, Elevated blood pressure reading without diagnosis of hypertension, unless patient has an established diagnosis of hypertension. Assign code 642.3x for transient hypertension of pregnancy.

9) Hypertension, Controlled

Assign appropriate code from categories 401-405. This diagnostic statement usually refers to an existing state of hypertension under control by therapy.

10) Hypertension, Uncontrolled

Uncontrolled hypertension may refer to untreated hypertension or hypertension not responding to current therapeutic regimen.

In either case, assign the appropriate code from categories

401-405 to designate the stage and type of hypertension. Code to the type of hypertension.

11) Elevated Blood Pressure

For a statement of elevated blood pressure without further specificity, assign code 796.2, Elevated blood pressure reading without diagnosis of hypertension, rather than a code from category 401.

b. Cerebral infarction/stroke/cerebrovascular accident (CVA)

The terms stroke and CVA are often used interchangeably to refer to a cerebral infarction. The terms stroke, CVA, and cerebral infarction NOS are all indexed to the default code 434.91, Cerebral artery occlusion, unspecified, with infarction. Code 436, Acute, but ill-defined, cerebrovascular disease, should not be used when the documentation states stroke or CVA.

See section I.C.18.d.3 for information on coding status post administration of tPA in a different facility within the last 24 hours.

c. Postoperative cerebrovascular accident

A cerebrovascular hemorrhage or infarction that occurs as a result of medical intervention is coded to 997.02, Iatrogenic cerebrovascular infarction or hemorrhage. Medical record documentation should clearly specify the cause- and-effect relationship between the medical intervention and the cerebrovascular accident in order to assign this code. A secondary code from the code range 430-432 or from a code from subcategories 433 or 434 with a fifth digit of "1" should also be used to identify the type of hemorrhage or infarct.

This guideline conforms to the use additional code note instruction at category 997. Code 436, Acute, but ill-defined, cerebrovascular disease, should not be used as a secondary code with code 997.02.

d. Late Effects of Cerebrovascular Disease

1) Category 438, Late Effects of Cerebrovascular disease

Category 438 is used to indicate conditions classifiable to categories 430-437 as the causes of late effects (neurologic deficits), themselves classified elsewhere. These "late effects" include neurologic deficits that persist after initial onset of conditions classifiable to 430-437. The neurologic deficits caused by cerebrovascular disease may be present from the onset or may arise at any time after the onset of the condition classifiable to 430-437.

2) Codes from category 438 with codes from 430-437

Codes from category 438 may be assigned on a health care record with codes from 430-437, if the patient has a current cerebrovascular accident (CVA) and deficits from an old CVA.

3) Code V12.54

Assign code V12.**54, Transient ischemic attack (TIA), and cerebral infarction without residual deficits** (and not a code from category 438) as an additional code for history of cerebrovascular disease when no neurologic deficits are present.

e. **Acute myocardial infarction (AMI)**

1) **ST elevation myocardial infarction (STEMI) and non ST elevation myocardial infarction (NSTEMI)**

   The ICD-9-CM codes for acute myocardial infarction (AMI) identify the site, such as anterolateral wall or true posterior wall. Subcategories 410.0-410.6 and 410.8 are used for ST elevation myocardial infarction (STEMI). Subcategory 410.7, Subendocardial infarction, is used for non ST elevation myocardial infarction (NSTEMI) and nontransmural MIs.

2) **Acute myocardial infarction, unspecified**

   Subcategory 410.9 is the default for the unspecified term acute myocardial infarction. If only STEMI or transmural MI without the site is documented, query the provider as to the site, or assign a code from subcategory 410.9.

3) **AMI documented as nontransmural or subendocardial but site provided**

   If an AMI is documented as nontransmural or subendocardial, but the site is provided, it is still coded as a subendocardial AMI. If NSTEMI evolves to STEMI, assign the STEMI code. If STEMI converts to NSTEMI due to thrombolytic therapy, it is still coded as STEMI.

See section I.C.18.d.3 for information on coding status post administration of tPA in a different facility within the last 24 hours.

8. **Chapter 8: Diseases of Respiratory System (460-519)**

   a. **Chronic Obstructive Pulmonary Disease [COPD] and Asthma**

   See I.C.17.f ventilator-associated pneumonia.

   1) **Conditions that comprise COPD and Asthma**

      The conditions that comprise COPD are obstructive chronic bronchitis, subcategory 491.2, and emphysema, category 492. All asthma codes are under category 493, Asthma. Code 496, Chronic airway obstruction, not elsewhere classified, is a nonspecific code that should only be used when the documentation in a medical record does not specify the type of COPD being treated.

   2) **Acute exacerbation of chronic obstructive bronchitis and asthma**

      The codes for chronic obstructive bronchitis and asthma distinguish between uncomplicated cases and those in acute exacerbation. An acute exacerbation is a worsening or a decompensation of a chronic condition. An acute exacerbation is not equivalent to an infection superimposed on a chronic condition, though an exacerbation may be triggered by an infection.

   3) **Overlapping nature of the conditions that comprise COPD and asthma**

      Due to the overlapping nature of the conditions that make up COPD and asthma, there are many variations in the way these conditions are documented. Code selection must be based on the terms as documented. When selecting the correct code for the documented type of COPD and asthma, it is essential to first review the index, and then verify the code in the tabular list. There are many instructional notes under the different COPD subcategories and codes. It is important that all such notes be reviewed to assure correct code assignment.

4) Acute exacerbation of asthma and status asthmaticus

An acute exacerbation of asthma is an increased severity of the asthma symptoms, such as wheezing and shortness of breath. Status asthmaticus refers to a patient's failure to respond to therapy administered during an asthmatic episode and is a life threatening complication that requires emergency care. If status asthmaticus is documented by the provider with any type of COPD or with acute bronchitis, the status asthmaticus should be sequenced first. It supersedes any type of COPD including that with acute exacerbation or acute bronchitis. It is inappropriate to assign an asthma code with 5th digit 2, with acute exacerbation, together with an asthma code with 5th digit 1, with status asthmatics. Only the 5th digit 1 should be assigned.

b. Chronic Obstructive Pulmonary Disease [COPD] and Bronchitis

1) Acute bronchitis with COPD

Acute bronchitis, code 466.0, is due to an infectious organism. When acute bronchitis is documented with COPD, code 491.22, Obstructive chronic bronchitis with acute bronchitis, should be assigned. It is not necessary to also assign code 466.0. If a medical record documents acute bronchitis with COPD with acute exacerbation, only code 491.22 should be assigned. The acute bronchitis included in code 491.22 supersedes the acute exacerbation. If a medical record documents COPD with acute exacerbation without mention of acute bronchitis, only code 491.21 should be assigned.

c. Acute Respiratory Failure

1) Acute respiratory failure as principal diagnosis

Code 518.81, Acute respiratory failure, may be assigned as a principal diagnosis when it is the condition established after study to be chiefly responsible for occasioning the admission to the hospital, and the selection is supported by the Alphabetic Index and Tabular List. However, chapter-specific coding guidelines (such as obstetrics, poisoning, HIV, newborn) that provide sequencing direction take precedence.

2) Acute respiratory failure as secondary diagnosis

Respiratory failure may be listed as a secondary diagnosis if it occurs after admission, or if it is present on admission, but does not meet the definition of principal diagnosis.

3) Sequencing of acute respiratory failure and another acute condition

When a patient is admitted with respiratory failure and another acute condition, (e.g., myocardial infarction, cerebrovascular accident, aspiration pneumonia), the principal diagnosis will not be the same in every situation. **This applies whether the other acute condition is a respiratory or nonrespiratory condition.** Selection of the principal diagnosis will be dependent on the circumstances of admission. If both the respiratory failure and the other acute condition are equally responsible for occasioning the admission to the hospital, and there are no chapter-specific sequencing rules, the guideline regarding two or more diagnoses that equally meet the definition for principal diagnosis *(Section II, C.)* may be applied in these situations.

If the documentation is not clear as to whether acute respiratory failure and another condition are equally responsible for occasioning the admission, query the provider for clarification.

d. Influenza due to identified avian influenza virus (avian influenza)

Code only confirmed cases of avian influenza. This is an exception to the hospital inpatient guideline Section II, H. (Uncertain Diagnosis).

In this context, "confirmation" does not require documentation of positive laboratory testing specific for avian influenza. However, coding should be based on the provider's diagnostic statement that the patient has avian influenza.

If the provider records "suspected or possible or probable avian influenza," the appropriate influenza code from category 487 should be assigned. Code 488, Influenza due to identified avian influenza virus, should not be assigned.

9. Chapter 9: Diseases of Digestive System (520-579)

Reserved for future guideline expansion

10. Chapter 10: Diseases of Genitourinary System (580-629)

a. Chronic kidney disease

1) Stages of chronic kidney disease (CKD)

The ICD-9-CM classifies CKD based on severity. The severity of CKD is designated by stages I–V. Stage II, code 585.2, equates to mild CKD; stage III, code 585.3, equates to moderate CKD; and stage IV, code 585.4, equates to severe CKD. Code 585.6, End stage renal disease (ESRD), is assigned when the provider has documented end-stage-renal disease (ESRD).

If both a stage of CKD and ESRD are documented, assign code 585.6 only.

2) Chronic kidney disease and kidney transplant status

Patients who have undergone kidney transplant may still have some form of CKD, because the kidney transplant may not fully restore kidney function. Therefore, the presence of CKD alone does not constitute a transplant complication. Assign the appropriate 585 code for the patient's stage of CKD and code V42.0. If a transplant complication such as failure or rejection is documented, see section I.C.17.f.**2**.b for information on coding complications of a kidney transplant. If the documentation is unclear as to whether the patient has a complication of the transplant, query the provider.

3) Chronic kidney disease with other conditions

Patients with CKD may also suffer from other serious conditions, most commonly diabetes mellitus and hypertension. The sequencing of the CKD code in relationship to codes for other contributing conditions is based on the conventions in the tabular list.

See I.C.3.a.4 for sequencing instructions for diabetes.

See I.C.4.a.1 for anemia in CKD.

See I.C.7.a.3 for hypertensive chronic kidney disease.

See I.C.17.f.2.b, Kidney transplant complications, for instructions on coding of documented rejection or failure.

11. Chapter 11: Complications of Pregnancy, Childbirth, and the Puerperium (630-679)

a. General Rules for Obstetric Cases

1) Codes from chapter 11 and sequencing priority

Obstetric cases require codes from chapter 11, codes in the range 630-679, Complications of Pregnancy, Childbirth, and the Puerperium. Chapter 11 codes have sequencing priority over codes from other chapters. Additional codes from other chapters may be used in conjunction with chapter 11 codes to further specify conditions. Should the provider document that the pregnancy is incidental to the encounter, then code V22.2 should be used in place of any chapter 11 codes. It is the provider's responsibility to state that the condition being treated is not affecting the pregnancy.

2) Chapter 11 codes used only on the maternal record

Chapter 11 codes are to be used only on the maternal record, never on the record of the newborn.

3) Chapter 11 fifth-digits

Categories 640-648, 651-676 have required fifth-digits, which indicate whether the encounter is antepartum, postpartum and whether a delivery has also occurred.

4) Fifth-digits, appropriate for each code

The fifth-digits, which are appropriate for each code number, are listed in brackets under each code. The fifth-digits on each code should all be consistent with each other. That is, should a delivery occur all of the fifth-digits should indicate the delivery.

b. Selection of OB Principal or First-listed Diagnosis

1) Routine outpatient prenatal visits

For routine outpatient prenatal visits when no complications are present codes V22.0, Supervision of normal first pregnancy, and V22.1, Supervision of other normal pregnancy, should be used as the first-listed diagnoses. These codes should not be used in conjunction with chapter 11 codes.

2) Prenatal outpatient visits for high-risk patients

For prenatal outpatient visits for patients with high-risk pregnancies, a code from category V23, Supervision of high-risk pregnancy, should be used as the principal or first-listed diagnosis. Secondary chapter 11 codes may be used in conjunction with these codes if appropriate.

3) Episodes when no delivery occurs

In episodes when no delivery occurs, the principal diagnosis should correspond to the principal complication of the pregnancy, which necessitated the encounter. Should more than one complication exist, all of which are treated or monitored, any of the complications codes may be sequenced first.

4) When a delivery occurs

When a delivery occurs, the principal diagnosis should correspond to the main circumstances or complication of the delivery. In cases of cesarean delivery, the selection of the principal diagnosis should correspond to the reason the cesarean delivery was performed unless the reason for admission/encounter was unrelated to the condition resulting in the cesarean delivery.

5) Outcome of delivery

An outcome of delivery code, V27.0-V27.9, should be included on every maternal record when a delivery has occurred. These codes are not to be used on subsequent records or on the newborn record.

c. Fetal Conditions Affecting the Management of the Mother

1) Codes from category 655

Known or suspected fetal abnormality affecting management of the mother, and category 656, Other fetal and placental problems affecting the management of the mother, are assigned only when the fetal condition is actually responsible for modifying the management of the mother, i.e., by requiring diagnostic studies, additional observation, special care, or termination of pregnancy. The fact that the fetal condition exists does not justify assigning a code from this series to the mother's record.

See I.C.18.d for suspected maternal and fetal conditions not found.

2) In utero surgery

In cases when surgery is performed on the fetus, a diagnosis code from category 655, Known or suspected fetal abnormalities affecting management of the mother, should be assigned identifying the fetal condition. Procedure code 75.36, Correction of fetal defect, should be assigned on the hospital inpatient record.

No code from Chapter 15, the perinatal codes, should be used on the mother's record to identify fetal conditions. Surgery performed in utero on a fetus is still to be coded as an obstetric encounter.

d. HIV Infection in Pregnancy, Childbirth and the Puerperium

During pregnancy, childbirth or the puerperium, a patient admitted because of an HIV-related illness should receive a principal diagnosis of 647.6X, Other specified infectious and parasitic diseases in the mother classifiable elsewhere, but complicating the pregnancy, childbirth or the puerperium, followed by 042 and the code(s) for the HIV-related illness(es).

Patients with asymptomatic HIV infection status admitted during pregnancy, childbirth, or the puerperium should receive codes of 647.6X and V08.

e. **Current Conditions Complicating Pregnancy**

Assign a code from subcategory 648.x for patients that have current conditions when the condition affects the management of the pregnancy, childbirth, or the puerperium. Use additional secondary codes from other chapters to identify the conditions, as appropriate.

f. **Diabetes mellitus in pregnancy**

Diabetes mellitus is a significant complicating factor in pregnancy. Pregnant women who are diabetic should be assigned code 648.0x, Diabetes mellitus complicating pregnancy, and a secondary code from category 250, Diabetes mellitus, **or category 249, Secondary diabetes** to identify the type of diabetes.

Code V58.67, Long-term (current) use of insulin, should also be assigned if the diabetes mellitus is being treated with insulin.

g. **Gestational diabetes**

Gestational diabetes can occur during the second and third trimester of pregnancy in women who were not diabetic prior to pregnancy. Gestational diabetes can cause complications in the pregnancy similar to those of pre-existing diabetes mellitus. It also puts the woman at greater risk of developing diabetes after the pregnancy. Gestational diabetes is coded to 648.8x, Abnormal glucose tolerance. Codes 648.0x and 648.8x should never be used together on the same record.

Code V58.67, Long-term (current) use of insulin, should also be assigned if the gestational diabetes is being treated with insulin.

h. **Normal Delivery, Code 650**

1) **Normal delivery**

    Code 650 is for use in cases when a woman is admitted for a full-term normal delivery and delivers a single, healthy infant without any complications antepartum, during the delivery, or postpartum during the delivery episode. Code 650 is always a principal diagnosis. It is not to be used if any other code from chapter 11 is needed to describe a current complication of the antenatal, delivery, or perinatal period. Additional codes from other chapters may be used with code 650 if they are not related to or are in any way complicating the pregnancy.

2) **Normal delivery with resolved antepartum complication**

    Code 650 may be used if the patient had a complication at some point during her pregnancy, but the complication is not present at the time of the admission for delivery.

3) **V27.0, Single liveborn, outcome of delivery**

    V27.0, Single liveborn, is the only outcome of delivery code appropriate for use with 650.

i. **The Postpartum and Peripartum Periods**

1) **Postpartum and peripartum periods**

   The postpartum period begins immediately after delivery and continues for six weeks following delivery. The peripartum period is defined as the last month of pregnancy to five months postpartum.

2) **Postpartum complication**

   A postpartum complication is any complication occurring within the six-week period.

3) **Pregnancy-related complications after 6 week period**

   Chapter 11 codes may also be used to describe pregnancy-related complications after the six-week period should the provider document that a condition is pregnancy related.

4) **Postpartum complications occurring during the same admission as delivery**

   Postpartum complications that occur during the same admission as the delivery are identified with a fifth digit of "2." Subsequent admissions/encounters for postpartum complications should be identified with a fifth digit of "4."

5) **Admission for routine postpartum care following delivery outside hospital**

   When the mother delivers outside the hospital prior to admission and is admitted for routine postpartum care and no complications are noted, code V24.0, Postpartum care and examination immediately after delivery, should be assigned as the principal diagnosis.

6) **Admission following delivery outside hospital with postpartum conditions**

   A delivery diagnosis code should not be used for a woman who has delivered prior to admission to the hospital. Any postpartum conditions and/or postpartum procedures should be coded.

j. **Code 677, Late effect of complication of pregnancy**

1) **Code 677**

   Code 677, Late effect of complication of pregnancy, childbirth, and the puerperium is for use in those cases when an initial complication of a pregnancy develops a sequelae requiring care or treatment at a future date.

2) **After the initial postpartum period**

   This code may be used at any time after the initial postpartum period.

3) **Sequencing of Code 677**

   This code, like all late effect codes, is to be sequenced following the code describing the sequelae of the complication.

Appendix A ICD-9-CM Official Guidelines for Coding and Reporting

k. Abortions

1) **Fifth-digits required for abortion categories**

   Fifth-digits are required for abortion categories 634-637. Fifth-digit 1, incomplete, indicates that all of the products of conception have not been expelled from the uterus. Fifth-digit 2, complete, indicates that all products of conception have been expelled from the uterus.

2) **Code from categories 640-648 and 651-659**

   A code from categories 640-648 and 651-659 may be used as additional codes with an abortion code to indicate the complication leading to the abortion.

   Fifth digit 3 is assigned with codes from these categories when used with an abortion code because the other fifth digits will not apply. Codes from the 660-669 series are not to be used for complications of abortion.

3) **Code 639 for complications**

   Code 639 is to be used for all complications following abortion. Code 639 cannot be assigned with codes from categories 634-638.

4) **Abortion with Liveborn Fetus**

   When an attempted termination of pregnancy results in a liveborn fetus assign code 644.21, Early onset of delivery, with an appropriate code from category V27, Outcome of Delivery. The procedure code for the attempted termination of pregnancy should also be assigned.

5) **Retained Products of Conception following an abortion**

   Subsequent admissions for retained products of conception following a spontaneous or legally induced abortion are assigned the appropriate code from category 634, Spontaneous abortion, or 635 Legally induced abortion, with a fifth digit of "1" (incomplete). This advice is appropriate even when the patient was discharged previously with a discharge diagnosis of complete abortion.

12. Chapter 12: Diseases Skin and Subcutaneous Tissue (680-709)

a. **Pressure ulcer stage codes**

   1) **Pressure ulcer stages**

      Two codes are needed to completely describe a pressure ulcer: A code from subcategory 707.0, Pressure ulcer, to identify the site of the pressure ulcer and a code from subcategory 707.2, Pressure ulcer stages.

      The codes in subcategory 707.2, Pressure ulcer stages, are to be used as an additional diagnosis with a code(s) from subcategory 707.0, Pressure Ulcer. Codes from 707.2, Pressure ulcer stages, may not be assigned as a principal or first-listed diagnosis. The pressure ulcer stage codes should only be used with pressure ulcers and not with other types of ulcers (e.g., stasis ulcer).

The ICD-9-CM classifies pressure ulcer stages based on severity, which is designated by stages I-IV and unstageable.

2) **Unstageable pressure ulcers**

   Assignment of code 707.25, Pressure ulcer, unstageable, should be based on the clinical documentation. Code 707.25 is used for pressure ulcers whose stage cannot be clinically determined (e.g., the ulcer is covered by eschar or has been treated with a skin or muscle graft) and pressure ulcers that are documented as deep tissue injury but not documented as due to trauma. This code should not be confused with code 707.20, Pressure ulcer, stage unspecified. Code 707.20 should be assigned when there is no documentation regarding the stage of the pressure ulcer.

3) **Documented pressure ulcer stage**

   Assignment of the pressure ulcer stage code should be guided by clinical documentation of the stage or documentation of the terms found in the index. For clinical terms describing the stage that are not found in the index, and there is no documentation of the stage, the provider should be queried.

4) **Bilateral pressure ulcers with same stage**

   When a patient has bilateral pressure ulcers (e.g., both buttocks) and both pressure ulcers are documented as being the same stage, only the code for the site and one code for the stage should be reported.

5) **Bilateral pressure ulcers with different stages**

   When a patient has bilateral pressure ulcers at the same site (e.g., both buttocks) and each pressure ulcer is documented as being at a different stage, assign one code for the site and the appropriate codes for the pressure ulcer stage.

6) **Multiple pressure ulcers of different sites and stages**

   When a patient has multiple pressure ulcers at different sites (e.g., buttock, heel, shoulder) and each pressure ulcer is documented as being at different stages (e.g., stage 3 and stage 4), assign the appropriate codes for each different site and a code for each different pressure ulcer stage.

7) **Patients admitted with pressure ulcers documented as healed**

   No code is assigned if the documentation states that the pressure ulcer is completely healed.

8) **Patients admitted with pressure ulcers documented as healing**

   Pressure ulcers described as healing should be assigned the appropriate pressure ulcer stage code based on the documentation in the medical record. If the documentation does not provide information about the stage of the healing pressure ulcer, assign code 707.20, Pressure ulcer stage, unspecified.

If the documentation is unclear as to whether the patient has a current (new) pressure ulcer or if the patient is being treated for a healing pressure ulcer, query the provider.

9) **Patient admitted with pressure ulcer evolving into another stage during the admission**

If a patient is admitted with a pressure ulcer at one stage and it progresses to a higher stage, assign the code for highest stage reported for that site.

13. **Chapter 13: Diseases of Musculoskeletal and Connective Tissue (710-739)**

   a. **Coding of Pathologic Fractures**

   1) **Acute Fractures vs. Aftercare**

   Pathologic fractures are reported using subcategory 733.1, when the fracture is newly diagnosed. Subcategory 733.1 may be used while the patient is receiving active treatment for the fracture. Examples of active treatment are: surgical treatment, emergency department encounter, evaluation and treatment by a new physician.

   Fractures are coded using the aftercare codes (subcategories V54.0, V54.2, V54.8 or V54.9) for encounters after the patient has completed active treatment of the fracture and is receiving routine care for the fracture during the healing or recovery phase. Examples of
   fracture aftercare are: cast change or removal, removal of external or internal fixation device, medication adjustment, and follow up visits following fracture treatment.

   Care for complications of surgical treatment for fracture repairs during the healing or recovery phase should be coded with the appropriate complication codes.

   Care of complications of fractures, such as malunion and nonunion, should be reported with the appropriate codes.

   See Section I. C. 17.b for information on the coding of traumatic fractures.

14. **Chapter 14: Congenital Anomalies (740-759)**

   a. **Codes in categories 740-759, Congenital Anomalies**

   Assign an appropriate code(s) from categories 740-759, Congenital Anomalies, when an anomaly is documented. A congenital anomaly may be the principal/first listed diagnosis on a record or a secondary diagnosis.

   When a congenital anomaly does not have a unique code assignment, assign additional code(s) for any manifestations that may be present. When the code assignment specifically identifies the congenital anomaly, manifestations that are an inherent component of the anomaly should not be coded separately. Additional codes should be assigned for manifestations that are not an inherent component.

Codes from Chapter 14 may be used throughout the life of the patient. If a congenital anomaly has been corrected, a personal history code should be used to identify the history of the anomaly. Although present at birth, a congenital anomaly may not be identified until later in life. Whenever the condition is diagnosed by the physician, it is appropriate to assign a code from codes 740-759.

For the birth admission, the appropriate code from category V30, Liveborn infants, according to type of birth should be sequenced as the principal diagnosis, followed by any congenital anomaly codes, 740759.

15. Chapter 15: Newborn (Perinatal) Guidelines (760-779)

For coding and reporting purposes the perinatal period is defined as before birth through the 28th day following birth. The following guidelines are provided for reporting purposes. Hospitals may record other diagnoses as needed for internal data use.

a. General Perinatal Rules

1) Chapter 15 Codes

They are <u>never</u> for use on the maternal record. Codes from Chapter 11, the obstetric chapter, are never permitted on the newborn record. Chapter 15 code may be used throughout the life of the patient if the condition is still present.

2) Sequencing of perinatal codes

Generally, codes from Chapter 15 should be sequenced as the principal/first-listed diagnosis on the newborn record, with the exception of the appropriate V30 code for the birth episode, followed by codes from any other chapter that provide additional detail. The "use additional code" note at the beginning of the chapter supports this guideline. If the index does not provide a specific code for a perinatal condition, assign code 779.89, Other specified conditions originating in the perinatal period, followed by the code from another chapter that specifies the condition. Codes for signs and symptoms may be assigned when a definitive diagnosis has not been established.

3) Birth process or community acquired conditions

If a newborn has a condition that may be either due to the birth process or community acquired and the documentation does not indicate which it is, the default is due to the birth process and the code from Chapter 15 should be used. If the condition is community-acquired, a code from Chapter 15 should not be assigned.

4) Code all clinically significant conditions

All clinically significant conditions noted on routine newborn examination should be coded. A condition is clinically significant if it requires:

- clinical evaluation; or
- therapeutic treatment; or

- diagnostic procedures; or
- extended length of hospital stay; or
- increased nursing care and/or monitoring; or
- has implications for future health care needs

Note: The perinatal guidelines listed above are the same as the general coding guidelines for "additional diagnoses", except for the final point regarding implications for future health care needs. Codes should be assigned for conditions that have been specified by the provider as having implications for future health care needs. Codes from the perinatal chapter should not be assigned unless the provider has established a definitive diagnosis.

b. Use of codes V30-V39

When coding the birth of an infant, assign a code from categories V30-V39, according to the type of birth. A code from this series is assigned as a principal diagnosis, and assigned only once to a newborn at the time of birth.

c. Newborn transfers

If the newborn is transferred to another institution, the V30 series is not used at the receiving hospital.

d. Use of category V29

1) **Assigning a code from category V29**

   Assign a code from category V29, Observation and evaluation of newborns and infants for suspected conditions not found, to identify those instances when a healthy newborn is evaluated for a suspected condition that is determined after study not to be present. Do not use a code from category V29 when the patient has identified signs or symptoms of a suspected problem; in such cases, code the sign or symptom.

   A code from category V29 may also be assigned as a principal code for readmissions or encounters when the V30 code no longer applies. Codes from category V29 are for use only for healthy newborns and infants for which no condition after study is found to be present.

2) **V29 code on a birth record**

   A V29 code is to be used as a secondary code after the V30, Outcome of delivery, code.

e. Use of other V codes on perinatal records

V codes other than V30 and V29 may be assigned on a perinatal or newborn record code. The codes may be used as a principal or first-listed diagnosis for specific types of encounters or for readmissions or encounters when the V30 code no longer applies.

See Section I.C.18 for information regarding the assignment of V codes.

f. Maternal Causes of Perinatal Morbidity

Codes from categories 760-763, Maternal causes of perinatal morbidity and mortality, are assigned only when the maternal condition has actually affected the fetus or newborn. The fact that the mother has an associated medical condition or experiences some complication of pregnancy, labor or delivery does not justify the routine assignment of codes from these categories to the newborn record.

g. Congenital Anomalies in Newborns

For the birth admission, the appropriate code from category V30, Liveborn infants according to type of birth, should be used, followed by any congenital anomaly codes, categories 740-759. Use additional secondary codes from other chapters to specify conditions associated with the anomaly, if applicable.

Also, see Section I.C.14 for information on the coding of congenital anomalies.

h. Coding Additional Perinatal Diagnoses

1) Assigning codes for conditions that require treatment

Assign codes for conditions that require treatment or further investigation, prolong the length of stay, or require resource utilization.

2) Codes for conditions specified as having implications for future health care needs

Assign codes for conditions that have been specified by the provider as having implications for future health care needs.

Note: This guideline should not be used for adult patients.

3) Codes for newborn conditions originating in the perinatal period

Assign a code for newborn conditions originating in the perinatal period (categories 760-779), as well as complications arising during the current episode of care classified in other chapters, only if the diagnoses have been documented by the responsible provider at the time of transfer or discharge as having affected the fetus or newborn.

i. Prematurity and Fetal Growth Retardation

Providers utilize different criteria in determining prematurity. A code for prematurity should not be assigned unless it is documented. The 5th digit assignment for codes from category 764 and subcategories 765.0 and 765.1 should be based on the recorded birth weight and estimated gestational age.

A code from subcategory 765.2, Weeks of gestation, should be assigned as an additional code with category 764 and codes from 765.0 and 765.1 to specify weeks of gestation as documented by the provider in the record.

j. Newborn sepsis

Code 771.81, Septicemia [sepsis] of newborn, should be assigned with a secondary code from category 041, Bacterial infections in conditions classified elsewhere and of unspecified site, to identify the organism. A code from category 038, Septicemia, should not be used on a newborn record. **Do not assign code 995.91, Sepsis, as c**ode 771.81 describes the sepsis. **If applicable, use additional codes** to identify severe sepsis (995.92) and any associated acute organ dysfunction.

16. **Chapter 16: Signs, Symptoms and Ill-Defined Conditions (780-799)**

    Reserved for future guideline expansion

17. **Chapter 17: Injury and Poisoning (800-999)**

    a. **Coding of Injuries**

    When coding injuries, assign separate codes for each injury unless a combination code is provided, in which case the combination code is assigned. Multiple injury codes are provided in ICD-9-CM, but should not be assigned unless information for a more specific code is not available. These codes are not to be used for normal, healing surgical wounds or to identify complications of surgical wounds.

    The code for the most serious injury, as determined by the provider and the focus of treatment, is sequenced first.

    1) **Superficial injuries**

        Superficial injuries such as abrasions or contusions are not coded when associated with more severe injuries of the same site.

    2) **Primary injury with damage to nerves/blood vessels**

        When a primary injury results in minor damage to peripheral nerves or blood vessels, the primary injury is sequenced first with additional code(s) from categories 950-957, Injury to nerves and spinal cord, and/or 900-904, Injury to blood vessels. When the primary injury is to the blood vessels or nerves, that injury should be sequenced first.

    b. **Coding of Traumatic Fractures**

    The principles of multiple coding of injuries should be followed in coding fractures. Fractures of specified sites are coded individually by site in accordance with both the provisions within categories 800-829 and the level of detail furnished by medical record content. Combination categories for multiple fractures are provided for use when there is insufficient detail in the medical record (such as trauma cases transferred to another hospital), when the reporting form limits the number of codes that can be used in reporting pertinent clinical data, or when there is insufficient specificity at the fourth-digit or fifth-digit level. More specific guidelines are as follows:

    1) **Acute Fractures vs. Aftercare**

        Traumatic fractures are coded using the acute fracture codes (800-829) while the patient is receiving active treatment for the fracture. Examples of active treatment are: surgical treatment, emergency department encounter, and evaluation and treatment by a new physician.

        Fractures are coded using the aftercare codes (subcategories V54.0, V54.1, V54.8, or V54.9) for encounters after the patient has completed active treatment of the fracture and is receiving routine care for the fracture during the healing or recovery phase. Examples of fracture aftercare are: cast change or removal,

removal of external or internal fixation device, medication adjustment, and follow up visits following fracture treatment.

Care for complications of surgical treatment for fracture repairs during the healing or recovery phase should be coded with the appropriate complication codes.

Care of complications of fractures, such as malunion and nonunion, should be reported with the appropriate codes.

Pathologic fractures are not coded in the 800-829 range, but instead are assigned to subcategory 733.1. *See Section I.C.13.a for additional information.*

2) Multiple fractures of same limb

Multiple fractures of same limb classifiable to the same three-digit or four-digit category are coded to that category.

3) Multiple unilateral or bilateral fractures of same bone

Multiple unilateral or bilateral fractures of same bone(s) but classified to different fourth-digit subdivisions (bone part) within the same three-digit category are coded individually by site.

4) Multiple fracture categories 819 and 828

Multiple fracture categories 819 and 828 classify bilateral fractures of both upper limbs (819) and both lower limbs (828), but without any detail at the fourth-digit level other than open and closed type of fractures.

5) Multiple fractures sequencing

Multiple fractures are sequenced in accordance with the severity of the fracture. The provider should be asked to list the fracture diagnoses in the order of severity.

c. Coding of Burns

Current burns (940-948) are classified by depth, extent and by agent (E code). Burns are classified by depth as first degree (erythema), second degree (blistering), and third degree (full-thickness involvement).

1) Sequencing of burn and related condition codes

Sequence first the code that reflects the highest degree of burn when more than one burn is present.

a. When the reason for the admission or encounter is for treatment of external multiple burns, sequence first the code that reflects the burn of the highest degree.

b. When a patient has both internal and external burns, the circumstances of admission govern the selection of the principal diagnosis or first-listed diagnosis.

c. When a patient is admitted for burn injuries and other related conditions such as smoke inhalation and/or respiratory failure, the circumstances of admission govern the selection of the principal or first-listed diagnosis.

2) **Burns of the same local site**

Classify burns of the same local site (three-digit category level, 940-947) but of different degrees to the subcategory identifying the highest degree recorded in the diagnosis.

3) **Non-healing burns**

Non-healing burns are coded as acute burns.

Necrosis of burned skin should be coded as a non-healed burn.

4) **Code 958.3, Posttraumatic wound infection**

Assign code 958.3, Posttraumatic wound infection, not elsewhere classified, as an additional code for any documented infected burn site.

5) **Assign separate codes for each burn site**

When coding burns, assign separate codes for each burn site. Category 946 Burns of Multiple specified sites, should only be used if the location of the burns are not documented. Category 949, Burn, unspecified, is extremely vague and should rarely be used.

6) **Assign codes from category 948, Burns**

Burns classified according to extent of body surface involved, when the site of the burn is not specified or when there is a need for additional data. It is advisable to use category 948 as additional coding when needed to provide data for evaluating burn mortality, such as that needed by burn units. It is also advisable to use category 948 as an additional code for reporting purposes when there is mention of a third-degree burn involving 20 percent or more of the body surface.

In assigning a code from category 948:

Fourth-digit codes are used to identify the percentage of total body surface involved in a burn (all degree).

Fifth-digits are assigned to identify the percentage of body surface involved in third-degree burn.

Fifth-digit zero (0) is assigned when less than 10 percent or when no body surface is involved in a third-degree burn.

Category 948 is based on the classic "rule of nines" in estimating body surface involved: head and neck are assigned nine percent, each arm nine percent, each leg 18 percent, the anterior trunk 18 percent, posterior trunk 18 percent, and genitalia one percent. Providers may change these percentage assignments where necessary to accommodate infants and children who have proportionately larger heads than adults and patients who have large buttocks, thighs, or abdomen that involve burns.

7) **Encounters for treatment of late effects of burns**

Encounters for the treatment of the late effects of burns (i.e., scars or joint contractures) should be coded to the residual condition (sequelae) followed by the appropriate late effect code (906.5-906.9). A late effect E code may also be used, if desired.

8) **Sequelae with a late effect code and current burn**

When appropriate, both a sequelae with a late effect code, and a current burn code may be assigned on the same record (when both a current burn and sequelae of an old burn exist).

d. **Coding of Debridement of Wound, Infection, or Burn**

Excisional debridement involves surgical removal or cutting away, as opposed to a mechanical (brushing, scrubbing, washing) debridement.

For coding purposes, excisional debridement is assigned to code 86.22.

Nonexcisional debridement is assigned to code 86.28.

e. **Adverse Effects, Poisoning and Toxic Effects**

The properties of certain drugs, medicinal and biological substances or combinations of such substances, may cause toxic reactions. The occurrence of drug toxicity is classified in ICD-9-CM as follows:

1) **Adverse Effect**

When the drug was correctly prescribed and properly administered, code the reaction plus the appropriate code from the E930-E949 series. Codes from the E930-E949 series must be used to identify the causative substance for an adverse effect of drug, medicinal and biological substances, correctly prescribed and properly administered. The effect, such as tachycardia, delirium, gastrointestinal hemorrhaging, vomiting, hypokalemia, hepatitis, renal failure, or respiratory failure, is coded and followed by the appropriate code from the E930-E949 series.

Adverse effects of therapeutic substances correctly prescribed and properly administered (toxicity, synergistic reaction, side effect, and idiosyncratic reaction) may be due to (1) differences among patients, such as age, sex, disease, and genetic factors, and (2) drug-related factors, such as type of drug, route of administration, duration of therapy, dosage, and bioavailability.

2) **Poisoning**

(a) **Error was made in drug prescription**

Errors made in drug prescription or in the administration of the drug by provider, nurse, patient, or other person, use the appropriate poisoning code from the 960-979 series.

(b) **Overdose of a drug intentionally taken**

If an overdose of a drug was intentionally taken or administered and resulted in drug toxicity, it would be coded as a poisoning (960-979 series).

(c) **Nonprescribed drug taken with correctly prescribed and properly administered drug**

If a nonprescribed drug or medicinal agent was taken in combination with a correctly prescribed and properly administered drug, any drug toxicity or other reaction resulting from the interaction of the two drugs would be classified as a poisoning.

(d) Interaction of drug(s) and alcohol

When a reaction results from the interaction of a drug(s) and alcohol, this would be classified as poisoning.

(e) Sequencing of poisoning

When coding a poisoning or reaction to the improper use of a medication (e.g., wrong dose, wrong substance, wrong route of administration) the poisoning code is sequenced first, followed by a code for the manifestation. If there is also a diagnosis of drug abuse or dependence to the substance, the abuse or dependence is coded as an additional code.

See Section I.C.3.a.6.b. if poisoning is the result of insulin pump malfunctions and Section I.C.19 for general use of E-codes.

3) Toxic Effects

(a) Toxic effect codes

When a harmful substance is ingested or comes in contact with a person, this is classified as a toxic effect. The toxic effect codes are in categories 980-989.

(b) Sequencing toxic effect codes

A toxic effect code should be sequenced first, followed by the code(s) that identify the result of the toxic effect.

(c) External cause codes for toxic effects

An external cause code from categories E860-E869 for accidental exposure, codes E950.6 or E950.7 for intentional self-harm, category E962 for assault, or categories E980-E982, for undetermined, should also be assigned to indicate intent.

f. Complications of care

1) Complications of care

(a) Documentation of complications of care

As with all procedural or postprocedural complications, code assignment is based on the provider's documentation of the relationship between the condition and the procedure.

2) Transplant complications

(a) Transplant complications other than kidney

Codes under subcategory 996.8, Complications of transplanted organ, are for use for both complications and rejection of transplanted organs. A transplant complication code is only assigned if the complication affects the function of the transplanted organ. Two codes are required to fully describe a transplant complication, the appropriate code from subcategory 996.8 and a secondary code that identifies the complication.

Pre-existing conditions or conditions that develop after the transplant are not coded as complications unless they affect the function of the transplanted organs.

See I.C.18.d.3) for transplant organ removal status.

See I.C.2.c for malignant neoplasm associated with transplanted organ.

(b) **Chronic kidney disease and kidney transplant complications**

Patients who have undergone kidney transplant may still have some form of chronic kidney disease (CKD) because the kidney transplant may not fully restore kidney function. Code 996.81 should be assigned for documented complications of a kidney transplant, such as transplant failure or rejection **or other transplant complication**. Code 996.81 should not be assigned for post kidney transplant patients who have chronic kidney (CKD) unless a transplant complication such as transplant failure or rejection is documented. If the documentation is unclear as to whether the patient has a complication of the transplant, query the provider.

For patients with CKD following a kidney transplant, but who do not have a complication such as failure or rejection, *see section I.C.10.a.2, Chronic kidney disease and kidney transplant status.*

3) **Ventilator associated pneumonia**

(a) **Documentation of Ventilator associated Pneumonia**

As with all procedural or postprocedural complications, code assignment is based on the provider's documentation of the relationship between the condition and the procedure.

Code 997.31, Ventilator associated pneumonia, should be assigned only when the provider has documented ventilator associated pneumonia (VAP). An additional code to identify the organism (e.g., Pseudomonas aeruginosa, code 041.7) should also be assigned. Do not assign an additional code from categories 480-484 to identify the type of pneumonia.

Code 997.31 should not be assigned for cases where the patient has pneumonia and is on a mechanical ventilator but the provider has not specifically stated that the pneumonia is ventilator-associated pneumonia.

If the documentation is unclear as to whether the patient has a pneumonia that is a complication attributable to the mechanical ventilator, query the provider.

(b) **Patient admitted with pneumonia and develops VAP**

A patient may be admitted with one type of pneumonia (e.g., code 481, Pneumococcal pneumonia) and subsequently develop VAP. In this instance, the principal diagnosis would be the

appropriate code from categories 480-484 for the pneumonia diagnosed at the time of admission. Code 997.31, Ventilator associated pneumonia, would be assigned as an additional diagnosis when the provider has also documented the presence of ventilator associated pneumonia.

g. SIRS due to Non-infectious Process

The systemic inflammatory response syndrome (SIRS) can develop as a result of certain non-infectious disease processes, such as trauma, malignant neoplasm, or pancreatitis. When SIRS is documented with a noninfectious condition, and no subsequent infection is documented, the code for the underlying condition, such as an injury, should be assigned, followed by code 995.93, Systemic inflammatory response syndrome due to noninfectious process without acute organ dysfunction, or 995.94, Systemic inflammatory response syndrome due to non-infectious process with acute organ dysfunction. If an acute organ dysfunction is documented, the appropriate code(s) for the associated acute organ dysfunction(s) should be assigned in addition to code 995.94. If acute organ dysfunction is documented, but it cannot be determined if the acute organ dysfunction is associated with SIRS or due to another condition (e.g., directly due to the trauma), the provider should be queried.

When the non-infectious condition has led to an infection that results in SIRS, *see Section I.C.1.b.12 for the guideline for sepsis and severe sepsis associated with a non-infectious process.*

18. Classification of Factors Influencing Health Status and Contact with Health Service (Supplemental V01-V84)

Note: The chapter specific guidelines provide additional information about the use of V codes for specified encounters.

a. Introduction

ICD-9-CM provides codes to deal with encounters for circumstances other than a disease or injury. The Supplementary Classification of Factors Influencing Health Status and Contact with Health Services (V01.0-V84.8) is provided to deal with occasions when circumstances other than a disease or injury (codes 001-999) are recorded as a diagnosis or problem.

There are four primary circumstances for the use of V codes:

1) A person who is not currently sick encounters the health services for some specific reason, such as to act as an organ donor, to receive prophylactic care, such as inoculations or health screenings, or to receive counseling on health related issues.

2) A person with a resolving disease or injury, or a chronic, long-term condition requiring continuous care, encounters the health care system for specific aftercare of that disease or injury (e.g., dialysis for renal disease; chemotherapy for malignancy; cast change). A diagnosis/symptom code should be used whenever a current, acute, diagnosis is being treated or a sign or symptom is being studied.

3) Circumstances or problems influence a person's health status but are not in themselves a current illness or injury.

4) Newborns, to indicate birth status

b. V codes use in any healthcare setting

V codes are for use in any healthcare setting. V codes may be used as either a first listed (principal diagnosis code in the inpatient setting) or secondary code, depending on the circumstances of the encounter. Certain V codes may only be used as first listed, others only as secondary codes.

See Section I.C.18.e, V Code Table.

c. V Codes indicate a reason for an encounter

They are not procedure codes. A corresponding procedure code must accompany a V code to describe the procedure performed.

d. Categories of V Codes

1) **Contact/Exposure**

Category V01 indicates contact with or exposure to communicable diseases. These codes are for patients who do not show any sign or symptom of a disease but have been exposed to it by close personal contact with an infected individual or are in an area where a disease is epidemic. These codes may be used as a first listed code to explain an encounter for testing, or, more commonly, as a secondary code to identify a potential risk.

2) **Inoculations and vaccinations**

Categories V03-V06 are for encounters for inoculations and vaccinations. They indicate that a patient is being seen to receive a prophylactic inoculation against a disease. The injection itself must be represented by the appropriate procedure code. A code from V03-V06 may be used as a secondary code if the inoculation is given as a routine part of preventive health care, such as a well-baby visit.

3) **Status**

Status codes indicate that a patient is either a carrier of a disease or has the sequelae or residual of a past disease or condition. This includes such things as the presence of prosthetic or mechanical devices resulting from past treatment. A status code is informative, because the status may affect the course of treatment and its outcome. A status code is distinct from a history code. The history code indicates that the patient no longer has the condition.

A status code should not be used with a diagnosis code from one of the body system chapters, if the diagnosis code includes the information provided by the status code. For example, code V42.1, Heart transplant status, should not be used with code 996.83, Complications of transplanted heart. The status code does not provide additional information. The complication code indicates that the patient is a heart transplant patient.

Appendix A ICD-9-CM Official Guidelines for Coding and Reporting

The status V codes/categories are:

V02 Carrier or suspected carrier of infectious diseases

Carrier status indicates that a person harbors the specific organisms of a disease without manifest symptoms and is capable of transmitting the infection.

V07.5X **Prophylactic use of agents affecting estrogen receptors and estrogen level**

This code indicates when a patient is receiving a drug that affects estrogen receptors and estrogen levels for prevention of cancer.

V08 Asymptomatic HIV infection status

This code indicates that a patient has tested positive for HIV but has manifested no signs or symptoms of the disease.

V09 Infection with drug-resistant microorganisms

This category indicates that a patient has an infection that is resistant to drug treatment.

Sequence the infection code first.

V21 Constitutional states in development

V22.2 Pregnant state, incidental

This code is a secondary code only for use when the pregnancy is in no way complicating the reason for visit. Otherwise, a code from the obstetric chapter is required.

V26.5x Sterilization status

V42 Organ or tissue replaced by transplant

V43 Organ or tissue replaced by other means

V44 Artificial opening status

V45 Other postsurgical states

Assign code V45.87, Transplant organ removal status, to indicate that a transplanted organ has been previously removed. This code should not be assigned for the encounter in which the transplanted organ is removed. The complication necessitating removal of the transplant organ should be assigned for that encounter.

See section I.C17.f.2. for information on the coding of organ transplant complications.

Assign code V45.88, Status post administration of tPA (rtPA) in a different facility within the last 24 hours prior to admission to the current facility, as a secondary diagnosis when a patient is received by transfer into a facility and documentation indicates they were administered

tissue plasminogen activator (tPA) within the last 24 hours prior to admission to the current facility.

This guideline applies even if the patient is still receiving the tPA at the time they are received into the current facility.

The appropriate code for the condition for which the tPA was administered (such as cerebrovascular disease or myocardial infarction) should be assigned first.

Code V45.88 is only applicable to the receiving facility record and not to the transferring facility record.

V46 Other dependence on machines

V49.6 Upper limb amputation status

V49.7 Lower limb amputation status

Note: Categories V42-V46, and subcategories V49.6, V49.7 are for use only if there are no complications or malfunctions of the organ or tissue replaced, the amputation site or the equipment on which the patient is dependent.

V49.81 Postmenopausal status

V49.82 Dental sealant status

V49.83 Awaiting organ transplant status

V58.6x Long-term (current) drug use

Codes from this subcategory indicates a patient's continuous use of a prescribed drug (including such things as aspirin therapy) for the long-term treatment of a condition or for prophylactic use. It is not for use for patients who have addictions to drugs. **This subcategory is not for use of medications for detoxification or maintenance programs to prevent withdrawal symptoms in patients with drug dependence (e.g., methadone maintenance for opiate dependence). Assign the appropriate code for the drug dependence instead.**

Assign a code from subcategory V58.6, Long-term (current) drug use, if the patient is receiving a medication for an extended period as a prophylactic **measure (such as for the prevention of deep vein thrombosis) or as treatment of a chronic condition (such as arthritis) or a disease requiring a lengthy course of treatment (such as cancer). Do not assign a code from subcategory V58.6 for medication being administered for a brief period of time to treat an acute illness or injury (such as a course of antibiotics to treat acute bronchitis).**

V83 Genetic carrier status

Genetic carrier status indicates that a person carries a gene, associated with a particular disease, which may be passed to offspring who may develop that disease. The person does not have the disease and is not at risk of developing the disease.

V84 Genetic susceptibility status

Genetic susceptibility indicates that a person has a gene that increases the risk of that person developing the disease.

Codes from category V84, Genetic susceptibility to disease, should not be used as principal or first-listed codes. If the patient has the condition to which he/she is susceptible, and that condition is the reason for the encounter, the code for the current condition should be sequenced first. If the patient is being seen for follow-up after completed treatment for this condition, and the condition no longer exists, a follow-up code should be sequenced first, followed by the appropriate personal history and genetic susceptibility codes. If the purpose of the encounter is genetic counseling associated with procreative management, a code from subcategory V26.3, Genetic counseling and testing, should be assigned as the first-listed code, followed by a code from category V84. Additional codes should be assigned for any applicable family or personal history.

See Section I.C. 18.d.14 for information on prophylactic organ removal due to a genetic susceptibility.

V86 Estrogen receptor status

V88 Acquired absence of other organs and tissue

4) History (of)

There are two types of history V codes, personal and family. Personal history codes explain a patient's past medical condition that no longer exists and is not receiving any treatment, but that has the potential for recurrence, and therefore may require continued monitoring. The exceptions to this general rule are category V14, Personal history of allergy to medicinal agents, and subcategory V15.0, Allergy, other than to medicinal agents. A person who has had an allergic episode to a substance or food in the past should always be considered allergic to the substance.

Family history codes are for use when a patient has a family member(s) who has had a particular disease that causes the patient to be at higher risk of also contracting the disease.

Personal history codes may be used in conjunction with follow-up codes and family history codes may be used in conjunction with screening codes to explain the need for a test or procedure. History codes are also acceptable on any medical record regardless of the reason for visit. A history of an illness, even if no longer present, is important information that may alter the type of treatment ordered.

The history V code categories are:

V10 Personal history of malignant neoplasm

V12 Personal history of certain other diseases

V13 Personal history of other diseases

>Except: V13.4, Personal history of arthritis, and V13.6, Personal history of congenital malformations. These conditions are life-long so are not true history codes.

V14 Personal history of allergy to medicinal agents

V15 Other personal history presenting hazards to health

>Except: V15.7, Personal history of contraception.

V16 Family history of malignant neoplasm

V17 Family history of certain chronic disabling diseases

V18 Family history of certain other specific diseases

V19 Family history of other conditions

V87 Other specified personal exposures and history presenting hazards to health

5) Screening

Screening is the testing for disease or disease precursors in seemingly well individuals so that early detection and treatment can be provided for those who test positive for the disease. Screenings that are recommended for many subgroups in a population include: routine mammograms for women over 40, a fecal occult blood test for everyone over 50, an amniocentesis to rule out a fetal anomaly for pregnant women over 35, because the incidence of breast cancer and colon cancer in these subgroups is higher than in the general population, as is the incidence of Down's syndrome in older mothers.

The testing of a person to rule out or confirm a suspected diagnosis because the patient has some sign or symptom is a diagnostic examination, not a screening. In these cases, the sign or symptom is used to explain the reason for the test.

A screening code may be a first listed code if the reason for the visit is specifically the screening exam. It may also be used as an additional code if the screening is done during an office visit for other health problems. A screening code is not necessary if the screening is inherent to a routine examination, such as a pap smear done during a routine pelvic examination.

Should a condition be discovered during the screening then the code for the condition may be assigned as an additional diagnosis.

The V code indicates that a screening exam is planned. A procedure code is required to confirm that the screening was performed.

The screening V code categories:

V28   Antenatal screening

V73-V82   Special screening examinations

6) Observation

There are **three** observation V code categories. They are for use in very limited circumstances when a person is being observed for a suspected condition that is ruled out. The observation codes are not for use if an injury or illness or any signs or symptoms related to the suspected condition are present. In such cases the diagnosis/symptom code is used with the corresponding E code to identify any external cause.

The observation codes are to be used as principal diagnosis only. The only exception to this is when the principal diagnosis is required to be a code from the V30, Live born infant, category. Then the V29 observation code is sequenced after the V30 code. Additional codes may be used in addition to the observation code but only if they are unrelated to the suspected condition being observed.

Codes from subcategory V89.0, Suspected maternal and fetal conditions not found, may either be used as a first listed or as an additional code assignment depending on the case. They are for use in very limited circumstances on a maternal record when an encounter is for a suspected maternal or fetal condition that is ruled out during that encounter (for example, a maternal or fetal condition may be suspected due to an abnormal test result). These codes should not be used when the condition is confirmed. In those cases, the confirmed condition should be coded. In addition, these codes are not for use if an illness or any signs or symptoms related to the suspected condition or problem are present. In such cases the diagnosis/symptom code is used.

Additional codes may be used in addition to the code from subcategory V89.0, but only if they are unrelated to the suspected condition being evaluated.

Codes from subcategory V89.0 may not be used for encounters for antenatal screening of mother. *See Section I.C.18.d., Screening).*

For encounters for suspected fetal condition that are inconclusive following testing and evaluation, assign the appropriate code from category 655, 656, 657 or 658.

The observation V code categories:

V29 Observation and evaluation of newborns for suspected condition not found

   For the birth encounter, a code from category V30 should be sequenced before the V29 code.

V71 Observation and evaluation for suspected condition not found

V89 Suspected maternal and fetal conditions not found

7) Aftercare

Aftercare visit codes cover situations when the initial treatment of a disease or injury has been performed and the patient requires continued care during the healing or recovery phase, or for the long-term consequences of the disease. The aftercare V code should not be used if treatment is directed at a current, acute disease or injury. The diagnosis code is to be used in these cases. Exceptions to this rule are codes V58.0, Radiotherapy, and codes from subcategory V58.1, Encounter for chemotherapy and immunotherapy for neoplastic conditions. These codes are to be first listed, followed by the diagnosis code when a patient's encounter is solely to receive radiation therapy or chemotherapy for the treatment of a neoplasm. Should a patient receive both chemotherapy and radiation therapy during the same encounter code V58.0 and V58.1 may be used together on a record with either one being sequenced first.

The aftercare codes are generally first listed to explain the specific reason for the encounter. An aftercare code may be used as an additional code when some type of aftercare is provided in addition to the reason for admission and no diagnosis code is applicable. An example of this would be the closure of a colostomy during an encounter for treatment of another condition.

Aftercare codes should be used in conjunction with any other aftercare codes or other diagnosis codes to provide better detail on the specifics of an aftercare encounter visit, unless otherwise directed by the classification. The sequencing of multiple aftercare codes is discretionary.

Certain aftercare V code categories need a secondary diagnosis code to describe the resolving condition or sequelae, for others, the condition is inherent in the code title.

Additional V code aftercare category terms include, fitting and adjustment, and attention to artificial openings.

Status V codes may be used with aftercare V codes to indicate the nature of the aftercare. For example code V45.81, Aortocoronary bypass status, may be used with code V58.73, Aftercare following surgery of the circulatory system, NEC, to indicate the surgery for which the aftercare is being performed. Also, a transplant status code may be used following code V58.44, Aftercare following organ transplant, to identify the organ transplanted. A status code should not be used when the aftercare code indicates the type of status, such as using V55.0, Attention to tracheostomy with V44.0, Tracheostomy status.

See Section I. B.16 Admissions/Encounter for Rehabilitation

The aftercare V category/codes:

V51   **Encounter for breast reconstruction following mastectomy**

V52   Fitting and adjustment of prosthetic device and implant

Appendix A ICD-9-CM Official Guidelines for Coding and Reporting

V53	Fitting and adjustment of other device
V54	Other orthopedic aftercare
V55	Attention to artificial openings
V56	Encounter for dialysis and dialysis catheter care
V57	Care involving the use of rehabilitation procedures
V58.0	Radiotherapy
V58.11	Encounter for antineoplastic chemotherapy
V58.12	Encounter for antineoplastic immunotherapy
V58.3x	Attention to dressings and sutures
V58.41	Encounter for planned post-operative wound closure
V58.42	Aftercare, surgery, neoplasm
V58.43	Aftercare, surgery, trauma
V58.44	Aftercare involving organ transplant
V58.49	Other specified aftercare following surgery
V58.7x	Aftercare following surgery
V58.81	Fitting and adjustment of vascular catheter
V58.82	Fitting and adjustment of non-vascular catheter
V58.83	Monitoring therapeutic drug
V58.89	Other specified aftercare

8) Follow-up

The follow-up codes are used to explain continuing surveillance following completed treatment of a disease, condition, or injury. They imply that the condition has been fully treated and no longer exists. They should not be confused with aftercare codes that explain current treatment for a healing condition or its sequelae. Follow-up codes may be used in conjunction with history codes to provide the full picture of the healed condition and its treatment. The follow-up code is sequenced first, followed by the history code.

A follow-up code may be used to explain repeated visits. Should a condition be found to have recurred on the follow-up visit, then the diagnosis code should be used in place of the follow-up code.

The follow-up V code categories:

V24	Postpartum care and evaluation
V67	Follow-up examination

9) Donor

Category V59 is the donor codes. They are used for living individuals who are donating blood or other body tissue. These codes are only for individuals donating for others, not for self donations. They are not for use to identify cadaveric donations.

10) Counseling

Counseling V codes are used when a patient or family member receives assistance in the aftermath of an illness or injury, or when support is required in coping with family or social problems. They are not necessary for use in conjunction with a diagnosis code when the counseling component of care is considered integral to standard treatment.

The counseling V categories/codes:

V25.0 General counseling and advice for contraceptive management

V26.3 Genetic counseling

V26.4 General counseling and advice for procreative management

V61.**X** Other family circumstances

V65.1 Person consulted on behalf of another person

V65.3 Dietary surveillance and counseling

V65.4 Other counseling, not elsewhere classified

11) Obstetrics and related conditions

See Section I.C.11., the Obstetrics guidelines for further instruction on the use of these codes.

V codes for pregnancy are for use in those circumstances when none of the problems or complications included in the codes from the Obstetrics chapter exist (a routine prenatal visit or postpartum care). Codes V22.0, Supervision of normal first pregnancy, and V22.1, Supervision of other normal pregnancy, are always first listed and are not to be used with any other code from the OB chapter.

The outcome of delivery, category V27, should be included on all maternal delivery records. It is always a secondary code.

V codes for family planning (contraceptive) or procreative management and counseling should be included on an obstetric record either during the pregnancy or the postpartum stage, if applicable.

Obstetrics and related conditions V code categories:

V22 Normal pregnancy

V23 Supervision of high-risk pregnancy

    Except: V23.2, Pregnancy with history of abortion. Code 646.3, Habitual aborter, from the OB chapter is required to indicate a history of abortion during a pregnancy.

V24 Postpartum care and evaluation

V25 Encounter for contraceptive management

    Except V25.0x

    (See Section I.C.18.d.11, Counseling)

V26 Procreative management Except V26.5x, Sterilization status, V26.3 and V26.4

(See Section I.C.18.d.11., Counseling)

V27 Outcome of delivery

V28 Antenatal screening

(See Section I.C.18.d.6., Screening)

12) Newborn, infant and child

See Section I.C.15, the Newborn guidelines for further instruction on the use of these codes.

Newborn V code categories:

V20 Health supervision of infant or child

V29 Observation and evaluation of newborns for suspected condition not found

(See Section I.C.18.d.7, Observation)

V30-V39 Liveborn infant according to type of birth

13) Routine and administrative examinations

The V codes allow for the description of encounters for routine examinations, such as, a general check-up, or, examinations for administrative purposes, such as, a pre-employment physical. The codes are not to be used if the examination is for diagnosis of a suspected condition or for treatment purposes. In such cases the diagnosis code is used. During a routine exam, should a diagnosis or condition be discovered, it should be coded as an additional code. Pre-existing and chronic conditions and history codes may also be included as additional codes as long as the examination is for administrative purposes and not focused on any particular condition.

Pre-operative examination V codes are for use only in those situations when a patient is being cleared for surgery and no treatment is given.

The V codes categories/code for routine and administrative examinations:

V20.2 Routine infant or child health check

Any injections given should have a corresponding procedure code.

V70 General medical examination

V72 Special investigations and examinations

Codes V72.5 and V72.6 may be used if the reason for the patient encounter is for routine laboratory/radiology testing in the absence of any signs, symptoms, or associated diagnosis. If routine testing is performed during the same encounter as a test to evaluate a sign, symptom, or diagnosis, it is appropriate to assign both the V code and the code describing the reason for the non-routine test.

Appendix A ICD-9-CM Official Guidelines for Coding and Reporting

14) Miscellaneous V codes

The miscellaneous V codes capture a number of other health care encounters that do not fall into one of the other categories. Certain of these codes identify the reason for the encounter, others are for use as additional codes that provide useful information on circumstances that may affect a patient's care and treatment.

Prophylactic Organ Removal

For encounters specifically for prophylactic removal of breasts, ovaries, or another organ due to a genetic susceptibility to cancer or a family history of cancer, the principal or first listed code should be a code from subcategory V50.4, Prophylactic organ removal, followed by the appropriate genetic susceptibility code and the appropriate family history code.

If the patient has a malignancy of one site and is having prophylactic removal at another site to prevent either a new primary malignancy or metastatic disease, a code for the malignancy should also be assigned in addition to a code from subcategory V50.4. A V50.4 code should not be assigned if the patient is having organ removal for treatment of a malignancy, such as the removal of the testes for the treatment of prostate cancer.

Miscellaneous V code categories/codes:

V07   Need for isolation and other prophylactic measures

Except for V07.5, Prophylactic use of agents affecting estrogen receptors and estrogen levels

V50   Elective surgery for purposes other than remedying health states

V58.5 Orthodontics

V60   Housing, household, and economic circumstances

V62   Other psychosocial circumstances

V63   Unavailability of other medical facilities for care

V64   Persons encountering health services for specific procedures, not carried out

V66   Convalescence and Palliative Care

V68   Encounters for administrative purposes

V69   Problems related to lifestyle

V85   Body Mass Index

15) Nonspecific V codes

Certain V codes are so non-specific, or potentially redundant with other codes in the classification, that there can be little justification for their use in the inpatient setting. Their use in the outpatient setting should be limited to those instances when there is no further documentation to permit more precise coding. Otherwise, any sign or symptom or any other reason for visit that is captured in another code should be used.

Appendix A ICD-9-CM Official Guidelines for Coding and Reporting

Nonspecific V code categories/codes:

V11   Personal history of mental disorder A code from the mental disorders chapter, with an in remission fifth-digit, should be used.

V13.4   Personal history of arthritis

V13.6   Personal history of congenital malformations

V15.7   Personal history of contraception

V23.2   Pregnancy with history of abortion

V40   Mental and behavioral problems

V41   Problems with special senses and other special functions

V47   Other problems with internal organs

V48   Problems with head, neck, and trunk

V49   Problems with limbs and other problems

Exceptions:

     V49.6   Upper limb amputation status

     V49.7   Lower limb amputation status

     V49.81   Postmenopausal status

     V49.82   Dental sealant status

     V49.83   Awaiting organ transplant status

V51.**8**   **Other a**ftercare involving the use of plastic surgery

V58.2   Blood transfusion, without reported diagnosis

V58.9   Unspecified aftercare

See Section IV.K. and Section IV.L. of the Outpatient guidelines.

Appendix A   ICD-9-CM Official Guidelines for Coding and Reporting

V CODE TABLE

October 1, 2008 (FY2009)

Items in bold indicate a new entry or change from the October 2007 table Items underlined have been moved within the table since November 2006

The V code table below contains columns for 1st listed, 1st or additional, additional only, and non-specific. Each code or category is listed in the left hand column and the allowable sequencing of the code or codes within the category is noted under the appropriate column.

As indicated by the footnote in the "1st Dx Only" column, the V codes designated as first-listed only are generally intended to be limited for use as a first-listed only diagnosis, but may be reported as an additional diagnosis in those situations when the patient has more than one encounter on a single day and the codes for the multiple encounters are combined, or when there is more than one V code that meets the definition of principal diagnosis (e.g., a patient is admitted to home healthcare for both aftercare and rehabilitation and they equally meet the definition of principal diagnosis). The V codes designated as first-listed only should not be reported if they do not meet the definition of principal or first-listed diagnosis.

See Section II and Section IV.A for information on selection of principal and first-listed diagnosis.

See Section II.C for information on two or more diagnoses that equally meet the definition for principal diagnosis.

Code(s)	Description	1st Dx Only[1]	1st or Add'l Dx[2]	Add'l Dx Only[3]	Non-Specific Diagnosis[4]
V01.X	Contact with or exposure to communicable diseases		X		
V02.X	Carrier or suspected carrier of infectious diseases		X		
V03.X	Need for prophylactic vaccination and inoculation against bacterial diseases		X		
V04.X	Need for prophylactic vaccination and inoculation against certain diseases		X		
V05.X	Need for prophylactic vaccination and inoculation against single diseases		X		
V06.X	Need for prophylactic vaccination and inoculation against combinations of diseases		X		
V07.0	**Isolation**		X		
V07.1	**Desensitization to allergens**		X		
V07.2	**Prophylactic immunotherapy**		X		
V07.3X	**Other prophylactic chemotherapy**		X		
V07.4	Hormone replacement therapy (postmenopausal)			X	
V07.5X	**Prophylactic use of agents affecting estrogen receptors and estrogen levels**			X	
V07.8	**Other specified prophylactic measure**		X		
V07.9	**Unspecified prophylactic measure**				X
V08	Asymptomatic HIV infection status		X		
V09.X	Infection with drug resistant organisms			X	
V10.X	Personal history of malignant neoplasm		X		

[1]Generally for use as first listed only but may be used as additional if patient has more than one encounter on one day or there is more than one reason for the encounter
[2]These codes may be used as first listed or additional codes
[3]These codes are only for use as additional codes
[4]These codes are primarily for use in the nonacute setting and should be limited to encounters for which no sign or symptom or reason for visit is documented in the record. Their use may be as either a first listed or additional code.

Appendix A ICD-9-CM Official Guidelines for Coding and Reporting

Code(s)	Description	1st Dx Only[1]	1st or Add'l Dx[2]	Add'l Dx Only[3]	Non-Specific Diagnosis[4]
V11.X	Personal history of mental disorder				X
V12.X	Personal history of certain other diseases		X		
V13.0X	Personal history of other disorders of urinary system		X		
V13.1	Personal history of trophoblastic disease		X		
V13.2X	Personal history of other genital system and obstetric disorders		X		
V13.3	Personal history of diseases of skin and subcutaneous tissue		X		
V13.4	Personal history of arthritis				X
V13.5X	Personal history of other musculoskeletal disorders		X		
V13.61	Personal history of hypospadias			X	
V13.69	Personal history of congenital malformations				X
V13.7	Personal history of perinatal problems		X		
V13.8	Personal history of other specified diseases		X		
V13.9	Personal history of unspecified disease				X
V14.X	Personal history of allergy to medicinal agents			X	
V15.0X	Personal history of allergy, other than to medicinal agents			X	
V15.1	Personal history of surgery to heart and great vessels			X	
V15.2X	**Personal history of surgery to other organs**			**X**	
V15.3	Personal history of irradiation			X	
V15.4X	Personal history of psychological trauma			X	
V15.5X	Personal history of injury			X	
V15.6	Personal history of poisoning			X	
V15.7	Personal history of contraception				X
V15.81	Personal history of noncompliance with medical treatment			X	
V15.82	Personal history of tobacco use			X	
V15.84	Personal history of exposure to asbestos			X	
V15.85	Personal history of exposure to potentially hazardous body fluids			X	
V15.86	Personal history of exposure to lead			X	
V15.87	Personal history of extracorporeal membrane oxygenation [ECMO]			X	
V15.88	History of fall		X		
V15.89	Other specified personal history presenting hazards to health			X	
V16.X	Family history of malignant neoplasm		X		
V17.X	Family history of certain chronic disabling diseases		X		
V18.X	Family history of certain other specific conditions		X		
V19.X	Family history of other conditions		X		
V20.X	Health supervision of infant or child	X			
V21.X	Constitutional states in development			X	
V22.0	Supervision of normal first pregnancy	X			
V22.1	Supervision of other normal pregnancy	X			
V22.2	Pregnancy state, incidental			X	
V23.X	Supervision of high-risk pregnancy		X		
V24.X	Postpartum care and examination	X			
V25.X	Encounter for contraceptive management		X		
V26.0	Tuboplasty or vasoplasty after previous sterilization		X		

[1]Generally for use as first listed only but may be used as additional if patient has more than one encounter on one day or there is more than one reason for the encounter
[2]These codes may be used as first listed or additional codes
[3]These codes are only for use as additional codes
[4]These codes are primarily for use in the nonacute setting and should be limited to encounters for which no sign or symptom or reason for visit is documented in the record. Their use may be as either a first listed or additional code.

Appendix A   ICD-9-CM Official Guidelines for Coding and Reporting

Code(s)	Description	1st Dx Only[1]	1st or Add'l Dx[2]	Add'l Dx Only[3]	Non-Specific Diagnosis[4]
V26.1	Artificial insemination		X		
V26.2X	Procreative management investigation and testing		X		
V26.3X	Procreative management, genetic counseling and testing		X		
V26.4X	Procreative management, genetic counseling and advice		X		
V26.5X	Procreative management, sterilization status			X	
V26.81	Encounter for assisted reproductive fertility procedure cycle	X			
V26.89	Other specified procreative management		X		
V26.9	Unspecified procreative management		X		
V27.X	Outcome of delivery			X	
V28.X	Encounter for antenatal screening of mother		X		
V29.X	Observation and evaluation of newborns for suspected condition not found		X		
V30.X	Single liveborn	X			
V31.X	Twin, mate liveborn	X			
V32.X	Twin, mate stillborn	X			
V33.X	Twin, unspecified	X			
V34.X	Other multiple, mates all liveborn	X			
V35.X	Other multiple, mates all stillborn	X			
V36.X	Other multiple, mates live- and stillborn	X			
V37.X	Other multiple, unspecified	X			
V39.X	Unspecified	X			
V40.X	Mental and behavioral problems				X
V41.X	Problems with special senses and other special functions				X
V42.X	Organ or tissue replaced by transplant			X	
V43.0	Organ or tissue replaced by other means, eye globe			X	
V43.1	Organ or tissue replaced by other means, lens			X	
V43.21	Organ or tissue replaced by other means, heart assist device			X	
V43.22	Fully implantable artificial heart status		X		
V43.3	Organ or tissue replaced by other means, heart valve			X	
V43.4	Organ or tissue replaced by other means, blood vessel			X	
V43.5	Organ or tissue replaced by other means, bladder			X	
V43.6X	Organ or tissue replaced by other means, joint			X	
V43.7	Organ or tissue replaced by other means, limb			X	
V43.8X	Other organ or tissue replaced by other means			X	
V44.X	Artificial opening status			X	
V45.0X	Cardiac device in situ			X	
V45.1X	Renal dialysis status			X	
V45.2	Presence of cerebrospinal fluid drainage device			X	
V45.3	Intestinal bypass or anastomosis status			X	
V45.4	Arthrodesis status			X	
V45.5X	Presence of contraceptive device			X	
V45.6X	States following surgery of eye and adnexa			X	

[1]Generally for use as first listed only but may be used as additional if patient has more than one encounter on one day or there is more than one reason for the encounter
[2]These codes may be used as first listed or additional codes
[3]These codes are only for use as additional codes
[4]These codes are primarily for use in the nonacute setting and should be limited to encounters for which no sign or symptom or reason for visit is documented in the record. Their use may be as either a first listed or additional code.

Appendix A ICD-9-CM Official Guidelines for Coding and Reporting

Code(s)	Description	1st Dx Only[1]	1st or Add'l Dx[2]	Add'l Dx Only[3]	Non-Specific Diagnosis[4]
V45.7X	Acquired absence of organ		X		
V45.8X	Other postprocedural status			X	
V46.0	Other dependence on machines, aspirator			X	
V46.11	Dependence on respiratory, status			X	
V46.12	Encounter for respirator dependence during power failure	X			
V46.13	Encounter for weaning from respirator [ventilator]	X			
V46.14	Mechanical complication of respirator [ventilator]		X		
V46.2	Other dependence on machines, supplemental oxygen			X	
V46.3	**Wheelchair dependence**			X	
V46.8	Other dependence on other enabling machines			X	
V46.9	Unspecified machine dependence				X
V47.X	Other problems with internal organs				X
V48.X	Problems with head, neck and trunk				X
V49.0	Deficiencies of limbs				X
V49.1	Mechanical problems with limbs				X
V49.2	Motor problems with limbs				X
V49.3	Sensory problems with limbs				X
V49.4	Disfigurements of limbs				X
V49.5	Other problems with limbs				X
V49.6X	Upper limb amputation status		X		
V49.7X	Lower limb amputation status		X		
V49.81	Asymptomatic postmenopausal status (age-related) (natural)		X		
V49.82	Dental sealant status			X	
V49.83	Awaiting organ transplant status			X	
V49.84	Bed confinement status		X		
V49.85	Dual sensory impairment			X	
V49.89	Other specified conditions influencing health status		X		
V49.9	Unspecified condition influencing health status				X
V50.X	Elective surgery for purposes other than remedying health states		X		
V51.0	**Encounter for breast reconstruction following mastectomy**	X			
V51.8	**Other aftercare involving the use of plastic surgery**				X
V52.X	Fitting and adjustment of prosthetic device and implant		X		
V53.X	Fitting and adjustment of other device		X		
V54.X	Other orthopedic aftercare		X		
V55.X	Attention to artificial openings		X		
V56.0	Extracorporeal dialysis	X			
V56.1	Encounter for fitting and adjustment of extracorporeal dialysis catheter		X		
V56.2	Encounter for fitting and adjustment of peritoneal dialysis catheter		X		
V56.3X	Encounter for adequacy testing for dialysis		X		
V56.8	Encounter for other dialysis and dialysis catheter care		X		

[1]Generally for use as first listed only but may be used as additional if patient has more than one encounter on one day or there is more than one reason for the encounter
[2]These codes may be used as first listed or additional codes
[3]These codes are only for use as additional codes
[4]These codes are primarily for use in the nonacute setting and should be limited to encounters for which no sign or symptom or reason for visit is documented in the record. Their use may be as either a first listed or additional code.

Appendix A ICD-9-CM Official Guidelines for Coding and Reporting

Code(s)	Description	1st Dx Only[1]	1st or Add'l Dx[2]	Add'l Dx Only[3]	Non-Specific Diagnosis[4]
V57.X	Care involving use of rehabilitation procedures	X			
V58.0	Radiotherapy	X			
V58.11	Encounter for antineoplastic chemotherapy	X			
V58.12	Encounter for antineoplastic immunotherapy	X			
V58.2	Blood transfusion without reported diagnosis				X
V58.3X	Attention to dressings and sutures		X		
V58.4X	Other aftercare following surgery		X		
V58.5	Encounter for orthodontics				X
V58.6X	Long term (current) drug use			X	
V58.7X	Aftercare following surgery to specified body systems, not elsewhere classified		X		
V58.8X	Other specified procedures and aftercare		X		
V58.9	Unspecified aftercare				X
V59.X	Donors	X			
V60.X	Housing, household, and economic circumstances			X	
V61.X	Other family circumstances		X		
V62.X	Other psychosocial circumstances			X	
V63.X	Unavailability of other medical facilities for care		X		
V64.X	Persons encountering health services for specified procedure, not carried out			X	
V65.X	Other persons seeking consultation without complaint or sickness		X		
V66.0	Convalescence and palliative care following surgery	X			
V66.1	Convalescence and palliative care following radiotherapy	X			
V66.2	Convalescence and palliative care following chemotherapy	X			
V66.3	Convalescence and palliative care following psychotherapy and other treatment for mental disorder	X			
V66.4	Convalescence and palliative care following treatment of fracture	X			
V66.5	Convalescence and palliative care following other treatment	X			
V66.6	Convalescence and palliative care following combined treatment	X			
V66.7	Encounter for palliative care			X	
V66.9	Unspecified convalescence	X			
V67.X	Follow-up examination		X		
V68.X	Encounters for administrative purposes	X			
V69.X	Problems related to lifestyle		X		
V70.0	Routine general medical examination at a health care facility	X			
V70.1	General psychiatric examination, requested by the authority	X			
V70.2	General psychiatric examination, other and unspecified	X			
V70.3	Other medical examination for administrative purposes	X			

[1] Generally for use as first listed only but may be used as additional if patient has more than one encounter on one day or there is more than one reason for the encounter
[2] These codes may be used as first listed or additional codes
[3] These codes are only for use as additional codes
[4] These codes are primarily for use in the nonacute setting and should be limited to encounters for which no sign or symptom or reason for visit is documented in the record. Their use may be as either a first listed or additional code.

Appendix A ICD-9-CM Official Guidelines for Coding and Reporting

Code(s)	Description	1st Dx Only[1]	1st or Add'l Dx[2]	Add'l Dx Only[3]	Non-Specific Diagnosis[4]
V70.4	Examination for medicolegal reasons	X			
V70.5	Health examination of defined subpopulations	X			
V70.6	Health examination in population surveys	X			
V70.7	Examination of participant in clinical trial		X		
V70.8	Other specified general medical examinations	X			
V70.9	Unspecified general medical examination	X			
V71.X	Observation and evaluation for suspected conditions not found	X			
V72.0	Examination of eyes and vision		X		
V72.1X	Examination of ears and hearing		X		
V72.2	Dental examination		X		
V72.3X	Gynecological examination		X		
V72.4X	Pregnancy examination or test		X		
V72.5	Radiological examination, NEC		X		
V72.6	Laboratory examination		X		
V72.7	Diagnostic skin and sensitization tests		X		
V72.81	Preoperative cardiovascular examination		X		
V72.82	Preoperative respiratory examination		X		
V72.83	Other specified preoperative examination		X		
V72.84	Preoperative examination, unspecified		X		
V72.85	Other specified examination		X		
V72.86	Encounter for blood typing		X		
V72.9	Unspecified examination				X
V73.X	Special screening examination for viral and chlamydial diseases		X		
V74.X	Special screening examination for bacterial and spirochetal diseases		X		
V75.X	Special screening examination for other infectious diseases		X		
V76.X	Special screening examination for malignant neoplasms		X		
V77.X	Special screening examination for endocrine, nutritional, metabolic and immunity disorders		X		
V78.X	Special screening examination for disorders of blood and blood-forming organs		X		
V79.X	Special screening examination for mental disorders and developmental handicaps		X		
V80.X	Special screening examination for neurological, eye, and ear diseases		X		
V81.X	Special screening examination for cardiovascular, respiratory, and genitourinary diseases		X		
V82.X	Special screening examination for other conditions		X		
V83.X	Genetic carrier status		X		
V84.X	Genetic susceptibility to disease			X	
V85	Body mass index			X	
V86	Estrogen receptor status			X	
V87.0X	**Contact with and (suspected) exposure to hazardous metals**		X		

[1]Generally for use as first listed only but may be used as additional if patient has more than one encounter on one day or there is more than one reason for the encounter
[2]These codes may be used as first listed or additional codes
[3]These codes are only for use as additional codes
[4]These codes are primarily for use in the nonacute setting and should be limited to encounters for which no sign or symptom or reason for visit is documented in the record. Their use may be as either a first listed or additional code.

Code(s)	Description	1st Dx Only[1]	1st or Add'l Dx[2]	Add'l Dx Only[3]	Non-Specific Diagnosis[4]
V87.1X	Contact with and (suspected) exposure to hazardous aromatic compounds		X		
V87.2	Contact with and (suspected) exposure to other potentially hazardous chemicals		X		
V87.3X	Contact with and (suspected) exposure to other potentially hazardous substances		X		
V87.4X	Personal history of drug therapy			X	
V88.0X	Acquired absence of cervix and uterus			X	
V89.0X	Suspected maternal and fetal anomalies not found		X		

[1] Generally for use as first listed only but may be used as additional if patient has more than one encounter on one day or there is more than one reason for the encounter
[2] These codes may be used as first listed or additional codes
[3] These codes are only for use as additional codes
[4] These codes are primarily for use in the nonacute setting and should be limited to encounters for which no sign or symptom or reason for visit is documented in the record. Their use may be as either a first listed or additional code.

19. Supplemental Classification of External Causes of Injury and Poisoning (E-codes, E800-E999)

Introduction: These guidelines are provided for those who are currently collecting E codes in order that there will be standardization in the process. If your institution plans to begin collecting E codes, these guidelines are to be applied. The use of E codes is supplemental to the application of ICD-9-CM diagnosis codes. E codes are never to be recorded as principal diagnoses (first-listed in non-inpatient setting) and are not required for reporting to CMS.

External causes of injury and poisoning codes (E codes) are intended to provide data for injury research and evaluation of injury prevention strategies. E codes capture how the injury or poisoning happened (cause), the intent (unintentional or accidental; or intentional, such as suicide or assault), and the place where the event occurred.

Some major categories of E codes include:

transport accidents

poisoning and adverse effects of drugs, medicinal substances and biologicals

accidental falls

accidents caused by fire and flames

accidents due to natural and environmental factors

late effects of accidents, assaults or self injury

assaults or purposely inflicted injury

suicide or self inflicted injury

These guidelines apply for the coding and collection of E codes from records in hospitals, outpatient clinics, emergency departments, other ambulatory care settings and provider offices, and nonacute care settings, except when other specific guidelines apply.

a. General E Code Coding Guidelines

1) **Used with any code in the range of 001-V89**

   An E code may be used with any code in the range of 001-**V89**, which indicates an injury, poisoning, or adverse effect due to an external cause.

2) **Assign the appropriate E code for all initial treatments**

   Assign the appropriate E code for the initial encounter of an injury, poisoning, or adverse effect of drugs, not for subsequent treatment.

   External cause of injury codes (E-codes) may be assigned while the acute fracture codes are still applicable. *See Section I.C.17.b.1 for coding of acute fractures.*

3) **Use the full range of E codes**

   Use the full range of E codes to completely describe the cause, the intent and the place of occurrence, if applicable, for all injuries, poisonings, and adverse effects of drugs.

4) **Assign as many E codes as necessary**

   Assign as many E codes as necessary to fully explain each cause. If only one E code can be recorded, assign the E code most related to the principal diagnosis.

5) **The selection of the appropriate E code**

   The selection of the appropriate E code is guided by the Index to External Causes, which is located after the alphabetical index to diseases and by Inclusion and Exclusion notes in the Tabular List.

6) **E code can never be a principal diagnosis**

   An E code can never be a principal (first listed) diagnosis.

7) **External cause code(s) with systemic inflammatory response syndrome (SIRS)**

   An external cause code is not appropriate with a code from subcategory 995.9, unless the patient also has an injury, poisoning, or adverse effect of drugs.

b. Place of Occurrence Guideline

Use an additional code from category E849 to indicate the Place of Occurrence for injuries and poisonings. The Place of Occurrence describes the place where the event occurred and not the patient's activity at the time of the event.

Do not use E849.9 if the place of occurrence is not stated.

c. Adverse Effects of Drugs, Medicinal and Biological Substances Guidelines

1) **Do not code directly from the Table of Drugs**

   Do not code directly from the Table of Drugs and Chemicals.

   Always refer back to the Tabular List.

2) **Use as many codes as necessary to describe**

   Use as many codes as necessary to describe completely all drugs, medicinal or biological substances.

3) If the same E code would describe the causative agent

If the same E code would describe the causative agent for more than one adverse reaction, assign the code only once.

4) If two or more drugs, medicinal or biological substances

If two or more drugs, medicinal or biological substances are reported, code each individually unless the combination code is listed in the Table of Drugs and Chemicals. In that case, assign the E code for the combination.

5) When a reaction results from the interaction of a drug(s)

When a reaction results from the interaction of a drug(s) and alcohol, use poisoning codes and E codes for both.

6) If the reporting format limits the number of E codes

If the reporting format limits the number of E codes that can be used in reporting clinical data, code the one most related to the principal diagnosis. Include at least one from each category (cause, intent, place) if possible.

If there are different fourth digit codes in the same three digit category, use the code for "Other specified" of that category. If there is no "Other specified" code in that category, use the appropriate "Unspecified" code in that category.

If the codes are in different three digit categories, assign the appropriate E code for other multiple drugs and medicinal substances.

7) Codes from the E930-E949 series

Codes from the E930-E949 series must be used to identify the causative substance for an adverse effect of drug, medicinal and biological substances, correctly prescribed and properly administered. The effect, such as tachycardia, delirium, gastrointestinal hemorrhaging, vomiting, hypokalemia, hepatitis, renal failure, or respiratory failure, is coded and followed by the appropriate code from the E930-E949 series.

d. Multiple Cause E Code Coding Guidelines

If two or more events cause separate injuries, an E code should be assigned for each cause. The first listed E code will be selected in the following order:

E codes for child and adult abuse take priority over all other E codes.

See Section I.C.19.e., Child and Adult abuse guidelines.

E codes for terrorism events take priority over all other E codes except child and adult abuse

E codes for cataclysmic events take priority over all other E codes except child and adult abuse and terrorism.

E codes for transport accidents take priority over all other E codes except cataclysmic events and child and adult abuse and terrorism.

The first-listed E code should correspond to the cause of the most serious diagnosis due to an assault, accident, or self-harm, following the order of hierarchy listed above.

e. **Child and Adult Abuse Guideline**

1) **Intentional injury**

    When the cause of an injury or neglect is intentional child or adult abuse, the first listed E code should be assigned from categories E960-E968, Homicide and injury purposely inflicted by other persons, (except category E967). An E code from category E967, Child and adult battering and other maltreatment, should be added as an additional code to identify the perpetrator, if known.

2) **Accidental intent**

    In cases of neglect when the intent is determined to be accidental E code E904.0, Abandonment or neglect of infant and helpless person, should be the first listed E code.

f. **Unknown or Suspected Intent Guideline**

1) **If the intent (accident, self-harm, assault) of the cause of an injury or poisoning is unknown**

    If the intent (accident, self-harm, assault) of the cause of an injury or poisoning is unknown or unspecified, code the intent as undetermined E980-E989.

2) **If the intent (accident, self-harm, assault) of the cause of an injury or poisoning is questionable**

    If the intent (accident, self-harm, assault) of the cause of an injury or poisoning is questionable, probable or suspected, code the intent as undetermined E980-E989.

g. **Undetermined Cause**

    When the intent of an injury or poisoning is known, but the cause is unknown, use codes: E928.9, Unspecified accident, E958.9, Suicide and self-inflicted injury by unspecified means, and E968.9, Assault by unspecified means.

    These E codes should rarely be used, as the documentation in the medical record, in both the inpatient outpatient and other settings, should normally provide sufficient detail to determine the cause of the injury.

h. **Late Effects of External Cause Guidelines**

1) **Late effect E codes**

    Late effect E codes exist for injuries and poisonings but not for adverse effects of drugs, misadventures and surgical complications.

2) **Late effect E codes (E929, E959, E969, E977, E989, or E999.1)**

    A late effect E code (E929, E959, E969, E977, E989, or E999.1) should be used with any report of a late effect or sequela resulting from a previous injury or poisoning (905-909).

3) Late effect E code with a related current injury

A late effect E code should never be used with a related current nature of injury code.

4) Use of late effect E codes for subsequent visits

Use a late effect E code for subsequent visits when a late effect of the initial injury or poisoning is being treated. There is no late effect E code for adverse effects of drugs. Do not use a late effect E code for subsequent visits for follow-up care (e.g., to assess healing, to receive rehabilitative therapy) of the injury or poisoning when no late effect of the injury has been documented.

i. Misadventures and Complications of Care Guidelines

1) Code range E870-E876

Assign a code in the range of E870-E876 if misadventures are stated by the provider.

2) Code range E878-E879

Assign a code in the range of E878-E879 if the provider attributes an abnormal reaction or later complication to a surgical or medical procedure, but does not mention misadventure at the time of the procedure as the cause of the reaction.

j. Terrorism Guidelines

1) Cause of injury identified by the Federal Government (FBI) as terrorism

When the cause of an injury is identified by the Federal Government (FBI) as terrorism, the first-listed E-code should be a code from category E979, Terrorism. The definition of terrorism employed by the FBI is found at the inclusion note at E979. The terrorism E-code is the only E-code that should be assigned. Additional E codes from the assault categories should not be assigned.

2) Cause of an injury is suspected to be the result of terrorism

When the cause of an injury is suspected to be the result of terrorism a code from category E979 should not be assigned. Assign a code in the range of E codes based circumstances on the documentation of intent and mechanism.

3) Code E979.9, Terrorism, secondary effects

Assign code E979.9, Terrorism, secondary effects, for conditions occurring subsequent to the terrorist event. This code should not be assigned for conditions that are due to the initial terrorist act.

4) Statistical tabulation of terrorism codes

For statistical purposes these codes will be tabulated within the category for assault, expanding the current category from E960-E969 to include E979 and E999.1.

Appendix A ICD-9-CM Official Guidelines for Coding and Reporting

SECTION II. SELECTION OF PRINCIPAL DIAGNOSIS

The circumstances of inpatient admission always govern the selection of principal diagnosis. The principal diagnosis is defined in the Uniform Hospital Discharge Data Set (UHDDS) as "that condition established after study to be chiefly responsible for occasioning the admission of the patient to the hospital for care."

The UHDDS definitions are used by hospitals to report inpatient data elements in a standardized manner. These data elements and their definitions can be found in the July 31, 1985, Federal Register (Vol. 50, No, 147), pp. 31038-40.

Since that time the application of the UHDDS definitions has been expanded to include all non-outpatient settings (acute care, short term, long term care and psychiatric hospitals; home health agencies; rehab facilities; nursing homes, etc).

In determining principal diagnosis the coding conventions in the ICD-9-CM, Volumes I and II take precedence over these official coding guidelines.

(See Section I.A., Conventions for the ICD-9-CM)

The importance of consistent, complete documentation in the medical record cannot be overemphasized. Without such documentation the application of all coding guidelines is a difficult, if not impossible, task.

A. Codes for symptoms, signs, and ill-defined conditions

Codes for symptoms, signs, and ill-defined conditions from Chapter 16 are not to be used as principal diagnosis when a related definitive diagnosis has been established.

B. Two or more interrelated conditions, each potentially meeting the definition for principal diagnosis.

When there are two or more interrelated conditions (such as diseases in the same ICD-9-CM chapter or manifestations characteristically associated with a certain disease) potentially meeting the definition of principal diagnosis, either condition may be sequenced first, unless the circumstances of the admission, the therapy provided, the Tabular List, or the Alphabetic Index indicate otherwise.

C. Two or more diagnoses that equally meet the definition for principal diagnosis

In the unusual instance when two or more diagnoses equally meet the criteria for principal diagnosis as determined by the circumstances of admission, diagnostic workup and/or therapy provided, and the Alphabetic Index, Tabular List, or another coding guidelines does not provide sequencing direction, any one of the diagnoses may be sequenced first.

D. Two or more comparative or contrasting conditions.

In those rare instances when two or more contrasting or comparative diagnoses are documented as "either/or" (or similar terminology), they are coded as if the diagnoses were confirmed and the diagnoses are sequenced according to the circumstances of the admission. If no further determination can be made as to which diagnosis should be principal, either diagnosis may be sequenced first.

E. A symptom(s) followed by contrasting/comparative diagnoses

When a symptom(s) is followed by contrasting/comparative diagnoses, the symptom code is sequenced first. All the contrasting/comparative diagnoses should be coded as additional diagnoses.

F. Original treatment plan not carried out

Sequence as the principal diagnosis the condition, which after study occasioned the admission to the hospital, even though treatment may not have been carried out due to unforeseen circumstances.

G. Complications of surgery and other medical care

When the admission is for treatment of a complication resulting from surgery or other medical care, the complication code is sequenced as the principal diagnosis. If the complication is classified to the 996-999 series and the code lacks the necessary specificity in describing the complication, an additional code for the specific complication should be assigned.

H. Uncertain Diagnosis

If the diagnosis documented at the time of discharge is qualified as "probable", "suspected", "likely", "questionable", "possible", or "still to be ruled out", or other similar terms indicating uncertainty, code the condition as if it existed or was established. The bases for these guidelines are the diagnostic workup, arrangements for further workup or observation, and initial therapeutic approach that correspond most closely with the established diagnosis.

Note: This guideline is applicable only to <u>inpatient admissions to</u> short-term, acute, long-term care and psychiatric hospitals.

I. Admission from Observation Unit

1. Admission Following Medical Observation

When a patient is admitted to an observation unit for a medical condition, which either worsens or does not improve, and is subsequently admitted as an inpatient of the same hospital for this same medical condition, the principal diagnosis would be the medical condition which led to the hospital admission.

2. Admission Following Post-Operative Observation

When a patient is admitted to an observation unit to monitor a condition (or complication) that develops following outpatient surgery, and then is subsequently admitted as an inpatient of the same hospital, hospitals should apply the Uniform Hospital Discharge Data Set (UHDDS) definition of principal diagnosis as "that condition established after study to be chiefly responsible for occasioning the admission of the patient to the hospital for care."

J. Admission from Outpatient Surgery

When a patient receives surgery in the hospital's outpatient surgery department and is subsequently admitted for continuing inpatient care at the same hospital, the following guidelines should be followed in selecting the principal diagnosis for the inpatient admission:

- If the reason for the inpatient admission is a complication, assign the complication as the principal diagnosis.

- If no complication, or other condition, is documented as the reason for the inpatient admission, assign the reason for the outpatient surgery as the principal diagnosis.

- If the reason for the inpatient admission is another condition unrelated to the surgery, assign the unrelated condition as the principal diagnosis.

Appendix A   ICD-9-CM Official Guidelines for Coding and Reporting

SECTION III. REPORTING ADDITIONAL DIAGNOSES

GENERAL RULES FOR OTHER (ADDITIONAL) DIAGNOSES

For reporting purposes the definition for "other diagnoses" is interpreted as additional conditions that affect patient care in terms of requiring:

clinical evaluation; or
therapeutic treatment; or
diagnostic procedures; or
extended length of hospital stay; or
increased nursing care and/or monitoring.

The UHDDS item #11-b defines Other Diagnoses as "all conditions that coexist at the time of admission, that develop subsequently, or that affect the treatment received and/or the length of stay. Diagnoses that relate to an earlier episode which have no bearing on the current hospital stay are to be excluded." UHDDS definitions apply to inpatients in acute care, short-term, long term care and psychiatric hospital setting. The UHDDS definitions are used by acute care short-term hospitals to report inpatient data elements in a standardized manner. These data elements and their definitions can be found in the July 31, 1985, Federal Register (Vol. 50, No, 147), pp. 31038-40.

Since that time the application of the UHDDS definitions has been expanded to include all non-outpatient settings (acute care, short term, long term care and psychiatric hospitals; home health agencies; rehab facilities; nursing homes, etc).

The following guidelines are to be applied in designating "other diagnoses" when neither the Alphabetic Index nor the Tabular List in ICD-9-CM provide direction. The listing of the diagnoses in the patient record is the responsibility of the attending provider.

A. Previous conditions

If the provider has included a diagnosis in the final diagnostic statement, such as the discharge summary or the face sheet, it should ordinarily be coded. Some providers include in the diagnostic statement resolved conditions or diagnoses and status-post procedures from previous admission that have no bearing on the current stay. Such conditions are not to be reported and are coded only if required by hospital policy.

However, history codes (V10-V19) may be used as secondary codes if the historical condition or family history has an impact on current care or influences treatment.

B. Abnormal findings

Abnormal findings (laboratory, x-ray, pathologic, and other diagnostic results) are not coded and reported unless the provider indicates their clinical significance. If the findings are outside the normal range and the attending provider has ordered other tests to evaluate the condition or prescribed treatment, it is appropriate to ask the provider whether the abnormal finding should be added.

Please note: This differs from the coding practices in the outpatient setting for coding encounters for diagnostic tests that have been interpreted by a provider.

C. Uncertain Diagnosis

If the diagnosis documented at the time of discharge is qualified as "probable", "suspected", "likely", "questionable", "possible", or "still to be ruled out" or other similar terms indicating uncertainty, code the condition as if it existed or was established. The bases for these guidelines are the diagnostic workup, arrangements for further workup or observation, and initial therapeutic approach that correspond most closely with the established diagnosis.

Note: This guideline is applicable only to <u>inpatient admissions to</u> short-term, acute, long-term care and psychiatric hospitals.

SECTION IV. DIAGNOSTIC CODING AND REPORTING GUIDELINES FOR OUTPATIENT SERVICES

These coding guidelines for outpatient diagnoses have been approved for use by hospitals/providers in coding and reporting hospital-based outpatient services and provider-based office visits.

Information about the use of certain abbreviations, punctuation, symbols, and other conventions used in the ICD-9-CM Tabular List (code numbers and titles), can be found in Section IA of these guidelines, under "Conventions Used in the Tabular List." Information about the correct sequence to use in finding a code is also described in Section I.

The terms encounter and visit are often used interchangeably in describing outpatient service contacts and, therefore, appear together in these guidelines without distinguishing one from the other.

Though the conventions and general guidelines apply to all settings, coding guidelines for outpatient and provider reporting of diagnoses will vary in a number of instances from those for inpatient diagnoses, recognizing that:

The Uniform Hospital Discharge Data Set (UHDDS) definition of principal diagnosis applies only to inpatients in acute, short-term, long-term care and psychiatric hospitals.

Coding guidelines for inconclusive diagnoses (probable, suspected, rule out, etc.) were developed for inpatient reporting and do not apply to outpatients.

A. Selection of first-listed condition

In the outpatient setting, the term first-listed diagnosis is used in lieu of principal diagnosis.

In determining the first-listed diagnosis the coding conventions of ICD-9-CM, as well as the general and disease specific guidelines take precedence over the outpatient guidelines.

Diagnoses often are not established at the time of the initial encounter/visit. It may take two or more visits before the diagnosis is confirmed.

The most critical rule involves beginning the search for the correct code assignment through the Alphabetic Index. Never begin searching initially in the Tabular List as this will lead to coding errors.

1. Outpatient Surgery

When a patient presents for outpatient surgery, code the reason for the surgery as the first-listed diagnosis (reason for the encounter), even if the surgery is not performed due to a contraindication.

2. Observation Stay

When a patient is admitted for observation for a medical condition, assign a code for the medical condition as the first-listed diagnosis.

When a patient presents for outpatient surgery and develops complications requiring admission to observation, code the reason for the surgery as the first reported diagnosis (reason for the encounter), followed by codes for the complications as secondary diagnoses.

B. Codes from 001.0 through V89

The appropriate code or codes from 001.0 through **V89** must be used to identify diagnoses, symptoms, conditions, problems, complaints, or other reason(s) for the encounter/visit.

C. Accurate reporting of ICD-9-CM diagnosis codes

For accurate reporting of ICD-9-CM diagnosis codes, the documentation should describe the patient's condition, using terminology which includes specific diagnoses as well as symptoms, problems, or reasons for the encounter. There are ICD-9-CM codes to describe all of these.

D. Selection of codes 001.0 through 999.9

The selection of codes 001.0 through 999.9 will frequently be used to describe the reason for the encounter. These codes are from the section of ICD-9-CM for the classification of diseases and injuries (e.g. infectious and parasitic diseases; neoplasms; symptoms, signs, and ill-defined conditions, etc.).

E. Codes that describe symptoms and signs

Codes that describe symptoms and signs, as opposed to diagnoses, are acceptable for reporting purposes when a diagnosis has not been established (confirmed) by the provider. Chapter 16 of ICD-9-CM, Symptoms, Signs, and Ill-defined conditions (codes 780.0-799.9) contain many, but not all codes for symptoms.

F. Encounters for circumstances other than a disease or injury

ICD-9-CM provides codes to deal with encounters for circumstances other than a disease or injury. The Supplementary Classification of factors Influencing Health Status and Contact with Health Services (V01.0-**V89**) is provided to deal with occasions when circumstances other than a disease or injury are recorded as diagnosis or problems. ***See Section I.C. 18 for information on V-codes***

G. Level of Detail in Coding

1. ICD-9-CM codes with 3, 4, or 5 digits

ICD-9-CM is composed of codes with either 3, 4, or 5 digits. Codes with three digits are included in ICD-9-CM as the heading of a category of codes that may be further subdivided by the use of fourth and/or fifth digits, which provide greater specificity.

2. Use of full number of digits required for a code

A three-digit code is to be used only if it is not further subdivided. Where fourth-digit subcategories and/or fifth-digit subclassifications are provided, they must be assigned. A code is invalid if it has not been coded to the full number of digits required for that code.

See also discussion under Section I.b.3., General Coding Guidelines, Level of Detail in Coding.

Appendix A ICD-9-CM Official Guidelines for Coding and Reporting

H. ICD-9-CM code for the diagnosis, condition, problem, or other reason for encounter/visit

List first the ICD-9-CM code for the diagnosis, condition, problem, or other reason for encounter/visit shown in the medical record to be chiefly responsible for the services provided. List additional codes that describe any coexisting conditions. In some cases the first-listed diagnosis may be a symptom when a diagnosis has not been established (confirmed) by the physician.

I. Uncertain diagnosis

Do not code diagnoses documented as "probable", "suspected," "questionable," "rule out," or "working diagnosis" or other similar terms indicating uncertainty. Rather, code the condition(s) to the highest degree of certainty for that encounter/visit, such as symptoms, signs, abnormal test results, or other reason for the visit. **Please note:** This differs from the coding practices used by short-term, acute care, long-term care and psychiatric hospitals.

J. Chronic diseases

Chronic diseases treated on an ongoing basis may be coded and reported as many times as the patient receives treatment and care for the condition(s)

K. Code all documented conditions that coexist

Code all documented conditions that coexist at the time of the encounter/visit, and require or affect patient care treatment or management. Do not code conditions that were previously treated and no longer exist. However, history codes (V10-V19) may be used as secondary codes if the historical condition or family history has an impact on current care or influences treatment.

L. Patients receiving diagnostic services only

For patients receiving diagnostic services only during an encounter/visit, sequence first the diagnosis, condition, problem, or other reason for encounter/visit shown in the medical record to be chiefly responsible for the outpatient services provided during the encounter/visit. Codes for other diagnoses (e.g., chronic conditions) may be sequenced as additional diagnoses.

For encounters for routine laboratory/radiology testing in the absence of any signs, symptoms, or associated diagnosis, assign V72.5 and V72.6. If routine testing is performed during the same encounter as a test to evaluate a sign, symptom, or diagnosis, it is appropriate to assign both the V code and the code describing the reason for the non-routine test.

For outpatient encounters for diagnostic tests that have been interpreted by a physician, and the final report is available at the time of coding, code any confirmed or definitive diagnosis(es) documented in the interpretation. Do not code related signs and symptoms as additional diagnoses.

Please note: This differs from the coding practice in the hospital inpatient setting regarding abnormal findings on test results.

M. Patients receiving therapeutic services only

For patients receiving therapeutic services only during an encounter/visit, sequence first the diagnosis, condition, problem, or other reason for encounter/visit shown in the medical record to be chiefly responsible for the outpatient services provided during the encounter/visit. Codes for other diagnoses (e.g., chronic conditions) may be sequenced as additional diagnoses.

The only exception to this rule is that when the primary reason for the admission/encounter is chemotherapy, radiation therapy, or rehabilitation, the appropriate V code for the service is listed first, and the diagnosis or problem for which the service is being performed listed second.

N. Patients receiving preoperative evaluations only

For patients receiving preoperative evaluations only, sequence **first** a code from category V72.8, Other specified examinations, to describe the pre-op consultations. Assign a code for the condition to describe the reason for the surgery as an additional diagnosis. Code also any findings related to the pre-op evaluation.

O. Ambulatory surgery

For ambulatory surgery, code the diagnosis for which the surgery was performed. If the postoperative diagnosis is known to be different from the preoperative diagnosis at the time the diagnosis is confirmed, select the postoperative diagnosis for coding, since it is the most definitive.

P. Routine outpatient prenatal visits

For routine outpatient prenatal visits when no complications are present, codes V22.0, Supervision of normal first pregnancy, or V22.1, Supervision of other normal pregnancy, should be used as the principal diagnosis. These codes should not be used in conjunction with chapter 11 codes.

APPENDIX I PRESENT ON ADMISSION REPORTING GUIDELINES

Introduction

These guidelines are to be used as a supplement to the *ICD-9-CM Official Guidelines for Coding and Reporting* to facilitate the assignment of the Present on Admission (POA) indicator for each diagnosis and external cause of injury code reported on claim forms (UB-04 and 837 Institutional).

These guidelines are not intended to replace any guidelines in the main body of the *ICD-9-CM Official Guidelines for Coding and Reporting*. The POA guidelines are not intended to provide guidance on when a condition should be coded, but rather, how to apply the POA indicator to the final set of diagnosis codes that have been assigned in accordance with Sections I, II, and III of the official coding guidelines. Subsequent to the assignment of the ICD-9-CM codes, the POA indicator should then be assigned to those conditions that have been coded.

As stated in the Introduction to the ICD-9-CM Official Guidelines for Coding and Reporting, a joint effort between the healthcare provider and the coder is essential to achieve complete and accurate documentation, code assignment, and reporting of diagnoses and procedures. The importance of consistent, complete documentation in the medical record cannot be overemphasized. Medical record documentation from any provider involved in the care and treatment of the patient may be used to support the determination of whether a condition was present on admission or not. In the context of the official coding guidelines, the term "provider" means a physician or any qualified healthcare practitioner who is legally accountable for establishing the patient's diagnosis.

These guidelines are not a substitute for the provider's clinical judgment as to the determination of whether a condition was/was not present on admission. The provider should be queried regarding

issues related to the linking of signs/symptoms, timing of test results, and the timing of findings.

General Reporting Requirements

All claims involving inpatient admissions to general acute care hospitals or other facilities that are subject to a law or regulation mandating collection of present on admission information.

Present on admission is defined as present at the time the order for inpatient admission occurs – conditions that develop during an outpatient encounter, including emergency department, observation, or outpatient surgery, are considered as present on admission.

POA indicator is assigned to principal and secondary diagnoses (as defined in Section II of the Official Guidelines for Coding and Reporting) and the external cause of injury codes.

Issues related to inconsistent, missing, conflicting or unclear documentation must still be resolved by the provider.

If a condition would not be coded and reported based on UHDDS definitions and current official coding guidelines, then the POA indicator would not be reported.

Reporting Options
Y – Yes
N – No
U – Unknown
W – Clinically undetermined
Unreported/Not used **(or "1" for Medicare usage)** – (Exempt from POA reporting)

For more specific instructions on Medicare POA indicator reporting options, refer to http://www.cms.hhs.gov/HospitalAcqCond/02_Statute_Regulations_Program_Instructions.asp#TopOfPage

Reporting Definitions
Y = present at the time of inpatient admission N = not present at the time of inpatient admission U = documentation is insufficient to determine if condition is present on admission W = provider is unable to clinically determine whether condition was present on admission or not

Timeframe for POA Identification and Documentation

There is no required timeframe as to when a provider (per the definition of "provider" used in these guidelines) must identify or document a condition to be present on admission. In some clinical situations, it may not be possible for a provider to make a definitive diagnosis (or a condition may not be recognized or reported by the patient) for a period of time after admission. In some cases it may be several days before the provider arrives at a definitive diagnosis. This does not mean that the condition was not present on admission. Determination of whether the condition was present on admission or not will be based on the applicable POA guideline as identified in this document, or on the provider's best clinical judgment.

If at the time of code assignment the documentation is unclear as to whether a condition was present on admission or not, it is appropriate to query the provider for clarification.

Assigning the POA Indicator

Condition is on the "Exempt from Reporting" List
Leave the "present on admission" field blank if the condition is on the list of ICD-9-CM codes for which this field is not applicable. This is the only circumstance in which the field may be left blank.

POA Explicitly Documented
Assign Y for any condition the provider explicitly documents as being present on admission.

Assign N for any condition the provider explicitly documents as not present at the time of admission.

Conditions Diagnosed Prior to Inpatient Admission
Assign "Y" for conditions that were diagnosed prior to admission (example: hypertension, diabetes mellitus, asthma)

Conditions Diagnosed During the Admission but Clearly Present Before Admission
Assign "Y" for conditions diagnosed during the admission that were clearly present but not diagnosed until after admission occurred.

Diagnoses subsequently confirmed after admission are considered present on admission if at the time of admission they are documented as suspected, possible, rule out, differential diagnosis, or constitute an underlying cause of a symptom that is present at the time of admission.

Condition Develops During Outpatient Encounter Prior to Inpatient Admission
Assign Y for any condition that develops during an outpatient encounter prior to a written order for inpatient admission.

Documentation does not Indicate Whether Condition was Present on Admission
Assign "U" when the medical record documentation is unclear as to whether the condition was present on admission. "U" should not be routinely assigned and used only in very limited circumstances. Coders are encouraged to query the providers when the documentation is unclear.

Documentation States That It Cannot be Determined Whether the Condition Was or Was Not Present on Admission
Assign "W" when the medical record documentation indicates that it cannot be clinically determined whether or not the condition was present on admission.

Chronic Condition with Acute Exacerbation During the Admission
If the code is a combination code that identifies both the chronic condition and the acute exacerbation, see POA guidelines pertaining to combination codes.

If the combination code only identifies the chronic condition and not the acute exacerbation (e.g., acute exacerbation of CHF), assign "Y."

Conditions Documented as Possible, Probable, Suspected, or Rule out At the Time of Discharge
If the final diagnosis contains a possible, probable, suspected, or rule out diagnosis, and this diagnosis was suspected at the time of inpatient admission, assign "Y."

If the final diagnosis contains a possible, probable, suspected, or rule out diagnosis, and this diagnosis was based on symptoms or clinical findings that were not present on admission, assign "N".

Conditions Documented as Impending or Threatened at the Time of Discharge

If the final diagnosis contains an impending or threatened diagnosis, and this diagnosis is based on symptoms or clinical findings that were present on admission, assign "Y".

If the final diagnosis contains an impending or threatened diagnosis, and this diagnosis is based on symptoms or clinical findings that were **not** present on admission, assign "N".

Acute and Chronic Conditions

Assign "Y" for acute conditions that are present at time of admission and N for acute conditions that are not present at time of admission.

Assign "Y" for chronic conditions, even though the condition may not be diagnosed until after admission.

If a single code identifies both an acute and chronic condition, see the POA guidelines for combination codes.

Combination Codes

Assign "N" if any part of the combination code was not present on admission (e.g., obstructive chronic bronchitis with acute exacerbation and the exacerbation was not present on admission; gastric ulcer that does not start bleeding until after admission; asthma patient develops status asthmaticus after admission)

Assign "Y" if all parts of the combination code were present on admission (e.g., patient with diabetic nephropathy is admitted with uncontrolled diabetes)

If the final diagnosis includes comparative or contrasting diagnoses, and both were present, or suspected, at the time of admission, assign "Y".

For infection codes that include the causal organism, assign "Y" if the infection (or signs of the infection) was present on admission, even though the culture results may not be known until after admission (e.g., patient is admitted with pneumonia and the provider documents pseudomonas as the causal organism a few days later).

Same Diagnosis Code for Two or More Conditions

When the same ICD-9-CM diagnosis code applies to two or more conditions during the same encounter (e.g. bilateral condition, or two separate conditions classified to the same ICD-9-CM diagnosis code):

Assign "Y" if all conditions represented by the single ICD-9-CM code were present on admission (e.g. bilateral fracture of the same bone, same site, and both fractures were present on admission)

Assign "N" if any of the conditions represented by the single ICD-9-CM code was not present on admission (e.g. dehydration with hyponatremia is assigned to code 276.1, but only one of these conditions was present on admission).

Obstetrical Conditions

Whether or not the patient delivers during the current hospitalization does not affect assignment of the POA indicator. The determining factor for POA assignment is whether the pregnancy complication or obstetrical condition described by the code was present at the time of admission or not.

If the pregnancy complication or obstetrical condition was present on admission (e.g., patient admitted in preterm labor), assign "Y".

If the pregnancy complication or obstetrical condition was not present on admission (e.g., 2nd degree laceration during delivery, postpartum hemorrhage that occurred during current hospitalization, fetal distress develops after admission), assign "N".

If the obstetrical code includes more than one diagnosis and any of the diagnoses identified by the code were not present on admission assign "N".

(e.g., Code 642.7, Pre-eclampsia or eclampsia superimposed on pre-existing hypertension).

If the obstetrical code includes information that is not a diagnosis, do not consider that information in the POA determination.

(e.g. Code 652.1x, Breech or other malpresentation successfully converted to cephalic presentation should be reported as present on admission if the fetus was breech on admission but was converted to cephalic presentation after admission (since the conversion to cephalic presentation does not represent a diagnosis, the fact that the conversion occurred after admission has no bearing on the POA determination).

Perinatal Conditions

Newborns are not considered to be admitted until after birth. Therefore, any condition present at birth or that developed in utero is considered present at admission and should be assigned "Y". This includes conditions that occur during delivery (e.g., injury during delivery, meconium aspiration, exposure to streptococcus B in the vaginal canal).

Congenital Conditions and Anomalies

Assign "Y" for congenital conditions and anomalies. Congenital conditions are always considered present on admission.

External Cause of Injury Codes

Assign "Y" for any E code representing an external cause of injury or poisoning that occurred prior to inpatient admission (e.g., patient fell out of bed at home, patient fell out of bed in emergency room prior to admission)

Assign "N" for any E code representing an external cause of injury or poisoning that occurred during inpatient hospitalization (e.g., patient fell out of hospital bed during hospital stay, patient experienced an adverse reaction to a medication administered after inpatient admission)

CATEGORIES AND CODES EXEMPT FROM DIAGNOSIS PRESENT ON ADMISSION REQUIREMENT

Effective Date: October 1, 2008

Note: "Diagnosis present on admission" for these code categories are exempt because they represent circumstances regarding the healthcare encounter or factors influencing health status that do not represent a current disease or injury or are always present on admission

137-139, Late effects of infectious and parasitic diseases

268.1, Rickets, late effect

326, Late effects of intracranial abscess or pyogenic infection

412, Old myocardial infarction

438, Late effects of cerebrovascular disease

Appendix A ICD-9-CM Official Guidelines for Coding and Reporting

650, Normal delivery

660.7, Failed forceps or vacuum extractor, unspecified

677, Late effect of complication of pregnancy, childbirth, and the puerperium

905-909, Late effects of injuries, poisonings, toxic effects, and other external causes

V02, Carrier or suspected carrier of infectious diseases

V03, Need for prophylactic vaccination and inoculation against bacterial diseases

V04, Need for prophylactic vaccination and inoculation against certain viral diseases

V05, Need for other prophylactic vaccination and inoculation against single diseases

V06, Need for prophylactic vaccination and inoculation against combinations of diseases

V07, Need for isolation and other prophylactic measures

V10, Personal history of malignant neoplasm

V11, Personal history of mental disorder

V12, Personal history of certain other diseases

V13, Personal history of other diseases

V14, Personal history of allergy to medicinal agents

V15.01-V15.09, Other personal history, Allergy, other than to medicinal agents

V15.1, Other personal history, Surgery to heart and great vessels

V15.2, Other personal history, Surgery to other major organs

V15.3, Other personal history, Irradiation

V15.4, Other personal history, Psychological trauma

V15.5, Other personal history, Injury

V15.6, Other personal history, Poisoning

V15.7, Other personal history, Contraception

V15.81, Other personal history, Noncompliance with medical treatment

V15.82, Other personal history, History of tobacco use

V15.88, Other personal history, History of fall

V15.89, Other personal history, Other

V15.9 Unspecified personal history presenting hazards to health

V16, Family history of malignant neoplasm

V17, Family history of certain chronic disabling diseases

V18, Family history of certain other specific conditions

V19, Family history of other conditions

V20, Health supervision of infant or child

V21, Constitutional states in development

V22, Normal pregnancy

V23, Supervision of high-risk pregnancy

V24, Postpartum care and examination

V25, Encounter for contraceptive management

V26, Procreative management

V27, Outcome of delivery

V28, Antenatal screening

V29, Observation and evaluation of newborns for suspected condition not found

V30-V39, Liveborn infants according to type of birth

V42, Organ or tissue replaced by transplant

V43, Organ or tissue replaced by other means

V44, Artificial opening status

V45, Other postprocedural states

V46, Other dependence on machines

V49.60-V49.77, Upper and lower limb amputation status

V49.81-V49.84, Other specified conditions influencing health status

V50, Elective surgery for purposes other than remedying health states

V51, Aftercare involving the use of plastic surgery

V52, Fitting and adjustment of prosthetic device and implant

V53, Fitting and adjustment of other device

V54, Other orthopedic aftercare

V55, Attention to artificial openings

V56, Encounter for dialysis and dialysis catheter care

V57, Care involving use of rehabilitation procedures

V58, Encounter for other and unspecified procedures and aftercare

V59, Donors

V60, Housing, household, and economic circumstances

V61, Other family circumstances

V62, Other psychosocial circumstances

V64, Persons encountering health services for specific procedures, not carried out

V65, Other persons seeking consultation

V66, Convalescence and palliative care

V67, Follow-up examination

V68, Encounters for administrative purposes

V69, Problems related to lifestyle

V70, General medical examination

V71, Observation and evaluation for suspected condition not found

V72, Special investigations and examinations

V73, Special screening examination for viral and chlamydial diseases

V74, Special screening examination for bacterial and spirochetal diseases

V75, Special screening examination for other infectious diseases

V76, Special screening for malignant neoplasms

V77, Special screening for endocrine, nutritional, metabolic, and immunity disorders

Appendix A ICD-9-CM Official Guidelines for Coding and Reporting

V78, Special screening for disorders of blood and blood-forming organs

V79, Special screening for mental disorders and developmental handicaps

V80, Special screening for neurological, eye, and ear diseases

V81, Special screening for cardiovascular, respiratory, and genitourinary diseases

V82, Special screening for other conditions

V83, Genetic carrier status

V84, Genetic susceptibility to disease

V85, Body Mass Index

V86, Estrogen receptor status

V87.4, Personal history of drug therapy

V88, Acquired absence of cervix and uterus

V89, Suspected maternal and fetal conditions not found

E800-E807, Railway accidents

E810-E819, Motor vehicle traffic accidents

E820-E825, Motor vehicle nontraffic accidents

E826-E829, Other road vehicle accidents

E830-E838, Water transport accidents

E840-E845, Air and space transport accidents

E846-E848, Vehicle accidents not elsewhere classifiable

E849.0-E849.6, Place of occurrence

E849.8-E849.9, Place of occurrence

E883.1, Accidental fall into well

E883.2, Accidental fall into storm drain or manhole

E884.0, Fall from playground equipment

E884.1, Fall from cliff

E885.0, Fall from (nonmotorized) scooter

E885.1, Fall from roller skates

E885.2, Fall from skateboard

E885.3, Fall from skis

E885.4, Fall from snowboard

E886.0, Fall on same level from collision, pushing, or shoving, by or with other person, In sports

E890.0-E89.9, Conflagration in private dwelling

E893.0, Accident caused by ignition of clothing, from controlled fire in private dwelling

E893.2, Accident caused by ignition of clothing, from controlled fire not in building or structure

E894, Ignition of highly inflammable material

E895, Accident caused by controlled fire in private dwelling

E897, Accident caused by controlled fire not in building or structure

E898.0-E898.1, Accident caused by other specified fire and flames

E917.0, Striking against or struck accidentally by objects or persons, in sports without subsequent fall

E917.1, Striking against or struck accidentally by objects or persons, caused by a crowd, by collective fear or panic without subsequent fall

E917.2, Striking against or struck accidentally by objects or persons, in running water without subsequent fall

E917.5, Striking against or struck accidentally by objects or persons, object in sports with subsequent fall

E917.6, Striking against or struck accidentally by objects or persons, caused by a crowd, by collective fear or panic with subsequent fall

E919.0-E919.1, Accidents caused by machinery

E919.3-E919.9, Accidents caused by machinery

E921.0-E921.9, Accident caused by explosion of pressure vessel

E922.0-E922.9, Accident caused by firearm and air gun missile

E924.1, Caustic and corrosive substances

E926.2, Visible and ultraviolet light sources

E927, Overexertion and strenuous movements

E928.0-E928.8, Other and unspecified environmental and accidental causes

E929.0-E929.9, Late effects of accidental injury

E959, Late effects of self-inflicted injury

E970-E978, Legal intervention

E979, Terrorism

E981.0-E981.8, Poisoning by gases in domestic use, undetermined whether accidentally or purposely inflicted

E982.0-E982.9, Poisoning by other gases, undetermined whether accidentally or purposely inflicted

E985.0-E985.7, Injury by firearms, air guns and explosives, undetermined whether accidentally or purposely inflicted

E987.0, Falling from high place, undetermined whether accidentally or purposely inflicted, residential premises

E987.2, Falling from high place, undetermined whether accidentally or purposely inflicted, natural sites

E989, Late effects of injury, undetermined whether accidentally or purposely inflicted

E990-E999, Injury resulting from operations of war

POA EXAMPLES

General Medical Surgical

1. Patient is admitted for diagnostic work-up for cachexia. The final diagnosis is malignant neoplasm of lung with metastasis.

   Assign "Y" on the POA field for the malignant neoplasm. The malignant neoplasm was clearly present on admission, although it was not diagnosed until after the admission occurred.

Appendix A ICD-9-CM Official Guidelines for Coding and Reporting

2. A patient undergoes outpatient surgery. During the recovery period, the patient develops atrial fibrillation and the patient is subsequently admitted to the hospital as an inpatient.

   Assign "Y" on the POA field for the atrial fibrillation since it developed prior to a written order for inpatient admission.

3. A patient is treated in observation and while in Observation, the patient falls out of bed and breaks a hip. The patient is subsequently admitted as an inpatient to treat the hip fracture.

   Assign "Y" on the POA field for the hip fracture since it developed prior to a written order for inpatient admission.

4. A patient with known congestive heart failure is admitted to the hospital after he develops decompensated congestive heart failure.

   Assign "Y" on the POA field for the congestive heart failure. The ICD-9-CM code identifies the chronic condition and does not specify the acute exacerbation.

5. A patient undergoes inpatient surgery. After surgery, the patient develops fever and is treated aggressively. The physician's final diagnosis documents "possible postoperative infection following surgery."

   Assign "N" on the POA field for the postoperative infection since final diagnoses that contain the terms "possible", "probable", "suspected" or "rule out" and that are based on symptoms or clinical findings that were not present on admission should be reported as "N".

6. A patient with severe cough and difficulty breathing was diagnosed during his hospitalization to have lung cancer.

   Assign "Y" on the POA field for the lung cancer. Even though the cancer was not diagnosed until after admission, it is a chronic condition that was clearly present before the patient's admission.

7. A patient is admitted to the hospital for a coronary artery bypass surgery. Postoperatively he developed a pulmonary embolism.

   Assign "N" on the POA field for the pulmonary embolism. This is an acute condition that was not present on admission.

8. A patient is admitted with a known history of coronary atherosclerosis, status post myocardial infarction five years ago is now admitted for treatment of impending myocardial infarction. The final diagnosis is documented as "impending myocardial infarction."

   Assign "Y" to the impending myocardial infarction because the condition is present on admission.

9. A patient with diabetes mellitus developed uncontrolled diabetes on day 3 of the hospitalization.

   Assign "N" to the diabetes code because the "uncontrolled" component of the code was not present on admission.

10. A patient is admitted with high fever and pneumonia. The patient rapidly deteriorates and becomes septic. The discharge diagnosis lists sepsis and pneumonia. The documentation is unclear as to whether the sepsis was present on admission or developed shortly after admission.

    Query the physician as to whether the sepsis was present on admission, developed shortly after admission, or it cannot be clinically determined as to whether it was present on admission or not.

11. A patient is admitted for repair of an abdominal aneurysm. However, the aneurysm ruptures after hospital admission.

    Assign "N" for the ruptured abdominal aneurysm. Although the aneurysm was present on admission, the "ruptured" component of the code description did not occur until after admission.

12. A patient with viral hepatitis B progresses to hepatic coma after admission.

    Assign "N" for the viral hepatitis B with hepatic coma because part of the code description did not develop until after admission.

13. A patient with a history of varicose veins and ulceration of the left lower extremity strikes the area against the side of his hospital bed during an inpatient hospitalization. It bleeds profusely. The final diagnosis lists varicose veins with ulcer and hemorrhage.

    Assign "Y" for the varicose veins with ulcer. Although the hemorrhage occurred after admission, the code description for varicose veins with ulcer does not mention hemorrhage.

14. The nursing initial assessment upon admission documents the presence of a decubitus ulcer. There is no mention of the decubitus ulcer in the physician documentation until several days after admission.

    Query the physician as to whether the decubitus ulcer was present on admission, or developed after admission. Both diagnosis code assignment and determination of whether a condition was present on admission must be based on provider documentation in the medical record (per the definition of "provider" found at the beginning of these POA guidelines and in the introductory section of the ICD-9-CM Official Guidelines for Coding and Reporting). If it cannot be determined from the provider documentation whether or not a condition was present on admission, the provider should be queried.

15. **A urine culture is obtained on admission. The provider documents urinary tract infection when the culture results become available a few days later.**

    Assign "Y" to the urinary tract infection since the diagnosis is based on test results from a specimen obtained on admission. It may not be possible for a provider to make a definitive diagnosis for a period of time after admission. There is no required timeframe as to when a provider must identify or document a condition to be present on admission.

16. **A patient tested positive for Methicillin resistant Staphylococcus (MRSA) on routine nasal culture on admission to the hospital. During the hospitalization, he underwent insertion of a central venous catheter and later developed an infection and was diagnosed with MRSA sepsis due to central venous catheter infection.**

    Assign "Y" to the positive MRSA colonization. Assign "N" for the MRSA sepsis due to central venous catheter infection since the patient did not have a MRSA infection at the time of admission.

Obstetrics

1. A female patient was admitted to the hospital and underwent a normal delivery.

Leave the "present on admission" (POA) field blank. Code 650, Normal delivery, is on the "exempt from reporting" list.

2. Patient admitted in late pregnancy due to excessive vomiting and dehydration. During admission patient goes into premature labor

   Assign "Y" for the excessive vomiting and the dehydration.

   Assign "N" for the premature labor

3. Patient admitted in active labor. During the stay, a breast abscess is noted when mother attempted to breast feed. Provider is unable to determine whether the abscess was present on admission

   Assign "W" for the breast abscess.

4. Patient admitted in active labor. After 12 hours of labor it is noted that the infant is in fetal distress and a Cesarean section is performed

   Assign "N" for the fetal distress.

5. **Pregnant female was admitted in labor and fetal nuchal cord entanglement was diagnosed. Physician is queried, but is unable to determine whether the cord entanglement was present on admission or not.**

   Assign "W" for the fetal nuchal cord entanglement.

Newborn

1. A single liveborn infant was delivered in the hospital via Cesarean section. The physician documented fetal bradycardia during labor in the final diagnosis in the newborn record.

   Assign " Y" because the bradycardia developed prior to the newborn admission (birth).

2. A newborn developed diarrhea which was believed to be due to the hospital baby formula.

   Assign " N" because the diarrhea developed after admission.

3. **A newborn born in the hospital, birth complicated by nuchal cord entanglement.**

   Assign "Y" for the nuchal cord entanglement on the baby's record. Any condition that is present at birth or that developed in utero is considered present at admission, including conditions that occur during delivery.

Appendix B

Medical Terminology

ablation	removal or destruction by cutting, chemicals, or electrocautery
abortion	termination of pregnancy
absence	without
actinotherapy	treatment of acne using ultraviolet rays
adenoidectomy	removal of adenoids
adipose	fatty
adrenals	glands, located at the top of the kidneys, that produce steroid hormones
albinism	lack of color pigment
allograft	homograft, same species graft
alopecia	condition in which hair falls out
amniocentesis	percutaneous aspiration of amniotic fluid
amniotic sac	sac containing the fetus and amniotic fluid
A-mode	one-dimensional ultrasonic display reflecting the time it takes a sound wave to reach a structure and reflect back; maps the structure's outline
anastomosis	surgical connection of two tubular structures, such as two pieces of the intestine
aneurysm	abnormal dilation of vessels, usually an artery
angina	sudden pain
angiography	radiography of the blood vessels
angioplasty	procedure in a vessel to dilate the vessel opening
anhidrosis	deficiency of sweat
anomaloscope	instrument used to test color vision
anoscopy	procedure that uses a scope to examine the anus
antepartum	before childbirth
anterior (ventral)	in front of
anterior segment	those parts of the eye in the front of and including the lens, orbit, extraocular muscles, and eyelid

anteroposterior	from front to back
antigen	a substance that produces a specific response
aortography	radiographic recording of the aorta
apex cardiography	recording of the movement of the chest wall
aphakia	absence of the lens of the eye
apicectomy	excision of a portion of the temporal bone
apnea	cessation of breathing
arthrocentesis	injection and/or aspiration of joint
arthrodesis	surgical immobilization of joint
arthrography	radiography of joint
arthroplasty	reshaping or reconstruction of joint
arthroscopy	use of scope to view inside joint
arthrotomy	incision into a joint
articular	pertains to joint
asphyxia	lack of oxygen
aspiration	use of a needle and a syringe to withdraw fluid
assignment	Medicare's payment for the service, which participating physicians agree to accept as payment in full
asthma	shortage of breath caused by contraction of bronchi
astigmatism	condition in which the refractive surfaces of the eye are unequal
atelectasis	incomplete expansion of lung, collapse
atherectomy	removal of plaque by percutaneous method
atrophy	wasting away
audiometry	hearing test
aural atresia	congenital absence of the external auditory canal
auscultation	listening to sounds within the body
autograft	from patient's own body
avulsion	ripping or tearing away of part either surgically or accidentally
axillary nodes	lymph nodes located in the armpit
bacilli	plural of bacillus, a rod-shaped bacterium
barium enema	radiographic contrast medium
beneficiary	person who benefits from health or life insurance
bifocal	two focuses in eyeglasses, one usually for close work and the other for improvement of distance vision
bilaminate skin	skin substitute usually made of silicone-covered nylon mesh
bilateral	occurring on two sides
biliary	refers to gallbladder, bile, or bile duct
bilobectomy	surgical removal of two lobes of a lung
biofeedback	process of giving a person self-information

Appendix B Medical Terminology

biometry	application of a statistical measure to a biologic fact
biopsy	removal of a small piece of living tissue for diagnostic purposes
block	frozen piece of a sample
brachytherapy	therapy using radioactive sources that are placed inside the body
bronchiole	smaller division of bronchial tree
bronchography	radiographic recording of the lungs
bronchoplasty	surgical repair of the bronchi
bronchoscopy	inspection of the bronchial tree using a bronchoscope
B-scan	two-dimensional display of tissues and organs
bulbocavernosus	muscle that constricts the vagina in a female and the urethra in a male
bulbourethral	gland with duct leading to the urethra
bundle of His	muscular cardiac fibers that provide the heart rhythm to the ventricles; blockage of this rhythm produces heart block
bundled codes	one code that represents a package of services
bunion	hallux valgus, abnormal increase in size of metatarsal head that results in displacement of the great toe
burr	drill used to create an entry into the cranium
bursa	fluid-filled sac that absorbs friction
bursitis	inflammation of bursa (joint sac)
bypass	to go around
calcaneal	pertaining to the heel bone
calculus	concretion of mineral salts, also called a stone
calycoplasty	surgical reconstruction of a recess of the renal pelvis
calyx	recess of the renal pelvis
cancellous	lattice-type structure, usually of bone
cardiopulmonary	refers to the heart and lungs
cardiopulmonary bypass	blood bypasses the heart through a heart-lung machine
cardioversion	electrical shock to the heart to restore normal rhythm
cardioverter-defibrillator	surgically placed device that directs an electrical shock to the heart to restore rhythm
carotid body	located on each side of the common carotid artery, often a site of tumor
cartilage	connective tissue
cataract	opaque covering on or in the lens
catheter	tube placed into the body to put fluid in or take fluid out
caudal	same as inferior; away from the head, or the lower part of the body

causalgia	burning pain
cauterization	destruction of tissue by the use of cautery
cavernosa	connection between the cavity of the penis and a vein
cavernosography	radiographic recording of a cavity, e.g., the pulmonary cavity or the main part of the penis
cavernosometry	measurement of the pressure in a cavity, e.g., the penis
central nervous system	brain and spinal cord
cervical	pertaining to the neck or to the cervix of the uterus
cervix uteri	rounded, cone-shaped neck of the uterus
cesarean	surgical opening through abdominal wall for delivery
cholangiography	radiographic recording of the bile ducts
cholangiopancreatography	ERCP, radiographic recording of the biliary system or pancreas
cholecystectomy	surgical removal of the gallbladder
cholecystoenterostomy	creation of a connection between the gallbladder and intestine
cholecystography	radiographic recording of the gallbladder
cholesteatoma	tumor that forms in middle ear
chondral	referring to the cartilage
chordee	condition resulting in the penis being bent downward
chorionic villus sampling	CVS, biopsy of the outermost part of the placenta
circumflex	a coronary artery that circles the heart
Cloquet's node	also called a gland; it is the highest of the deep groin lymph nodes
closed fracture repair	not surgically opened with/without manipulation and with/without traction
closed treatment	fracture site that is not surgically opened and visualized
coccyx	caudal extremity of vertebral column
collagen	protein substance of skin
Colles' fracture	fracture at lower end of radius that displaces the bone posteriorly
colonoscopy	fiberscopic examination of the entire colon that may include part of the terminal ileum
colostomy	artificial opening between the colon and the abdominal wall
component	part
computed axial tomography	CAT or CT, procedure by which selected planes of tissue are pinpointed through computer enhancement, and images may be reconstructed by analysis of variance in absorption of the tissue
conjunctiva	the lining of the eyelids and the covering of the sclera
contraction	drawn together

Appendix B   Medical Terminology

contralateral	opposite side
cordectomy	surgical removal of the vocal cord(s)
cordocentesis	procedure to obtain a fetal blood sample; also called a percutaneous umbilical blood sampling
corneosclera	cornea and sclera of the eye
corpectomy	removal of vertebrae
corpora cavernosa	the two cavities of the penis
corpus uteri	uterus
crackle	abnormal sound when breathing (heard on auscultation)
craniectomy	permanent, partial removal of skull
craniotomy	opening of the skull
cranium	that part of the skeleton that encloses the brain
curettage	scraping of a cavity using a spoon-shaped instrument
curette	spoon-shaped instrument used to scrape a cavity
cutdown	incision into a vessel for placement of a catheter
cyanosis	bluish discoloration
cystocele	herniation of the bladder into the vagina
cystography	radiographic recording of the urinary bladder
cystolithectomy	removal of a calculus (stone) from the urinary bladder
cystolithotomy	cystolithectomy
cystometrogram	CMG, measurement of the pressures and capacity of the urinary bladder
cystoplasty	surgical reconstruction of the bladder
cystorrhaphy	suture of the bladder
cystoscopy	use of a scope to view the bladder
cystostomy	surgical creation of an opening into the bladder
cystotomy	incision into the bladder
cystourethroplasty	surgical reconstruction of the bladder and urethra
cystourethroscopy	use of a scope to view the bladder and urethra
dacryocystography	radiographic recording of the lacrimal sac or tear duct sac
dacryostenosis	narrowing of the lacrimal duct
debridement	cleansing of or removal of dead tissue from a wound
deductible	amount the patient is liable for before the payer begins to pay for covered services
delayed flap	pedicle of skin with blood supply that is separated from origin over time
delivery	childbirth
dermabrasion	planing of the skin by means of sander, brush, or sandpaper

dermatologist	physician who treats conditions of the skin
dermatoplasty	surgical repair of skin
dialysis	filtration of blood
dilation	expansion
diskectomy	removal of a vertebral disk
diskography	radiographic recording of an intervertebral joint
dislocation	placement in a location other than the original location
distal	farther from the point of attachment or origin
diverticulum	protrusion in the wall of an organ
Doppler	ultrasonic measure of blood movement
dosimetry	scientific calculation of radiation emitted from various radioactive sources
drainage	free flow or withdrawal of fluids from a wound or cavity
duodenography	radiographic recording of the duodenum or first part of the small intestine
dysphagia	difficulty swallowing
dysphonia	speech impairment
dyspnea	shortness of breath, difficult breathing
dysuria	painful urination
echocardiography	radiographic recording of the heart or heart walls or surrounding tissues
echoencephalography	ultrasound of the brain
echography	ultrasound procedure in which sound waves are bounced off an internal organ and the resulting image is recorded
ectopic	pregnancy outside the uterus (i.e., in the fallopian tube)
edema	swelling due to abnormal fluid collection in the tissue spaces
elective surgery	nonemergency procedure
electrocardiogram	ECG, written record of the electrical action of the heart
electrocautery	cauterization by means of heated instrument
electrocochleography	test to measure the eighth cranial nerve (hearing test)
electrode	lead attached to a generator that carries the electrical current from the generator to the atria or ventricles
electroencephalogram	EEG, written record of the electrical action of the brain
electromyogram	EMG, written record of the electrical activity of the skeletal muscles
electronic claim submission	claims prepared and submitted via a computer
electronic signature	identification system of a computer
electro-oculogram	EOG, written record of the electrical activity of the eye

Appendix B Medical Terminology

electrophysiology	study of the electrical system of the heart, including the study of arrhythmias
embolectomy	removal of blockage (embolism) from vessel
emphysema	air accumulated in organ or tissue
encephalography	radiographic recording of the subarachnoid space and ventricles of the brain
endarterectomy	incision into an artery to remove the inner lining so as to eliminate disease or blockage
endomyocardial	pertaining to the inner and middle layers of the heart
endopyelotomy	procedure involving the bladder and ureters, including the insertion of a stent into the renal pelvis
endoscopy	inspection of body organs or cavities using a lighted scope that may be inserted through an existing opening or through a small incision
enterolysis	releasing of adhesions of intestine
enucleation	removal of an organ or organs from a body cavity
epicardial	over the heart
epidermolysis	loosening of the epidermis
epidermomycosis	superficial fungal infection
epididymectomy	surgical removal of the epididymis
epididymis	tube located at the top of the testes that stores sperm
epididymography	radiographic recording of the epididymis
epididymovasostomy	creation of a new connection between the vas deferens and epididymis
epiglottidectomy	excision of the covering of the larynx
episclera	connective covering of sclera
epistaxis	nose bleed
epithelium	surface covering of internal and external organs of the body
erythema	redness of skin
escharotomy	surgical incision into necrotic (dead) tissue
eventration	protrusion of the bowel through an opening in the abdomen
evisceration	pulling the viscera outside of the body through an incision
evocative	tests that are administered to evoke a predetermined response
exenteration	removal of an organ all in one piece
exophthalmos	protrusion of the eyeball
exostosis	bony growth
exstrophy	condition in which an organ is turned inside out
extracorporeal	occurring outside of the body
false aneurysm	sac of clotted blood that has completely destroyed the vessel and is being contained by the tissue that surrounds the vessel

fasciectomy	removal of a band of fibrous tissue
Federal Register	official publication of all "Presidential Documents," "Rules and Regulations," "Proposed Rules," and "Notices"; government-instituted national changes are published in the *Federal Register*
fee schedule	services and payment allowed for each service
femoral	pertaining to the bone from the pelvis to knee
fenestration	creation of a new opening in the inner wall of the middle ear
fissure	cleft or groove
fistula	abnormal opening from one area to another area or to the outside of the body
fluoroscopy	procedure for viewing the interior of the body using x-rays and projecting the image onto a television screen
fracture	break in a bone
free full-thickness graft	graft of epidermis and dermis that is completely removed from donor area
fulguration	use of electrical current to destroy tissue
fundoplasty	repair of the bottom of the bladder
furuncle	nodule in the skin caused by *Staphylococci* entering through hair follicle
ganglion	knot
gastrointestinal	pertaining to the stomach and intestine
gastroplasty	operation on the stomach for repair or reconfiguration
gastrostomy	artificial opening between the stomach and the abdominal wall
gatekeeper	a physician who manages a patient's access to health care
glaucoma	eye diseases that are characterized by an increase of intraocular pressure
globe	eyeball
glottis	true vocal cords
gonioscopy	use of a scope to examine the angles of the eye
Group Practice Model	an organization of physicians who contract with a Health Maintenance Organization to provide services to the enrollees of the HMO
grouper	computer used to input the principal diagnosis and other critical information about a patient and then provide the correct DRG code
Health Maintenance Organization	HMO, a healthcare delivery system in which an enrollee is assigned a primary care physician who manages all the healthcare needs of the enrollee
hematoma	mass of blood that forms outside the vessel
hemodialysis	cleansing of the blood outside of the body
hemolysis	breakdown of red blood cells

Appendix B Medical Terminology

hemoptysis	bloody sputum
hepatography	radiographic recording of the liver
hernia	organ or tissue protruding through the wall or cavity that usually contains it
histology	study of structure of tissue and cells
homograft	allograft, same species graft
hormone	chemical substance produced by the body's endocrine glands
hydrocele	sac of fluid
hyperopia	farsightedness, eyeball is too short from front to back
hypogastric	lowest middle abdominal area
hyposensitization	decreased sensitivity
hypothermia	low body temperature; sometimes induced during surgical procedures
hypoxemia	low level of oxygen in the blood
hypoxia	low level of oxygen in the tissue
hysterectomy	surgical removal of the uterus
hysterorrhaphy	suturing of the uterus
hysterosalpingography	radiographic recording of the uterine cavity and fallopian tubes
hysteroscopy	visualization of the canal and cavity of the uterus using a scope placed through the vagina
ichthyosis	skin disorder characterized by scaling
ileostomy	artificial opening between the ileum and the abdominal wall
ilium	portion of hip
imbrication	overlapping
immunotherapy	therapy to increase immunity
incarcerated	regarding hernias, a constricted, irreducible hernia that may cause obstruction of an intestine
incise	to cut into
Individual Practice Association	IPA, an organization of physicians who provide services for a set fee; Health Maintenance Organizations often contract with the IPA for services to their enrollees
inferior	away from the head or the lower part of the body; also known as caudalingual
inguinofemoral	referring to the groin and thigh
inofemoral	referring to the groin and thigh
internal/external fixation	application of pins, wires, and/or screws placed externally or internally to immobilize a body part
intracardiac	inside the heart

intramural	within the organ wall
intramuscular	into a muscle
intrauterine	inside the uterus
intravenous	into a vein
intravenous pyelography	IVP, radiographic recording of the urinary system
introitus	opening or entrance to the vagina from the uterus
intubation	insertion of a tube
intussusception	slipping of one part of the intestine into another part
invasive	entering the body, breaking skin
iontophoresis	introduction of ions into the body
ischemia	deficient blood supply due to obstruction of the circulatory system
island pedicle flap	contains a single artery and vein that remains attached to origin temporarily or permanently
isthmus	connection of two regions or structures
isthmus, thyroid	tissue connection between right and left thyroid lobes
isthmusectomy	surgical removal of the isthmus
jejunostomy	artificial opening between the jejunum and the abdominal wall
jugular nodes	lymph nodes located next to the large vein in the neck
keratomalacia	softening of the cornea associated with a deficiency of vitamin A
keratoplasty	surgical repair of the cornea
Kock pouch	surgical creation of a urinary bladder from a segment of the ileum
kyphosis	humpback
labyrinth	inner connecting cavities, such as the internal ear
labyrinthitis	inner ear inflammation
lacrimal	related to tears
lamina	flat plate
laminectomy	surgical excision of the lamina
laparoscopy	exploration of the abdomen and pelvic cavities using a scope placed through a small incision in the abdominal wall
laryngeal web	congenital abnormality of connective tissue between the vocal cords
laryngectomy	surgical removal of the larynx
laryngography	radiographic recording of the larynx
laryngoplasty	surgical repair of the larynx
laryngoscope	fiberoptic scope used to view the inside of the larynx

Appendix B Medical Terminology

laryngoscopy	direct visualization and examination of the interior of larynx with a laryngoscope
laryngotomy	incision into the larynx
lateral	away from the midline of the body (to the side)
lavage	washing out
leukoderma	depigmentation of skin
leukoplakia	white patch on mucous membrane
ligament	fibrous band of tissue that connects cartilage or bone
ligation	binding or tying off, as in constricting the blood flow of a vessel or binding fallopian tubes for sterilization
lipocyte	fat cell
lipoma	fatty tumor
lithotomy	incision into an organ or a duct for the purpose of removing a stone
lithotripsy	crushing of a stone by sound waves or force
lobectomy	surgical excision of lobe of the lung
lordosis	anterior curve of spine
lumbodynia	pain in the lumbar area
lunate	one of the wrist (carpal) bones
lymph node	station along the lymphatic system
lymphadenectomy	excision of a lymph node or nodes
lymphadenitis	inflammation of a lymph node
lymphangiography	radiographic recording of the lymphatic vessels and nodes
lymphangiotomy	incision into a lymphatic vessel
lysis	releasing
magnetic resonance imaging	MRI, procedure that uses nonionizing radiation to view the body in a cross-sectional view
Major Diagnostic Categories	MDC, the division of all principal diagnoses into 25 mutually exclusive principal diagnosis areas within the DRG system
mammography	radiographic recording of the breasts
Managed Care Organization	MCO, a group that is responsible for the health care services offered to an enrolled group of persons
manipulation	movement by hand
manipulation or reduction	alignment of a fracture or joint dislocation to its normal position
mastoidectomy	removal of the mastoid bone
Maximum Actual Allowable Charge	MAAC, limitation on the total amount that can be charged by physicians who are not participants in Medicare
meatotomy	surgical enlargement of the opening of the urinary meatus

medial	toward the midline of the body
Medical Volume Performance Standards	MVPS, government's estimate of how much growth is appropriate for nationwide physician expenditures paid by the Part B Medicare program
Medicare Economic Index	MEI, government mandated index that ties increases in the Medicare prevailing charges to economic indicators
Medicare Fee Schedule	MFS, schedule that listed the allowable charges for Medicare services; was replaced by the Medicare reasonable charge payment system
Medicare Risk HMO	a Medicare-funded alternative to the standard Medicare supplemental coverage
melanin	dark pigment of skin
melanoma	tumor of epidermis, malignant and black in color
Ménière's disease	condition that causes dizziness, ringing in the ears, and deafness
M-mode	one-dimensional display of movement of structures
modality	treatment method
Mohs' surgery or Mohs' micrographic surgery	removal of skin cancer in layers by a surgeon who also acts as pathologist during surgery
monofocal	eyeglasses with one vision correction
multipara	more than one pregnancy
muscle	organ of contraction for movement
muscle flap	transfer of muscle from origin to recipient site
myasthenia gravis	syndrome characterized by muscle weakness
myelography	radiographic recording of the subarachnoid space of the spine
myopia	nearsightedness, eyeball too long from front to back
myringotomy	incision into tympanic membrane
nasal button	synthetic circular disk used to cover a hole in the nasal septum
nasopharyngoscopy	use of a scope to visualize the nose and pharynx
National Provider Identifier	NPI, a 10-digit number assigned to a physician by Medicare
nephrectomy, paraperitoneal	kidney transplant
nephrocutaneous fistula	a channel from the kidney to the skin
nephrolithotomy	removal of a kidney stone through an incision made into the kidney
nephrorrhaphy	suturing of the kidney
nephrostolithotomy	creation of an artificial channel to the kidney
nephrostolithotomy, percutaneous	procedure to establish an artificial channel between the skin and the kidney
nephrostomy	creation of a channel into the renal pelvis of the kidney
nephrostomy, percutaneous	creation of a channel from the skin to the renal pelvis

Appendix B Medical Terminology

nephrotomy	incision into the kidney
neurovascular flap	contains artery, vein, and nerve
noninvasive	not entering the body, not breaking skin
nuclear cardiology	diagnostic specialty that uses radiologic procedures to aid in diagnosis of cardiologic conditions
nystagmus	rapid involuntary eye movements
ocular adnexa	orbit, extraocular muscles, and eyelid
olecranon	elbow bone
Omnibus Budget Reconciliation Act of 1989	OBRA, act that established new rules for Medicare reimbursement
oophorectomy	surgical removal of the ovary(ies)
opacification	area that has become opaque (milky)
open fracture repair	surgical opening (incision) over or remote opening as access to a fracture site
open treatment	fracture site that is surgically opened and visualized
ophthalmodynamometry	test of the blood pressure of the eye
ophthalmology	body of knowledge regarding the eyes
ophthalmoscopy	examination of the interior of the eye by means of a scope, also known as funduscopy
optokinetic	movement of the eyes to objects moving in the visual field
orchiectomy	castration, removal of the testes
orchiopexy	surgical procedure to release undescended testes and fixate them within the scrotum
order	shows subordination of one thing to another; family or class
orthopnea	difficulty in breathing, needing to be in erect position to breathe
orthoptic	corrective; in the correct place
osteoarthritis	degenerative condition of articular cartilage
osteoclast	absorbs or removes bone
osteotomy	cutting into bone
otitis media	noninfectious inflammation of the middle ear; serous otitis media produces liquid drainage (not purulent) and suppurative otitis media produces purulent (pus) matter
otoscope	instrument used to examine the internal and external ear
oviduct	fallopian tube
papilledema	swelling of the optic disk (papilla)
paraesophageal hiatus hernia	hernia that is near the esophagus
parathyroid	produces a hormone to mobilize calcium from the bones to the blood
paronychia	infection around nail

Part A	Medicare's Hospital Insurance; covers hospital/facility care
Part B	Medicare's Supplemental Medical Insurance; covers physician services and durable medical equipment that are not paid for under Part A
participating provider program	Medicare providers who have agreed in advance to accept assignment on all Medicare claims, now termed Quality Improvement Organizations (QIO)
patella	knee cap
pedicle	growth attached with a stem
Peer Review Organizations	PROs, groups established to review hospital admission and care
pelviolithotomy	pyeloplasty
penoscrotal	referring to the penis and scrotum
percussion	tapping with sharp blows as a diagnostic technique
percutaneous	through the skin
percutaneous fracture repair	repair of a fracture by means of pins and wires inserted through the fracture site
percutaneous skeletal fixation	considered neither open nor closed; the fracture is not visualized, but fixation is placed across the fracture site under x-ray imaging
pericardiocentesis	procedure in which a surgeon withdraws fluid from the pericardial space by means of a needle inserted percutaneously
pericardium	membranous sac enclosing heart and ends of great vessels
perineum	area between the vulva and anus; also known as the pelvic floor
peripheral nerves	12 pairs of cranial nerves, 31 pairs of spinal nerves, and autonomic nervous system; connects peripheral receptors to the brain and spinal cord
peritoneal	within the lining of the abdominal cavity
peritoneoscopy	visualization of the abdominal cavity using one scope placed through a small incision in the abdominal wall and another scope placed in the vagina
pharyngolaryngectomy	surgical removal of the pharynx and larynx
phlebotomy	cutting into a vein
phonocardiogram	recording of heart sounds
photochemotherapy	treatment by means of drugs that react to ultraviolet radiation or sunlight
physics	scientific study of energy
pilosebaceous	pertains to hair follicles and sebaceous glands
placenta	a structure that connects the fetus and mother during pregnancy
plethysmography	determining the changes in volume of an organ part or body
pleura	covers the lungs and lines the thoracic cavity
pleurectomy	surgical excision of the pleura

Appendix B Medical Terminology

pleuritis	inflammation of the pleura
pneumonocentesis	surgical puncturing of a lung to withdraw fluid
pneumonolysis	surgical separation of the lung from the chest wall to allow the lung to collapse
pneumonostomy	surgical procedure in which the chest cavity is exposed and the lung is incised
pneumonotomy	incision of the lung
pneumoplethysmography	determining the changes in the volume of the lung
posterior (dorsal)	in back of
posterior segment	those parts of the eye behind the lens
posteroanterior	from back to front
postpartum	after childbirth
Preferred Provider Organization	PPO, a group of providers who form a network and who have agreed to provide services to enrollees at a discounted rate
priapism	painful condition in which the penis is constantly erect
primary care physician	PCP, physician who oversees a patient's care within a managed care organization
primary diagnosis	chief complaint of a patient in outpatient setting
primipara	first pregnancy
prior approval	also known as a prior authorization, the payer's approval of care
proctosigmoidoscopy	fiberscopic examination of the sigmoid colon and rectum
Professional Standards Review Organization	PSRO, voluntary physicians' organization designed to monitor the necessity of hospital admissions, treatment costs, and medical records of hospitals
prognosis	probable outcome of an illness
prostatotomy	incision into the prostate
Provider Identification Number	PIN, assigned to physicians by payers for use in claims submission
pyelography	radiographic recording of the kidneys, renal pelvis, ureters, and bladder
qualitative	measuring the presence or absence of
Quality Improvement Organizations	QIO, consists of a national network of 53 entities that work with consumers, physicians, hospitals, and caregivers to refine care delivery systems
quantitative	measuring the presence or absence of and the amount of
rad	radiation-absorbed dose, the energy deposited in patient's tissues
radiation oncology	branch of medicine concerned with the application of radiation to a tumor site for treatment (destruction) of cancerous tumors
radiograph	film on which an image is produced through exposure to x-radiation

radiologist	physician who specializes in the use of radioactive materials in the diagnosis and treatment of disease and illness
radiology	branch of medicine concerned with the use of radioactive substances for diagnosis and therapy
rales	coarse sound on inspiration, also known as crackle (heard on auscultation)
real time	two-dimensional display of both the structures and the motion of tissues and organs, with the length of time also recorded as part of the study
reduction	replacement to normal position
Relative Value Unit	RVU, unit value that has been assigned for each service
Resource-Based Relative Value Scale	RBRVS, scale designed to decrease Medicare expenditures, redistribute physician payment, and ensure quality health care at reasonable rates
resource intensity	refers to the relative volume and type of diagnostic, therapeutic, and bed services used in the management of a particular illness
retrograde	moving backward or against the usual direction of flow
rhinoplasty	surgical repair of nose
rhinorrhea	nasal mucous discharge
salpingectomy	surgical removal of the uterine tube
salpingostomy	creation of a fistula into the uterine tube
scan	mapping of emissions of radioactive substances after they have been introduced into the body; the density can determine normal or abnormal conditions
sclera	outer covering of the eye
scoliosis	lateral curve of the spine
sebaceous gland	secretes sebum
seborrhea	excess sebum secretion
sebum	oily substance
section	slice of a frozen block
segmentectomy	surgical removal of a portion of a lung
septoplasty	surgical repair of the nasal septum
serum	blood from which the fibrinogen has been removed
severity of illness	refers to the levels of loss of function and mortality that may be experienced by patients with a particular disease
shunt	an artificial passage
sialography	radiographic recording of the salivary duct and branches
sialolithotomy	surgical removal of a stone of the salivary gland or duct
sinography	radiographic recording of the sinus or sinus tract
sinusotomy	surgical incision into a sinus

Appendix B Medical Terminology

skeletal traction	application of pressure to the bone by means of pins and/or wires inserted into the bone
skin traction	application of pressure to the bone by means of tape applied to the skin
skull	entire skeletal framework of the head
somatic nerve	sensory or motor nerve
specimen	sample of tissue or fluid
spirometry	measurement of breathing capacity
splenectomy	excision of the spleen
splenography	radiographic recording of the spleen
splenoportography	radiographic procedure to allow visualization of the splenic and portal veins of the spleen
split-thickness graft	all epidermis and some of dermis
spondylitis	inflammation of vertebrae
Staff Model	a Health Maintenance Organization that directly employs the physicians who provide services to enrollees
steatoma	fat mass in sebaceous gland
stem cell	immature blood cell
stereotaxis	method of identifying a specific area or point in the brain
strabismus	extraocular muscle deviation resulting in unequal visual axes
stratified	layered
stratum (strata)	layer
subcutaneous	tissue below the dermis, primarily fat cells that insulate the body
subluxation	partial dislocation
subungual	beneath the nail
superior	toward the head or the upper part of the body; also known as cephalic
supination	supine position
supine	lying on the back
Swan-Ganz catheter	a catheter that measures pressure in the heart
sympathetic nerve	part of the peripheral nervous system that controls automatic body function and sympathetic nerves activated under stress
symphysis	natural junction
synchondrosis	union between two bones (connected by cartilage)
tachypnea	quick, shallow breathing
tarsorrhaphy	suturing together of the eyelids
Tax Equity and Fiscal Responsibility Act	TEFRA, act that contains language to reward cost-conscious healthcare providers

tendon	attaches a muscle to a bone
tenodesis	suturing of a tendon to a bone
tenorrhaphy	suture repair of tendon
thermogram	written record of temperature variation
third-party payer	insurance company or entity that is liable for another's health care services
thoracentesis	surgical puncture of the thoracic cavity, usually using a needle, to remove fluids
thoracic duct	collection and distribution point for lymph, and the largest lymph vessel located in the chest
thoracoplasty	surgical procedure that removes rib(s) and thereby allows the collapse of a lung
thoracoscopy	use of a lighted endoscope to view the pleural spaces and thoracic cavity or to perform surgical procedures
thoracostomy	incision into the chest wall and insertion of a chest tube
thoracotomy	surgical incision into the chest wall
thromboendarterectomy	procedure to remove plaque or clot formations from a vessel by percutaneous method
thymectomy	surgical removal of the thymus
thymus	gland that produces hormones important to the immune response
thyroglossal duct	connection between the thyroid and the tongue
thyroid	part of the endocrine system that produces hormones that regulate metabolism
thyroidectomy	surgical removal of the thyroid
tinnitus	ringing in the ears
titer	measure of a laboratory analysis
tocolysis	repression of uterine contractions
tomography	procedure that allows viewing of a single plane of the body by blurring out all but that particular level
tonography	recording of changes in intraocular pressure in response to sustained pressure on the eyeball
tonometry	measurement of pressure or tension
total pneumonectomy	surgical removal of an entire lung
tracheostomy	creation of an opening into trachea
tracheotomy	incision into trachea
traction	application of pressure to maintain normal alignment
transcutaneous	entering by way of the skin
transesophageal echocardiogram	TEE, echocardiogram performed by placing a probe down the esophagus and sending out sound waves to obtain images of the heart and its movement

Appendix B Medical Terminology

transmastoid	creates an opening in the mastoid for drainage antrostomy
transplantation	grafting of tissue from one source to another
transseptal	through the septum
transtracheal	across the trachea
transureteroureterostomy	surgical connection of one ureter to the other ureter
transurethral resection, prostate	procedure performed through the urethra by means of a cystoscopy to remove part or all of the prostate
transvenous	through a vein
transvesical ureterolithotomy	removal of a ureter stone (calculus) through the bladder
trephination	surgical removal of a disk of bone
trocar needle	needle with a tube on the end; used to puncture and withdraw fluid from a cavity
tubercle	lesion caused by infection of tuberculosis
tumescence	state of being swollen
tunica vaginalis	covering of the testes
tympanolysis	freeing of adhesions of the tympanic membrane
tympanometry	test of the inner ear using air pressure
tympanostomy	insertion of ventilation tube into tympanum
ultrasound	technique using sound waves to determine the density of the outline of tissue
unbundling	reporting with multiple codes that which can be reported with one code
unilateral	occurring on one side
uptake	absorption of a radioactive substance by body tissues; recorded for diagnostic purposes in conditions such as thyroid disease
ureterectomy	surgical removal of a ureter, either totally or partially
ureterocolon	pertaining to the ureter and colon
ureterocutaneous fistula	channel from the ureter to exterior skin
ureteroenterostomy	creation of a connection between the intestine and the ureter
ureterolithotomy	removal of a stone from the ureter
ureterolysis	freeing of adhesions of the ureter
ureteroneocystostomy	surgical connection of the ureter to a new site on the bladder
ureteropyelography	ureter and bladder radiography
ureterotomy	incision into the ureter
urethrocystography	radiography of the bladder and urethra
urethromeatoplasty	surgical repair of the urethra and meatus
urethropexy	fixation of the urethra by means of surgery
urethroplasty	surgical repair of the urethra

urethrorrhaphy	suturing of the urethra
urethroscopy	use of a scope to view the urethra
urography	same as pyelography; radiographic recording of the kidneys, renal pelvis, ureters, and bladder
uveal	vascular tissue of the choroid, ciliary body, and iris
varices	varicose veins
varicocele	swelling of a scrotal vein
vas deferens	tube that carries sperm from the epididymis to the urethra
vasectomy	removal of segment of vas deferens
vasogram	recording of the flow in the vas deferens
vasotomy	incision in the vas deferens
vasorrhaphy	suturing of the vas deferens
vasovasostomy	reversal of a vasectomy
vectorcardiogram	VCG, continuous recording of electrical direction and magnitude of the heart
venography	radiographic recording of the veins and tributaries
vertebrectomy	removal of vertebra
vertigo	dizziness
vesicostomy	surgical creation of a connection of the viscera of the bladder to the skin
vesicovaginal fistula	creation of a tube between the vagina and the bladder
vesiculectomy	excision of the seminal vesicle
vesiculography	radiographic recording of the seminal vesicles
vesiculotomy	incision into the seminal vesicle
viscera	an organ in one of the large cavities of the body
volvulus	twisted section of the intestine
vomer	flat bones of the nasal septum
xanthoma	tumor composed of cells containing lipid material, yellow in color
xenograft	different species graft
xeroderma	dry, discolored, scaly skin
xeroradiography	photoelectric process of radiographs

Appendix C

Combining Forms

abdomin/o	abdomen
acetabul/o	hip socket
acr/o	height/extremities
aden/o	in relationship to a gland
adenoid/o	adenoids
adip/o	fat
adren/o, adrenal/o	adrenal gland
albin/o	white
albumin/o	albumin
alveol/o	alveolus
ambly/o	dim
amni/o	amnion
an/o	anus
andr/o	male
andren/o	adrenal gland
andrenal/o	adrenal gland
angi/o	vessel
ankyl/o	bent, fused
aort/o	aorta
aponeur/o	tendon type
appendic/o	appendix
aque/o	water
arche/o	first
arter/o, arteri/o	artery
arthr/o	joint
atel/o	incomplete
ather/o	plaque
atri/o	atrium

audi/o	hearing
aut/o	self
axill/o	armpit
azot/o	urea
balan/o	glans penis
bi/o	life
bil/i	bile
bilirubin/o	bile pigment
blephar/o	eyelid
brachi/o	arm
bronch/o	bronchus
bronchi/o	bronchus
bronchiol/o	bronchiole
burs/o	fluid-filled sac in a joint
calc/o, calc/i	calcium
cardi/o	heart
carp/o	carpals (wrist bones)
cauter/o	burn
cec/o	cecum
celi/o	abdomen
cephal/o	head
cerebell/o	cerebellum
cerebr/o	cerebrum
cervic/o	neck/cervix
chol/e	gall/bile
cholangio/o	bile duct
cholecyst/o	gallbladder
choledoch/o	common bile duct
cholester/o	cholesterol
chondr/o	cartilage
chori/o	chorion
clavic/o, clavicul/o	clavicle (collar bone)
col/o	colon
colp/o	vagina
coni/o	dust
conjunctiv/o	conjunctiva

Appendix C Combining Forms

cor/o, core/o	pupil
corne/o	cornea
coron/o	heart
cortic/o	cortex
cost/o	rib
crani/o	cranium (skull)
crin/o	secrete
crypt/o	hidden
culd/o	cul-de-sac
cutane/o	skin
cyan/o	blue
cycl/o	ciliary body
cyst/o	bladder
dacry/o	tear
dacryocyst/o	prefix meaning pertaining to the lacrimal sac
dent/i	tooth
derm/o, dermat/o	skin
diaphragmat/o	diaphragm
dips/o	thirst
disk/o	intervertebral disk
diverticul/o	diverticulum
duoden/o	duodenum
dur/o	dura mater
encephal/o	brain
enter/o	small intestine
eosin/o	rosy
epididym/o	epididymis
epiglott/o	epiglottis
episi/o	vulva
erythr/o, erythem/o	red
esophag/o	esophagus
essi/o, esthesi/o	sensation
estr/o	female
femor/o	thighbone
fet/o	fetus
fibul/o	fibula

galact/o	milk
gangli/o	ganglion
ganglion/o	ganglion
gastr/o	stomach
gingiv/o	gum
glomerul/o	glomerulus
gloss/o	tongue
gluc/o	sugar
glyc/o	sugar
glycos/o	sugar
gonad/o	ovaries and testes
gyn/o	female
gynec/o	female
hepat/o	liver
herni/o	hernia
heter/o	different
hidr/o	sweat
home/o	same
hormon/o	hormone
humer/o	humerus (upper arm bone)
hydr/o	water
hymen/o	hymen
hyster/o	uterus
ichthy/o	dry/scaly
ile/o	ileus
ili/o	ilium (upper pelvic bone)
immun/o	immune
inguin/o	groin
ir/o	iris
irid/o	iris
ischi/o	ischium (posterior pelvic bone)
jaund/o	yellow
jejun/o	jejunum
kal/i	potassium
kerat/o	hard, cornea

Appendix C Combining Forms

kinesi/o	movement
kyph/o	hump
lacrim/o	tear
lact/o	milk
lamin/o	lamina
lapar/o	abdomen
laryng/o	larynx
lingu/o	tongue
lip/o	fat
lith/o	stone
lob/o	lobe
lord/o	curve
lumb/o	lower back
lute/o	yellow
lymph/o	lymph
lymphaden/o	lymph gland
mamm/o	breast
mandibul/o	mandible (lower jawbone)
mast/o	breast
maxill/o	maxilla (upper jawbone)
meat/o	meatus
melan/o	black
men/o	menstruation, month
mening/o, meningi/o	meninges
menisc/o, menisci/o	meniscus
ment/o	mind
metacarp/o	metacarpals (hand)
metatars/o	metatarsals (foot)
metr/o	uterus, measure
metr/i	uterus
mon/o	one
muc/o	mucus
my/o, muscul/o	muscle
myc/o	fungus

myel/o	bone marrow, spinal cord
myring/o	ear drum
myx/o	mucus
nas/o	nose
nat/a, nat/i	birth
natr/o	sodium
necr/o	death
nephr/o	kidney
neur/o	nerve
noct/i	night
ocul/o	eye
olecran/o	olecranon (elbow)
olig/o	scant, few
onych/o	nail
oo/o	egg
oophor/o	ovary
ophthalm/o	eye
opt/o	eye, vision
optic/o	eye
or/o	mouth
orch/i, orch/o, orchi/o, orchid/o	testicle
orth/o	straight
oste/o	bone
ot/o	ear
ov/o	egg
ovari/o	ovary
ovul/o	ovulation
ox/i, ox/o	oxygen
oxy/o	oxygen
pachy/o	thick
palat/o	palate
palpebr/o	eyelid
pancreat/o	pancreas

Appendix C Combining Forms

papill/o	optic nerve
patell/o	patella (kneecap)
pelv/i	pelvis (hip)
pericardi/o	pericardium
perine/o	perineum
peritone/o	peritoneum
petr/o	stone
phac/o	eye lens
phak/o	eye lens
phalang/o	phalanges (finger or toe)
pharyng/o	pharynx
phas/o	speech
phleb/o	vein
phren/o	mind, diaphragm
phys/o	growing
pil/o	hair
pituitar/o	pituitary gland
pleur/o	pleura
pneumat/o	lung/air
pneumon/o	lung/air
poli/o	gray matter
polyp/o	polyp
pont/o	pons
proct/o	rectum
prostat/o	prostate gland
psych/o	mind
pub/o	pubis
pulmon/o	lung
pupill/o	pupil
py/o	pus
pyel/o	renal pelvis
pylor/o	pylorus
quadr/i	four
rachi/o	spine
radi/o	radius (lower arm)
radic/o, radicul/o	nerve root
rect/o	rectum

ren/o	kidney
retin/o	retina
rhin/o	nose
rhiz/o	nerve root
rhytid/o	wrinkle
rube/o	red
sacr/o	sacrum
salping/o	uterine tube, Fallopian tube
scapul/o	scapula (shoulder)
scler/o	sclera
scoli/o	bent
seb/o	sebum/oil
semin/i	semen
sept/o	septum
sial/o	saliva
sigmoid/o	sigmoid colon
sinus/o	sinus
somat/o	body
son/o	sound
sperm/o, spermat/o	sperm
sphygm/o	pulse
spir/o	breath
splen/o	spleen
spondyl/o	vertebra
staped/o	middle ear, stapes
staphyl/o	clusters
steat/o	fat
ster/o, stere/o	solid, having three dimensions
stern/o	sternum (breast bone)
steth/o	chest
stomat/o	mouth
strept/o	twisted chain
synovi/o	synovial joint membrane
tars/o	tarsal (ankle)
ten/o	tendon

Appendix C Combining Forms

tend/o, tendin/o	tendon (connective tissue)
test/o	testicle
thorac/o	thorax
thromb/o	clot
thym/o	thymus gland
thyr/o, thyroid/o	thyroid gland
tibi/o	shin bone
toc/o	childbirth
tonsill/o	tonsil
top/o	place
tox/o, toxic/o	poison
trache/o	trachea
trich/o	hair
tympan/o	ear drum
uln/o	ulna (lower arm bone)
ungu/o	nail
ur/o	urine
ureter/o	ureter
urethr/o	urethra
urin/o	urine
uter/o	uterus
uve/o	uvea
uvul/o	uvula
vagin/o	vagina
valv/o, valvul/o	valve
vas/o, vascul/o	vessel
ven/o	vein
ventricul/o	ventricle
vertebr/o	vertebra
vesic/o	bladder
vesicul/o	seminal vesicles
vitre/o	glass/glassy
vulv/o	vulva
xanth/o	yellow
xer/o	dry

Appendix D

Prefixes

a-	not
an-	not
ante-	before
audi-	hearing
bi-	two
brady-	slow
de-	lack of
dys-	difficult, painful
ecto-	outside
endo-	in
epi-	on/upon
eso-	inward
eu-	good/normal
exo-	outward
extra-	outside
hemi-	half
hyper-	excess, over
hypo-	under
in-	into
inter-	between
intra-	within
meta-	change, after
multi-	many
neo-	new
nulli-, nulti-	none
oxy-	sharp, oxygen
pan-	all
para-	beside

Appendix D   Prefixes

per-	through
peri-	surrounding
poly-	many
post-	after
primi-	first
pseudo-	false
quadri-	four
retro-	behind
sub-	under
supra-	above
sym-	together
syn-	together
tachy-	fast
tetra-	four
tri-	three
tropin-	act upon
uni-	one

Appendix E

Suffixes

-agon	assemble
-algesia	pain sensation
-algia	pain
-ar	pertaining to
-arche	beginning
-ary	pertaining to
-asthenia	weakness
-blast	embryonic
-capnia	carbon dioxide
-cele	hernia
-centesis	puncture to remove (drain)
-chezia	defecation
-clast, -clasia, -clasis	break
-coccus	spherical bacterium
-cyesis	pregnancy
-desis	fusion
-dilation	widening, expanding
-drome	run
-dynia	pain
-eal	pertaining to
-ectasis	stretching
-ectomy	removal
-edema	swelling
-emia	blood
-esthesis	feeling
-gram	record
-graph	recording instrument
-graphy	recording process

Appendix E Suffixes

-gravida	pregnancy
-ia	condition
-iatrist	physician specialist
-iatry	medical treatment
-ical	pertaining to
-ictal	pertaining to
-in	a substance
-ine	a substance
-itis	inflammation
-listhesis	slipping
-lithiasis	condition of stones
-lysis	separation
-malacia	softening
-megaly	enlargement
-meta	change
-meter	measurement; instrument that measures
-metry	measurement of
-oid	resembling
-oma	tumor
-omia	smell
-one	hormone
-opia	vision
-opsy	view of
-orrhexis	rupture
-osis	condition
-oxia	oxygen
-para	woman who has given birth
-paresis	incomplete paralysis
-parous	to bear
-penia	deficient
-pexy	fixation
-phagia	eating
-phonia	sound
-phylaxis	protection
-physis	to grow
-plasty	repair
-plegia	paralysis

-pnea	breathing
-poiesis	production
-poly	many
-porosis	passage
-retro	behind
-rrhagia	bursting of blood
-rrhaphy	suture
-rrhea	discharge
-schisis	split
-sclerosis	hardening
-scopy	to examine
-spasm	contraction of muscle
-steat/o	fat
-stenosis	blockage, narrowing
-stomy	opening
-thorax	chest
-tocia	labor
-tom/o	to cut
-tome	an instrument that cuts
-tomy	cutting, incision
-tripsy	crush
-tropia	to turn
-tropin	act upon
-uria	urine
-version	turning

Appendix F

Abbreviations

ABG	arterial blood gas
ABN	Advanced Beneficiary Notice used by CMS to notify beneficiary of payment of provider services
ACL	anterior cruciate ligament
AD	right ear
AFB	acid-fast bacillus
AFI	amniotic fluid index
AGA	appropriate for gestational age
AGCUS	atypical glandular cells of undetermined significance
AKA	above-knee amputation
ANS	autonomic nervous system
APCs	Ambulatory Payment Classifications, patient classification that provides a payment system for outpatients
ARDS	adult respiratory distress syndrome
ARF	acute renal failure
ARM	artificial rupture of membrane
AS	left ear
ASCUS	atypical squamous cells of undetermined significance
ASCVD	arteriosclerotic cardiovascular disease
ASD	atrial septal defect
ASHD	arteriosclerotic heart disease
AU	both ears
AV	atrioventricular
BCC	benign cellular changes
BiPAP	bi-level positive airway pressure
BKA	below-knee amputation
BP	blood pressure
BPD	biparietal diameter

BPH	benign prostatic hypertrophy
BPP	biophysical profile
BUN	blood urea nitrogen
BV	bacterial vaginosis
bx	biopsy
C1-C7	cervical vertebrae
ca	cancer
CABG	coronary artery bypass graft
CBC	complete blood (cell) count
CF	conversion factor, national dollar amount that is applied to all services paid on the Medicare Fee Schedule basis
CHF	congestive heart failure
CHL	crown-to-heel length
CK	creatine kinase
CMS	Centers for Medicare and Medicaid Services, formerly HCFA, Health Care Financing Administration
CNM	certified nurse midwife
CNS	central nervous system
COB	coordination of benefits, management of payment between two or more third-party payers for a service
COPD	chronic obstructive pulmonary disease
CPAP	continuous positive airway pressure
CPD	cephalopelvic disproportion
CPK	creatine phosphokinase
CPP	chronic pelvic pain
CSF	cerebrospinal fluid
CTS	carpal tunnel syndrome
CVA	stroke/cerebrovascular accident
CVI	cerebrovascular insufficiency
D&C	dilation and curettage
D&E	dilation and evacuation
derm	dermatology
DHHS	Department of Health and Human Services
DLCO	diffuse capacity of lungs for carbon monoxide
DRGs	Diagnosis Related Groups, disease classification system that relates the type of inpatients a hospital treats (case mix) to the costs incurred by the hospital
DSE	dobutamine stress echocardiography

Appendix F Abbreviations

DUB	dysfunctional uterine bleeding
ECC	endocervical curettage
EDC	estimated date of confinement
EDD	estimated date of delivery
EDI	electronic data interchange, exchange of data between multiple computer terminals
EEG	electroencephalogram
EFM	electronic fetal monitoring
EFW	estimated fetal weight
EGA	estimated gestational age
EGD	esophagogastroduodenoscopy
EGJ	esophagogastric junction
EMC	endometrial curettage
EOB	explanation of benefits, remittance advice
EPO	Exclusive Provider Organization, similar to a Health Maintenance Organization except that the providers of the services are not prepaid, but rather are paid on a fee-for-service basis
EPSDT	Early and Periodic Screening, Diagnosis, and Treatment
ERCP	endoscopic retrograde cholangiopancreatography
ERT	estrogen replacement therapy
ESRD	end-stage renal disease
FAS	fetal alcohol syndrome
FEF	forced expiratory flow
FEV_1	forced expiratory volume in 1 second
$FEV_1:FVC$	maximum amount of forced expiratory volume in 1 second
FHR	fetal heart rate
FI	fiscal intermediary, financial agent acting on behalf of a third-party payer
FRC	functional residual capacity
FSH	follicle-stimulating hormone
FVC	forced vital capacity
fx	fracture
GERD	gastroesophageal reflux disease
GI	gastrointestinal
H or E	hemorrhage or exudate
HCFA	Health Care Financing Administration, now known as Centers for Medicare and Medicaid Services (CMS)
HCVD	hypertensive cardiovascular disease
HD	hemodialysis

HDL	high-density lipoprotein
HEA	hemorrhage, exudate, aneurysm
HHN	hand-held nebulizer
HJR	hepatojugular reflux
H&P	history and physical
HPV	human papillomavirus
HSG	hysterosalpingogram
HSV	herpes simplex virus
I&D	incision and drainage
IO	intraocular
IOL	intraocular lens
IPAP	inspiratory positive airway pressure
IRDS	infant respiratory distress syndrome
IVF	in vitro fertilization
IVP	intravenous pyelogram
JBP	jugular blood pressure
KUB	kidneys, ureter, bladder
L1-L5	lumbar vertebrae
LBBB	left bundle branch block
LEEP	loop electrosurgical excision procedure
LGA	large for gestational age
LLQ	left lower quadrant
LP	lumbar puncture
LUQ	left upper quadrant
LVH	left ventricular hypertrophy
MAT	multifocal atrial tachycardia
MDI	metered dose inhaler
MI	myocardial infarction
MRI	magnetic resonance imaging
MSLT	multiple sleep latency testing
MVV	maximum voluntary ventilation
NCPAP	nasal continuous positive airway pressure
NSR	normal sinus rhythm
OA	osteoarthritis
OD	right eye
OS	left eye
OU	each eye

Appendix F Abbreviations

PAC	premature atrial contraction
PAT	paroxysmal atrial tachycardia
PAWP	pulmonary artery wedge pressure
PCWP	pulmonary capillary wedge pressure
PEAP	positive end-airway pressure
PEEP	positive end-expiratory pressure
PEG	percutaneous endoscopic gastrostomy
PERL	pupils equal and reactive to light
PERRL	pupils equal, round, and reactive to light
PERRLA	pupils equal, round, and reactive to light and accommodation
PFT	pulmonary function test
pH	symbol for acid/base level
PICC	peripherally inserted central catheter
PID	pelvic inflammatory disease
PND	paroxysmal nocturnal dyspnea
PNS	peripheral nervous system
PROM	premature rupture of membranes
PSA	prostate-specific antigen
PST	paroxysmal supraventricular tachycardia
PSVT	paroxysmal supraventricular tachycardia
PT	prothrombin time
PTCA	percutaneous transluminal coronary angioplasty
PTT	partial thromboplastin time
PVC	premature ventricular contraction
RA	remittance advice, explanation of services
RA	rheumatoid arthritis
RBBB	right bundle branch block
RDS	respiratory distress syndrome
REM	rapid eye movement
RLQ	right lower quadrant
RSR	regular sinus rhythm
RUQ	right upper quadrant
RV	respiratory volume
RVG	*Relative Value Guide*
RVH	right ventricular hypertrophy
RVS	relative value studies, list of procedures with unit values assigned to each
RV:TLC	ratio of respiratory volume to total lung capacity

Appendix F Abbreviations

SHG	sonohysterogram
sp gr	specific gravity
SROM	spontaneous rupture of membranes
subcu, subq, SC, SQ	subcutaneous
SUI	stress urinary incontinence
SVT	supraventricular tachycardia
T1-T12	thoracic vertebrae
TAH	total abdominal hysterectomy
TEE	transesophageal echocardiography
TENS	transcutaneous electrical nerve stimulation
TIA	transient ischemic attack
TLC	total lung capacity
TLV	total lung volume
TM	tympanic membrane
TMJ	temporomandibular joint
TPA	tissue plasminogen activator
TSH	thyroid-stimulating hormone
TST	treadmill stress test
TURBT	transurethral resection of bladder tumor
TURP	transurethral resection of prostate
UA	urinalysis
UCR	usual, customary, and reasonable—third-party payers' assessment of the reimbursement for health care services: usual, that which would ordinarily be charged for the service; customary, the cost of that service in that locale; and reasonable, as assessed by the payer
UPJ	ureteropelvic junction
URI	upper respiratory infection
UTI	urinary tract infection
V/Q	ventilation/perfusion scan
VBAC	vaginal birth after cesarean
WBC	white blood (cell) count

Appendix G

Further Text Resources

ANATOMY AND PHYSIOLOGY

Book Title	Author	Imprint	Copyright Date	ISBN
The Anatomy and Physiology Learning System, 3rd Edition	Applegate	Saunders	2006	978-1-4160-2586-3
Gray's Anatomy for Students, 2nd Edition	Drake, Vogl, Mitchell	Churchill Livingstone	2009	978-0-443-06952-9
Anthony's Textbook of Anatomy and Physiology, 19th Edition	Thibodeau, Patton	Mosby	2010	978-0-323-05539-0

CODING

Book Title	Author	Imprint	Copyright Date	ISBN
Step-by-Step Medical Coding, 2009 Edition	Buck	Saunders	2009	978-1-4160-4566-3
2009 ICD-9-CM, Volumes 1 & 2 (Professional Edition)	Buck	Saunders	2009	978-1-4160-4448-2
2009 ICD-9-CM, Volumes 1, 2, & 3 (Professional Edition)	Buck	Saunders	2009	978-1-4160-4450-5
2009 HCPCS Level II (Professional Edition)	Buck	Saunders	2009	978-1-4160-5203-6
The Next Step, Advanced Medical Coding, 2009 Edition	Buck	Saunders	2009	978-1-4160-5679-9
The Extra Step: Facility-Based Coding Practice	Buck	Saunders	2006	978-1-4160-3450-6
The Extra Step: Physician-Based Coding Practice	Buck	Saunders	2009	978-1-4160-6162-5
CCS Coding Exam Review 2009: The Certification Step	Buck	Saunders	2009	978-1-4160-3686-9
The Evaluation and Management Step: An Auditing Tool, 2009 Edition	Buck	Saunders	2009	978-1-4160-6724-5
ICD-9-CM Coding: Theory and Practice, 2009 Edition	Lovaasen, Schwerdtfeger	Saunders	2009	978-1-4160-5881-6

Copyright © 2009, 2008, 2007, 2006, 2005, 2004 by Saunders, an imprint of Elsevier Inc. All rights reserved.

PATHOPHYSIOLOGY

Book Title	Author	Imprint	Copyright Date	ISBN-13
Pathology for the Health Professions, 3rd Edition	Damjanov	Saunders	2006	978-1-4160-0031-0
Essentials of Human Diseases and Conditions, 4th Edition	Frazier, Drzymkowski	Saunders	2008	978-1-4160-4714-8
Pathophysiology for the Health Related Professions, 3rd Edition	Gould	Saunders	2006	978-1-4160-0210-9
The Human Body in Health and Illness, 3rd Edition	Herlihy	Saunders	2007	978-1-4160-2885-7
The Human Body in Health and Disease, 5th Edition	Thibodeau, Patton	Mosby	2010	978-0-323-05492-8

MEDICAL TERMINOLOGY

Book Title	Author	Imprint	Copyright Date	ISBN-13
The Language of Medicine, 8th Edition	Chabner	Saunders	2007	978-1-4160-3492-6
Jablonski's Dictionary of Medical Acronyms & Abbreviations, 6th edition	Jablonski	Saunders	2009	978-1-4160-5899-1
Exploring Medical Language, 7th Edition	LaFleur, Brooks	Mosby	2008	978-0-323-04950-4
Building a Medical Vocabulary (with Spanish Translations), 7th Edition	Leonard	Saunders	2009	978-1-4160-5627-0
Quick & Easy Medical Terminology, 5th Edition	Leonard	Saunders	2007	978-1-4160-2494-1
Mastering Healthcare Terminology, 3rd Edition	Shiland	Mosby	2010	978-0-323-05506-2
Dorland's Illustrated Medical Dictionary, 31st Edition		Saunders	2007	978-1-4160-2364-7

INTRODUCTION TO COMPUTER

Book Title	Author	Imprint	Copyright Date	ISBN-13
Computerized Medical Office Procedures: A Worktext, 2nd Edition	Larsen	Saunders	2008	978-1-4160-4834-3

BASICS OF WRITING/MEDICAL TRANSCRIPTION

Book Title	Author	Imprint	Copyright Date	ISBN-13
Medical Transcription Guide: Do's and Don'ts, 3rd Edition	Diehl	Saunders	2005	978-0-7216-0684-2
Diehl & Fordney's Medical Transcribing: Techniques and Procedures, 6th Edition	Diehl	Saunders	2007	978-1-4160-2347-0

Appendix G Further Text Resources

COMPREHENSION BUILDING/STUDY SKILLS

Book Title	Author	Imprint	Copyright Date	ISBN-13
Career Development for Health Professionals: Success in School and on the Job, 2nd Edition	Haroun	Saunders	2006	978-0-7216-0609-5

BASIC MATH

Book Title	Author	Imprint	Copyright Date	ISBN-13
Basic Mathematics for the Health-Related Professions	Doucette	Saunders	2000	978-0-7216-7938-9
Using Maths in Health Sciences	Gunn	Churchill Livingstone	2001	978-0-443-07074-7

MEDICAL BILLING/INSURANCE

Book Title	Author	Imprint	Copyright Date	ISBN-13
Health Insurance Today: A Practical Approach, 2nd Edition	Beik	Saunders	2009	978-1-4160-5320-0
Medical Insurance Made Easy: Understanding the Claim Cycle, 2nd Edition	Brown	Saunders	2006	978-0-7216-0556-2
Insurance Handbook for the Medical Office, 10th Edition	Fordney	Saunders	2008	978-1-4160-3666-1

Index

Note: Page numbers followed by f refer to figures.

A

Abdominal aortic aneurysm, endovascular repair of, 354
Abdominal pain, 178, 202
ABG. *See* Arterial blood gas
Ablation, 90
ABN. *See* Advanced Beneficiary Notice
Abnormal menstruation types, 108
Abortion, 422, A-35
   with liveborn fetus, A-36
   methods, 119
   services, 371
   types, 118
Above-knee amputation (AKA), 2, 43
Abruptio placentae, 117
Absorption atelectasis, 66
Abuse, 285
   medicare fraud and, 284
Accessory organs, 98, 123, 164. *See also* Digestive system
Accessory sinuses, 55, 347
ACE (angiotensin-converting enzyme) inhibitors, 156
Acetabulum, 34
Achilles tendon, 40
Acid-fast bacillus (AFB), 59
Acidosis, respiratory, 66
ACL. *See* Anterior cruciate ligament
Acne vulgaris, 18
Acquired immunodeficiency syndrome (AIDS), 25
Acromegaly, 220
Actinic keratosis, 24
Actinotherapy, 397
Active wound care management, 398
Acute bronchitis, with COPD, A-30
Acute fractures vs. Aftercare, A-36, A-41
Acute infection, of B cells, 203
Acute lymphocytic leukemia, treatment for, 205
Acute myelogenous leukemia (AML), 204
Acute myocardial infarction (AMI), unspecified, A-29
Acute necrotizing fasciitis, 21
Acute organ dysfunction, A-16
Acute pericarditis, 92
Acute poststreptococcal glomerulonephritis (APSGN)
   cause, 153
   treatment, 154
Acute pyelonephritis
   cause, 152
   illustration, 151f
   symptoms, 152
   treatment, 152

Acute renal failure (ARF), 144, 149
Acute respiratory failure, 65, A-30
Acute superficial gastritis, 174
Addison's disease
   cause, 224
   symptoms, 224
   treatment, 225
Adenomyosis, 112
Adjacent tissue transfer, rearrangement, 335
Adrenal glands, 212
   disorders, 224
Adrenal insufficiency, primary, 224
Adrenal medulla, 225
Adult respiratory distress syndrome (ARDS), 59, 66, 186
Advanced Beneficiary Notice (ABN), reimbursement terminology, 286
Adverse effect, A-43
AFB. *See* Acid-fast bacillus
AFI. *See* Amniotic fluid index
Aftercare, A-50
   acute fractures vs., A-36, A-41
AGA. *See* Appropriate for gestational age
AIDS, 237
Air-conducting structure, 55
AKA. *See* Above-knee amputation
Alcohol, 175
Aldosterone, 212
Allergen immunotherapy, 393
Allergic contact dermatitis, 13
   diagnosis and treatment, 14
   manifestations, 14
   potential causes, 13
Allergy testing, 393
Allograft, 336
Alphabetic index, 403
   and tabular list, use of, A-9
Alveolar ducts, 56
Alzheimer's disease, 237
Amblyopia, 263
Ambulatory blood pressure, monitoring, 359
Amenorrhea, 107
American Health Information Management Association (AHIMA), A-1
American Hospital Association (AHA), A-1
Amniocentesis, 370
Amniotic fluid index (AFI), 101
A-mode, 379
Amphiarthrosis, 36

Index

Amyotrophic lateral sclerosis (ALS), 238
Analgesia, 321
Anastomosis, 167
Ancillary service, reimbursement terminology, 286
"And" codes, A-9
Androgen, 212, 226
Anemia
   aplastic, 201
   with chemotherapy, immunotherapy and radiation therapy, A-19
   in chronic kidney disease, A-22
   with malignancy, A-19
   in neoplastic disease, A-22
Anesthesia, 321–322
Anesthesiologist, 321
Aneurysm, 354
   cerebral, 244
   false, 87
   symptoms, 245
   treatment, 245
   true, 87
Angioma, 249
Angioplasty
   and atherectomy, 355
Ankylosing spondylitis (AS), treatment for, 50
Anorexia, 176
ANS. *See* Autonomic nervous system
Antacids, 176
Antepartum, medical term, 102, 370
Antepartum care, 369
Anterior cruciate ligament (ACL), 43
Antibiotic therapy, 24
Antibiotics, 133, 151, 176
Anti-inflammatory medications, 181
Antimicrobial therapy, for acute necrotizing fasciitis, 21
Antimotility agents, 181
Aorta, 76
Aortic regurgitation (AR), 92
Aortic valve stenosis, 91, 92
Aplastic anemia, 201
Apnea, 65
Appendicitis, 178
Appendicular skeleton, 34
Appropriate for gestational age (AGA), 101
ARDS. *See* Adult respiratory distress syndrome
ARF. *See* Acute renal failure
ARM. *See* Artificial rupture of membrane
Arterial blood gas (ABG), 59
Arteries and veins, 353. *See also* Circulatory system
Arteriosclerotic cardiovascular disease (ASCVD), 79
Arteriosclerotic heart disease (ASHD), 79
Arteriovenous fistula, repair, 355
Arthralgia, 202
Arthritis, infectious and septic, 50
Arthrodesis, 343
Arthroscopy, 345
Articulations, 36
Artificial rupture of membrane (ARM), 101
ASCVD. *See* Arteriosclerotic cardiovascular disease
ASD. *See* Atrial septal defect
ASHD. *See* Arteriosclerotic heart disease
Aspiration, 66, 331
Aspirin, 175
Assignment, reimbursement terminology, 286
Asthma, A-29
Astigmatism, medical term, 258, 263
Astrocytoma, 249
Atelectasis, 66
Atherectomy, angioplasty and, 355
Athlete's foot, 23
Atopic dermatitis, 13
Atrial fibrillation, 90, 222
Atrial septal defect (ASD), 79
Atrioventricular, 79
Atrioventricular node (AVN), 77
Atrophy
   illustration, 10f
   lesions, pathophysiology, 11
Attending physician, reimbursement terminology, 286
Aura, 246
Auscultation, 80
Autogenous grafts, 343
Autonomic nervous system (ANS), 232–233
Avian influenza virus, A-31
Axial skeleton, 30

B

B cells, acute infection of, 203
B vitamins, 238
Bacteria, 388
Bacterial impetigo, 19
Bacterial sepsis and septicemia, A-27
Bacterial vaginosis (BV), 101
Balanitis, 133
Basal cell carcinoma, 25
Base units, 321
Basophilia, 203
Below-knee amputation (BKA), 43
Beneficiary, reimbursement terminology, 286
Benign lesions, 111, 332
Benign prostatic hyperplasia/hypertrophy (BPH), 124, 135
Benign tumors, 24
Beta blockers, 156
Bicuspid, 76
Bi-level positive airway pressure (BiPAP), 59
Bilobectomy, 349
Biophysical profile, 101
Biopsy (Bx), 5, 332
   codes, 364
BiPAP. *See* Bi-level positive airway pressure
Biparietal diameter (BD), 101
Birthday rule, reimbursement terminology, 286
BKA. *See* Below-knee amputation
Bladder, subheading, 363
Bladder carcinoma
   risks, 155
   symptoms, 155
   treatment, 155
Blood, 73, 247
Blood cultures, negative or inconclusive, A-17
Blood pressure
   classification of, 86f
   elevated, A-28
   readouts, 77
Blood urea nitrogen (BUN), 144
Blood vessels, 76, 249
Body, planes of, 377f
Boils, 20
Bone marrow, 360

Index

Bone tumors, origin of, 51
Bones
  cancellous, 29
  classification of, 29
  compact, 29
  cortical, 29
  disorders, 48
  and joint studies, 380
  long, 29
  structure of, 30f
Bowen's disease, 134
BPD. *See* Biparietal diameter
BPH. *See* Benign prostatic hyperplasia/hypertrophy
BPP. *See* Biophysical profile
Brachiocephalic vascular family with vessels, 354f
Bradycardia, 90
Brain, 230
  and spinal cord, 230f
  tumors of, 249
Brain abscess
  symptoms, 246
  treatment, 246
Brainstem, 231
BRCA-1, 112, 114
BRCA-2, 112
Breast, 98
  carcinoma of, 112
  mammography, subsection, 380
  procedures, 339
  structure of, 98f
Breech, 119
Bronchial tree, minute branches of, 56
Bronchiectasis, 66
Bronchioles, 56
Bronchiolitis, 66
Bronchitis, COPD and, A-30
B-scan, 379
Buerger's disease, 89
Bulla
  illustration, 10f
  lesions, pathophysiology, 9
BUN. *See* Blood urea nitrogen
Bundle of His, 77
Burkitt's lymphoma, 207
Burns local treatment, 337
BV. *See* Bacterial vaginosis
Bx. *See* Biopsy

C

C. trachomatis, 132
C1-C7. *See* Cervical vertebrae
CABG. *See* Coronary artery bypass graft
Cancellous bones, 29
Cancer, 5
  endometrial, 113
  of esophagus, 173
  of liver, 182
  of oral cavity, 172
  of penis, 134–135
  of prostate
    stages, 137
    symptoms, 136
    treatment, 137
  of scrotum, 132
  of testes, 131
Candida albicans, 23, 133

Candidiasis, 23, 171
  treatment for, 109
Canker sore, 171
Capillaries, 74
Carcinoma. *See also* Basal cell carcinoma; Squamous cell carcinoma
  of breast, 112
  of cervix, 113
  of fallopian tubes, 115
  of ovary, 114
  of uterus, 113
  of vagina, 116
  of vulva, 116
Cardiac catheterization, 358
  components of coding, 359
Cardiac muscle, 37
Cardiography, 358
Cardiology coding terminology, 350
Cardiomyopathy, types of, 93
Cardiovascular
  anatomy and terminology, 73–77
  combining forms, 77
  in medicine section, 357, 392–393
  pathophysiology, 85
  prefixes, 78
  in radiology section, 359
  suffixes, 79
  in surgery section, 350
Cardioverter-defibrillator
  pacemakers and, 351
Care plan oversight services, 318
Carotid body, 372
Carpal tunnel syndrome (CTS), 43
Casting and strapping, 344
Cataracts, 374
  classified by morphology, 265
  examples of classification, 266
  symptoms, 266
  treatment, 266
Category II codes, supplemental tracking codes, 300
Causalgia, medical term, 5, 133
Celiac disease, 177
Cellular structures, 73
Cellulitis, 20
Centers for Medicare and Medicaid Services (CMS), 287, 310f, A-1
Central nervous system (CNS), 233, 394
  disorders, 243
  divisions of, 230
Central venous access (CVA) procedures, 355
Cephalopelvic disproportion (CPD), 101
Cerebellum, 231
Cerebral cortex, 254
Cerebral infarction, A-28
Cerebrospinal fluid (CSF), 233
  shunt, 373
Cerebrovascular accident (CVA), 233, 244, A-28
Cerebrovascular disease
  hypertensive, A-27
  late effects of, A-28
Cerebrovascular insufficiency (CVI), 79
Cerebrum, 231
Certified nurse midwife (CNM), 101
Certified registered nurse anesthetist, 321
  reimbursement terminology, 286
Cervical dilator, insertion of, 370

Index

Cervical vertebrae, 43
Cervix, 97
   carcinoma of, 113
   symptoms, 114
   treatment, 114
Cervix uteri, 367
Chamber walls, 75
Chambers
   lower, 74
   upper, 74
Chapter-specific coding guidelines, A-12
Chemotherapy, 112, 155, 396–397, A-19
   Kaposi's sarcoma and, 25
CHF. *See* Congestive heart failure
Chief complaint (CC), 304
Child and adult abuse guideline, A-65
CHL. *See* Crown-to-heel length
Chlamydia, 109–110
Cholangitis, 185
Cholecystitis, 185
Cholelithiasis, 185–186
Chondroblastoma, 51
Chondrosarcoma, 52
Chorea, 238
Choroid, 254
Chronic atrophic gastritis, 174
   antral, 175
   atrophic, 175
Chronic diseases, 69, A-72
   anemia of, A-22
Chronic glaucoma, 266
Chronic kidney disease (CKD)
   anemia of, A-22
   hypertensive, A-26, A-27
   and kidney transplant, A-31
   stages of, A-31
Chronic lymphocytic leukemia (CLL), 205
Chronic myelogenous leukemia (CML), 205
Chronic obstructive pulmonary disease (COPD), 59, 68
   and asthma, A-29
   and bronchitis, A-30
Chronic pain, A-25
Chronic pelvic pain (CPP), 101
Chronic pyelonephritis, 152
Chronic renal failure
   cause, 150
   stages, 149
   symptoms, 150
   treatment, 150
Cicatrix, pathophysiology, 13
Circulatory system, 73
   arteries of, 74f
   veins of, 75f
Cirrhosis, 184–185
CK. *See* Creatine kinase
"Clean claim", reimbursement terminology, 286
Cleft lip, and cleft palate, 171
Cleft palate, 171, 171f
Clot, 247
CMS. *See* Centers for Medicare and Medicaid Services
CMS-1500 health insurance claim form, 298f, 328
CNM. *See* Certified nurse midwife
CNS. *See* Central nervous system
Coal tar, 16
Coarctation of aorta (CoA), 93
COB. *See* Coordination of benefits

Code graft, 335
Coding of burns, A-41
Coinsurance, reimbursement terminology, 287
Colonoscopy, 362
Colorectal cancer, 181
Combination code, A-11
Compact bones, 29
Compliance plan, reimbursement terminology, 287
Component coding, 376
Component modifiers, 377
Comprehensive examination, 308
Computed axial tomography (CAT), 378
Conchae, 55
Concurrent care, reimbursement terminology, 287
Concussion, 247
Conduction system, 76
Congenital anomalies, A-37
Congenital disorders, 156
Congenital heart defects, 93
Congenital neurologic disorders, 241
Congestive heart failure (CHF), 79, 89
Conjunctiva, 254
Conjunctivitis, 264
Conscious sedation, 321
Constrictive pericarditis, 93
Consultation services, 315
Continuous positive airway pressure (CPAP), 59
Contusion, 247
Conversion factor, 322
Coordination of benefits (COB), reimbursement terminology, 287
Coordination of care, 311
Co-payment, reimbursement terminology, 288
COPD. *See* Chronic obstructive pulmonary disease
Cor pulmonale, 67
Cornea, 253–254
Coronary artery bypass graft (CABG), 79, 352
   arterial, 353
   venous, 352
Coronary artery disease (CAD), 85
Corpus uteri, 367
Cortical bones, 29
Cortisol, 212
Cough, 65
Counseling, 311, A-52
CPAP. *See* Continuous positive airway pressure
CPD. *See* Cephalopelvic disproportion
CPK. *See* Creatine phosphokinase
CPP. *See* Chronic pelvic pain
CPT, ICD-9-CM, and HCPCS coding, overview of, 295–470
CPT codes, 296–297
   appendices of, 301
   code descriptions, 299
   types of, 296
CPT modifier, 299
CPT/HCPCS level I modifiers, 323
Cranial, 30
Cranial nerve tumors, 250
Craniectomy, 372
Creatine kinase (CK), 79
Creatine phosphokinase (CPK), 79
Critical care services, 315–316
CRNA. *See* Certified Registered Nurse Anesthetist
Crohn's disease, 177–178
Crown-to-heel length (CHL), 101

Index

Crust
    illustration, 10f
    lesions, pathophysiology, 11
Cryotherapy, squamous cell carcinoma and, 25
Cryptorchidism, 129
CSF. See Cerebrospinal fluid
CTS. See Carpal tunnel syndrome
Cuboidal bones, 29
Curettage, 370
Curvatures, spinal, 49
Cushing syndrome, 224
CVA. See Cerebrovascular accident
CVI. See Cerebrovascular insufficiency
Cyclosporin, 16
Cystitis
    bacterial
        cause, 150
        symptoms, 150
        systemic signs, 150
        treatment, 151
    nonbacterial, 151
Cytopathology, 386

D

Decubitis ulcer, 11
Deductible, reimbursement terminology, 288
Dehydration, management of, due to malignancy, A-19
Delivery, medical term, 102, 370
Dementias, classified by causative factor, 237
Denial, reimbursement terminology, 288
Department of Health and Human Services (DHHS), A-1
Depression, 243
Dermatitis
    allergic contact, 13
    irritant contact, 14
    seborrheic, 15
Dermatology, 5
Dermis, 2
Destruction, 337, 365
Detailed examination, 307
DHHS. See Department of Health and Human Services
Diabetes codes, A-21
Diabetes insipidus, 221
Diabetes mellitus, 219, A-20
    acute complications, 219
    chronic complications, 219
    in gestational diabetes, 220, A-22
    and insulin, A-21
    in pregnancy, A-33
    symptoms, 219
    types of, 219
Diabetic ketoacidosis, 219
Diabetic macular edema, A-21
Diabetic retinopathy, A-21
Diagnosis codes, ICD-9-CM, 296, 401f
Dialysis, 391
Diaper dermatitis
    causes of, 18
    treatment for, 19
Diaphragm
    anatomy and terminology, 191
    mediastinum and, 191f
    subsection, 361
Diaphragmatic hernia, 173
Diaphysis, 29
Diarthrosis, types, 36

Diencephalon, 231
Diffuse capacity of lungs for carbon monoxide (DLCO), 59
Digestive system, 163f
    anatomy and terminology, 161–165
    combining forms, 165
    diseases of, A-31
    function, 161
    pathophysiology, 171
    subsection, 361
    suffixes, 166–167
Digital rectal examination (DRE), 135
Dilation
    and curettage, 101
    and evacuation, 101
    medical term, 102, 145
Diplopia, 263
Dislocations, 48, 341
Disorders
    joint, 49
    of pancreas, 186
    papulosquamous, 15
    of prostate gland, 135
Diverticulitis, 180
Diverticulosis, 180
DLCO. See Diffuse capacity of lungs for carbon monoxide
Dobutamine stress echocardiography (DSE), 79
Documentation, reimbursement terminology, 288
Domiciliary, rest home, or custodial care services, 316
Donor, A-52
Drugs
    and chemicals, table of, 405
    overdose of, A-44
    testing, 383
DSE. See Dobutamine stress echocardiography
Duodenal ulcers, 178
Duodenum, 164
    disorders, 174
Durable medical equipment, reimbursement terminology, 288
Dwarfism, 220
Dysfunctional uterine bleeding (DUB), 108
Dysmenorrhea
    primary, 107
    secondary, 107
Dyspnea, 65, 222

E

E codes, 424, A-63
E. coli, 130, 152
Ear
    bones, middle, 30
    both, 257
    divisions of, 31f, 255
    infections, 267
    left, 257
    right, 257
    structure of, 31f
Eburnation, sclerosis of bone, 49
ECC. See Endocervical curettage
Echocardiography, 358
Eclampsia, 117
Ectopic pregnancy, in fallopian tube, 118
EDC. See Estimated date of confinement
EDI. See Electronic data interchange
EEG. See Electroencephalogram
EFM. See Electronic fetal monitoring

Index

EFW. See Estimated fetal weight
EGA. See Estimated gestational age
EGD. See Esophagogastroduodenoscopy
EGJ. See Esophagogastric junction
Electroencephalogram (EEG), 233
Electronic analysis, 359
   Electronic data interchange, A-120
   reimbursement terminology, 288
Electronic fetal monitoring (EFM), 101
Electrophysiology, 350
E/M codes
   factors selecting, 302
   use of, 312
E/M services, selection of level of, 312
Embolectomy
   and thrombectomy, 353
Embolism, 88
   pulmonary, 67
EMC. See Endometrial curettage
Emergency department services, 315
Emphysema, 69
Employer identification number, reimbursement terminology, 288
Empyema, 67
Encephalitis, 245
Encounter form superbill, reimbursement terminology, 288
Endocarditis, infective, 90
Endocardium, 75
Endocervical curettage (ECC), 101
Endocrine glands, 211
Endocrine system
   anatomy and terminology, 211–213
   combining forms, 213
   illustration, 211f
   pathophysiology, 219
   prefixes, 214
   subsection, 371
   suffixes, 214
Endometrial cancer, 113
Endometrial curettage (EMC), 102
Endometriosis
   causes, 108
   risks, 109
   treatment, 109
Endometrium, 97
   repair of, 98
Endoscopic retrograde cholangiopancreatography (ERCP), 166
Endoscopy, 345, 366
   laparoscopy and, 362
Endosteum, 29
End-stage renal disease (ESRD), 144
   physician services, 391
EOB. See Explanation of benefits
Eosinophilia, 202
   cause, 203
Ependymoma, 249
Epicardium, 75
Epidermis, 2
Epididymis
   disorders of, 129
Epididymitis, 129
   symptoms, 130
   treatment, 130
   types, 129

Epilepsies
   causes, 246
   treatment, 247
   types, 246
Epiphyseal line, 29
Epiphysis, 29
Epispadias, 132
Epithelial tumors, 115
Eponychium, 2
ERCP. See Endoscopic retrograde cholangiopancreatography
Erosion
   illustration, 10f
   lesions, pathophysiology, 11
ERT. See Estrogen replacement therapy
Erysipelas
   cause, 20
   lesions, 21
Erythrocytes, 73
Esophageal disorders, 172
Esophagitis
   acute, 172
   chronic, 173
Esophagogastric junction (EGJ), 166
Esophagogastroduodenoscopy (EGD), 166, 361
Esophagogastroscopy, 361
Esophagoscopy, 361
Esophagus, 163
ESRD. See End-stage renal disease
Estimated date of confinement (EDC), 101
Estimated date of delivery (EDD), 101
Estimated fetal weight (EFW), 101
Estimated gestational age (EGA), 102
Estrogen hypersecretion, 226
Estrogen replacement therapy (ERT), 102
Estropia, 264
Evaluation and management (E/M) section (99201-99499), 302
Examination elements, 308f
Excision, 341, 348, 365, 367
   repair, 349
Exotropia, 264
Explanation of benefits (EOB), reimbursement terminology, 288
External fixation, 342
Extrauterine, 118
Extremities, 39
   lower, 34, 40
   upper, 34
Eye
   each, 258
   layers of, 253
   left, 258, 263
   and ocular adnexa, 253, 374
   right, 258
Eyelids, 374

F

Fallopian tubes, 97
   carcinoma, of, 115
   ectopic pregnancy in, 118
   primary, 115
   symptoms, 115
   treatment, 116
FAS. See Fetal alcohol syndrome
Federal register, 282
   example of, 283

Fee schedule, reimbursement terminology, 288
FEF. See Forced expiratory flow
Female genital system
   anatomy and terminology, 97–99
   pathophysiology, 107
   subsection, 365
Female reproductive system, 97f
   combining forms, 99
   prefixes, 100
   suffixes, 101
Femur, 34
Fetal alcohol syndrome (FAS), 102
Fetal conditions, affecting management of mother, A-33
Fetal heart rate, 102
FEV_1. See Forced expiratory volume in 1 second
Fever, rheumatic, 91
Fibrillation, 90
Fibroid, 111
Fibroma, 111
Fibromyalgia syndrome, primary, 51
Fibromyoma, 111
Fibrous lesions, encase heart, 93
Fissure
   illustration, 10f
   lesions, pathophysiology, 11
Fistulectomy codes, hemorrhoidectomy and, 362
Fixator, as joint stabilizer, 38
Flaps, 335. See also Muscles
Fluid replacement, for acute necrotizing fasciitis, 21
Fluids, 254
Flutter, treatment, 90
Follicle-stimulating hormone (FSH), 102
Folliculitis, 20
Follow-up days, reimbursement terminology, 288
Forced expiratory flow (FEF), 59
Forced expiratory volume in 1 second (FEV_1), 59
Forced vital capacity (FVC), 59
Fractures, 43, 44
   classification of, 47
   treatment
      closed, 340
      open, 340
      percutaneous, 341
FRC. See Functional residual capacity
FSH. See Follicle-stimulating hormone
Functional residual capacity (FRC), 59
Fundus, 97
Fungal, 23
Furuncles, 20
FVC. See Forced vital capacity

G

Gallbladder
   containing gallstones, 185f
   disorders of, 182, 185
Gamma globulin, 183
Gastric cancer, 176
Gastritis, 174
Gastrocnemius, 40
Gastroenterology, 392
Gastroesophageal reflux disease (GERD), 166
   treatment, 174
Gastrointestinal (GI), 166, 167
Genital herpes, 110
Genital warts, 110

Genitalia, external, 123
Genitourinary system, diseases of, A-31
GERD. See Gastroesophageal reflux disease
Germ cell tumors, 114, 249
Gestation, 99
   fetal, 369
Gestational diabetes mellitus, 220, A-34
GI. See Gastrointestinal
Gigantism, 220, 221f
Glands, 2
Glaucoma, 266
Glia, 229
Glioblastoma, 249
Glomerular disorders, 152
Glomerulonephritis
   cause, 152
   treatment, 153
Glucagons, 212
Goiter, 222f
   cause for, 221
Gonadal stromal tumors, 115
Gonads, 123
Gonorrhea, 110, 133
Gout, 50
Gouty arthritis, 50
Grafts, 335
   autogenous, 343
Granulocytosis, 202
Group A beta-hemolytic streptococcus, 19
Guillain-Barré syndrome, 241

H

Hand-held nebulizer, 59
HCPCS anatomical modifiers, examples of, 328
HCPCS coding, 399
HCPCS modifiers, level II, 300, 328
HCPCS National Level II index, 400
HCVD. See Hypertensive cardiovascular disease
Head injury, 247
Health Insurance Portability and Accountability Act (HIPAA), A-1
Health Maintenance Organization, 286
Hearing loss, 255. See also Sensorineural hearing
   conductive, 267
   ototoxic, 268
Heart, 74
   and chronic kidney disease, hypertensive, A-15
   disease, 91
   disorders, 89
   electrical system of, 77f
   internal view of, 76f
   muscle, 37
Heart block, bradycardia and, 90
Heart rhythms, abnormal, 90
Heart wall, disorders, 92
Hemangioblastoma, 249
Hematoma, 6, 80, 247
Hematopoietic organ, 195
Hemic system
   anatomy and terminology, 195
   combining forms, 195
   pathophysiology, 201
   prefixes, 197
   subsection, 360
   suffixes, 197

Index

Hemodialysis (HD), 144
   service, 391
Hemolytic anemia, treatment, 202
Hemoptysis, 65
Hemorrhoidectomy, and fistulectomy codes, 362
Hepatitis, 184
Hepatitis A (HAV), 182
Hepatitis B (HBV), 183
Hepatitis C (HCV), 183
Hepatitis D (HDV), 183
Hepatitis E (HEV), 183
Hepatitis G (HGV), 183
Hepatojugular reflux (HJR), 166
Hernia, 362
   sliding and paraesophageal, 173
Herpes simplex virus (HSV), 25, 102
   type 1 (HSV-1), 21, 172
   type 2 (HSV-2), 21
Herpes zoster, 22
HHN. See Hand-held nebulizer
Hiatal hernia
   symptoms, 173
   types, 173
HIPPA. See Health Insurance Portability and Accountability Act
History elements, 307f
History of present illness (HPI), 304
HIV codes, selection and sequencing of, A-12
HIV infection, in pregnancy, childbirth and puerperium, A-13, A-33
HJR. See Hepatojugular reflux
HMO, reimbursement terminology, 288
Hodgkin's disease
   presentation, 206
   symptoms, 206
   treatment, 206
Home services, 317
Hordeolum, medical term, 258, 264
Hormonal disorders, 107
Hospital care, 314
Hospital discharge services, 314
Hospital inpatient services, types of, 314
Hospital observation status, 313
HPV. See Human papillomavirus
HSG. See Hysterosalpingogram
HSV. See Herpes simplex virus
Human chorionic gonadotropin (HCG), 99
Human immunodeficiency virus (HIV), 25
   asymptomatic, A-13
   infections, A-12
Human papillomavirus (HPV), 22, 102
Huntington's disease, 238
Hydatidiform mole, 118
Hydration, 394
Hydrocele
   illustrations, 130f
   symptoms, 130
Hydrocephalus, 241
Hydronephrosis, 155–156
Hyperaldosteronism, 225
Hyperbilirubinemia, 182
Hypercapnia, 65
Hypercholesterolemia, 153
Hypercoagulability, 153
Hypercortisolism, 224
Hyperopia, medical term, 258, 263

Hyperparathyroidism, 223
Hyperpituitarism, 220
Hypertension (HTN), A-26
   controlled, A-27
   essential, or NOS, A-26
   with heart disease, A-26
   secondary, A-27
   table, A-26
   transient, A-27
   treatment for, 86
   uncontrolled, A-28
Hypertensive cardiovascular disease (HCVD), 79
Hypertensive retinopathy, A-27
Hyperthyroidism, treatment, 222
Hypertropia, 264
Hyperventilation, 65
Hypoalbuminemia, 153
Hypodermis, 2
Hypomenorrhea, 108
Hypoparathyroidism
   symptoms, 223
   treatment, 224
Hypophysis glands, 211
Hypopituitarism, 220
Hypospadias, 132
Hypotension, 87
Hypothalamus, 213
Hypothyroidism, 222
   treatment, 223
   types, 222
Hypotropia, 264
Hypoventilation, 65
Hysterosalpingogram (HSG), 102

I

ICD-9-CM, 402
   with 3, 4, or 5 digits, A-71
   conventions for, A-7
   format of, 402
   on insurance forms, 401
   overview of, 401
   uses of, 401, 407
ICD-9-CM official guidelines for coding and reporting, A-1
Iliac aneurysm, endovascular repair of, 354
Immune globulins, 388
Immunotherapy, A-19
Improper union, 48
In vitro fertilization, 102, 368
Incision, and drainage, 5
Infant respiratory distress syndrome, 59
Infections, 109, 171, 264
   causes, 172
   ear, 267
   and parasitic diseases, A-12
   treatment, 172
Infectious arthritis, 50
Infectious disease, 68
Infectious mononucleosis, 203
Infectious pleural effusion, 67
Inferior vena cava, 76
Inflammation, 109
   thrombophlebitis cause of, 88
Inflammatory bowel disease, 177
Inflammatory disorders, pathophysiology, 13
Infusion, 394

Index

Injection, 395
Injury, in musculoskeletal systems, 47
Inspiratory positive airway pressure (IPAP), 59
Insulin, A-22
Insulin pump malfunction, A-22
Insulin-dependent diabetes mellitus, 219
Integumentary system, 3f
   anatomy and terminology, 2
   combining forms, 3
   pathophysiology, 9
   prefixes, 4
   suffixes, 5
Intensive care service, continuing, 320
Interleukin-2 inhibitors, 16
Intersex surgery, subsection, 365
Intestinal disorders, 177
Intestine
   large, 164, 180
   small, 164
Intracoronary brachytherapy, 358
Intraocular lens (IOL), 258
Intravenous pyelogram (IVP), 144
Invalid claim, reimbursement terminology, 288
IOL. *See* Intraocular lens
IPAP. *See* Inspiratory positive airway pressure
IRDS. *See* Infant respiratory distress syndrome
Iron deficiency anemia, 201
Irreversible ischemia, 85
Irritant contact dermatitis
   conditions associated with, 14
   progress, 14
   response, 14
   treatment, 14–15
Ischemia, 85
Ischemic heart disease, 85
Ischium, 34
Itching, 19
IVP. *See* Intravenous pyelogram

J

Jaundice, 182
Joints, 36
   disorders, 49

K

Kaposi's sarcoma, 172
   treatment for, 25
Keloids, pathophysiology, 12
Keratin plates, 2
Keratitis, 264
Keratoacanthoma, 24
Keratosis, 24
Ketoacidosis, 219
Kickbacks, 285
Kidney, 141
   disease, chronic, A-31
   illustration, 142f
   stones
     symptoms, 154
     treatment, 155
   structure, 142
   subheading, 363
   transplant, complications, A-45
   ureter, bladder, 121, 144
Kyphosis, medical term, 44, 49

L

Lactase deficiency, 177
Laparoscopy
   and endoscopy, 362
   hysteroscopy, 368
Large for gestational age (LGA), 102
Large intestine, 164
Larynx, 55, 348
Laser therapy, 132
LEEP. *See* Loop electrosurgical excision procedure
Left bundle branch block, 79
Left lower quadrant (LLQ), 167
Left upper quadrant (LUQ), 167
Left ventricular hypertrophy (LVH), 79
Leiomyomas, 111
Lens, 254
Lesions
   biopsy/removal of, 339
   calculating size of, 333f
   in integumentary system, 9
   of skin, 10
Leukemia, 204
Leukocytopenia, cause, 203
Leukocytosis, cause, 203
LGA. *See* Large for gestational age
Lichen planus
   lesions, 17
   treatment for, 18
Ligaments, 37
   disorders, 51
Lithotripsy, 167, 186
Liveborn fetus, abortion with, A-36
Liver, disorders of, 182
LLQ. *See* Left lower quadrant
Lobectomy, 349, 372
   medical term, 61, 215
Loop electrosurgical excision procedure, 102
Lordosis, 49
Lower respiratory infection (LRI), 68
Lower respiratory tract (LRT), 55
Lumbar puncture, 233
Lund-Browder chart, for estimating extent of burns on children, 338
Lungs, 57
   and pleura, 349
LUQ. *See* Left upper quadrant
LVH. *See* Left ventricular hypertrophy
Lymph, 195
Lymph nodes, 132
   and lymphatic channels subheading, 361
Lymphadenitis, 205
Lymphadenopathy, 205
Lymphangitis, medical term, 198, 205
Lymphatic system, 196f
   anatomy and terminology, 195
   combining forms, 195
   pathophysiology, 201
   prefixes, 197
   suffixes, 197
Lymphocytic leukemia, acute, 204

M

Macular degeneration, types of, 265
Macule
   illustration, 10f
   lesions, pathophysiology, 9

Index

Malabsorption, 48
Male genital system
   anatomy and terminology, 123–124
   combining forms, 124
   disorders of, 129
   pathophysiology, 129
   subsection, 364
   suffixes, 124
Malignant lesions, 112
Malignant lymphoma, 206
Malignant melanoma, 25
Malignant tumors, 24, 155, 176
Malposition, of fetus, 118–119
Malpresentation, of fetus, 118–119
Managed Health Care, 285
Manipulation, 341, 367
Marsupialization, 366
Mastectomy, 112
Master glands, 211
MAT. *See* Multifocal atrial tachycardia
MDI. *See* Metered dose inhaler
MDM. *See* Medical decision making
Mechanoreceptors, 256
Meckel's diverticulum, 178
Mediastinum
   anatomy and terminology, 191
   and diaphragm, 191f, 193
   subsection, 361
Medical coding, introduction to, 296
Medical decision making (MDM)
   complexity, 308
   elements for, 311f
   high-complexity, 309
   low-complexity, 309
   moderate-complexity, 309
   straightforward, 309
Medical record, reimbursement terminology, 288
Medical team conferences, 317
Medicare
   basic structure, 278–279
   covers, 279
   funding for, 279
   officiating office, 279
Medicare fraud, and abuse, 284
Medicine section, 387
Medulloblastoma, 250
Ménière's disease, 268
Meningioma, 250
Meningocele, 242f
Menometrorrhagia, 108
Menorrhagia, 108
Menorrhea, 108
Menstrual, disorders, 107
Menstruation
   abnormal, 108
   and pregnancy, 98
Mental disorders, 241, A-23
Metaphysis, 29
Metered dose inhaler (MDI), 60
Metrorrhagia, 108
MI. *See* Myocardial infarction
Mitral regurgitation, 92
Mitral valve stenosis, 92
M-mode, 379
Modifiers, 299
Modifying unit, 322

Mohs' micrographic surgery, 6, 339
Moles, 24
Monocytosis, 203
Mononucleosis, infectious, 203
Motor neuron disease, 238
Mouth, anatomic structures of, 161f
Movements, terms of, 39
Multifocal atrial tachycardia (MAT), 79
Multiple fractures, A-41
Multiple modifiers, 328
Multiple myeloma, 52
Multiple sclerosis, 239
Muscles
   action, 38
   capabilities, 38
   disorders, 51
   movement, 38
   names of, 39
   tumors, 52
   types of, 36
Muscular dystrophy, familial disorder, 51
Muscular system
   anterior view, 38f
   functions, 36
   posterior view of, 37f
Musculoskeletal systems
   anatomy and terminology, 29–42
   combining forms, 40
   pathophysiology, 47
   prefixes, 42
   subsection, 340
   suffixes, 42
Myasthenia gravis (MG)
   symptoms, 239
   treatment, 240
Mycobacterium tuberculosis, 68
Mycoses, 23
Myelinated axon, 229f
Myelocystocele, 242f
Myeloma, multiple, 207
Myelomeningocele, 242f
Myocardial infarction (MI), A-77
Myocardial ischemia, 85
Myocardium, 75, 93
Myoma, 111
Myometrium, 97
Myopia, medical term, 259, 263

N

Nails, 2
Nasal turbinates, superior, inferior, and middle, 56
National Center for Health Statistics (NCHS), A-1
National correct coding initiative, 281
National Fee Schedule (NFS), 284
National Provider Identification, 279
   reimbursement terminology, 288
Neonatal critical care, inpatient, 319
Neoplasms, general guidelines, A-18
Neoplastic disease, anemia in, A-22
Nephroblastoma, 157
Nephrolithiasis, 154
Nephron loss, stages of, 150
Nephrosclerosis, 156
Nephrosis, 153
Nephrotic syndrome, 153

Nervous system
  anatomy and terminology, 229
  cells of, 229
  combining forms, 232
  pathophysiology, 237
  prefixes, 232
  primary cells of, 229
  and sense organs, diseases of, A-23
  subsection, 372
  suffixes, 233
Neurons, 229
Neuropathy, 220f
Neutrophils, 202
Nevi. See Moles
Newborn care services, 319
Newborns, A-37
  congenital anomalies in, A-39
  infant and child, A-53
Niacin, 238
Nociceptors, 256
Nodule
  illustration, 10f
  lesions, pathophysiology, 9
Nonbacterial, 136
Noncoronary bypass grafts, 355
Noncovered services, reimbursement terminology, 288
Non-face-to-face physician services, 318
Non-healing burns, A-42
Non-Hodgkin lymphoma, 109, 206–207
Non-infectious process, SIRS due to, A-45
Non-insulin-dependent diabetes mellitus, 219
Non-invasive intervention, 88
Noninvasive vascular diagnostic studies, 393
Nonprescribed drug, A-44
Nonviral hepatitis, 184
Normal delivery, A-34
Normal sinus rhythm, 79
Nose, 55
Nuclear medicine, subsection, 382
Nursing facility services, 316
Nutritional degenerative disease, 238
Nystagmus, 263

O

Obstetric care, routine global, 371
Obstetric cases, general rules for, A-32
Obstruction, 179
Obstructs vessel, 88
Ocular adnexa, 253
Office of the Inspector General, 285
Olfactory sense receptors, 255
Oligodendrocytoma, 249
Oligomenorrhea, 108
Onychomycosis, 23
Ophthalmologic services, 392
Ophthalmology, 392
Opiates, 19
Optic chiasm, 254
Optic nerve fibers, 254
Oral cavity, disorders of, 171
Orchitis, 129
Organ systems (OS), 305
Organs, 141
  accessory, 123
  essential, in male genital system, 123
Orofacial cleft, 171

Ossicles, 255
Osteitis deformans, 49
Osteoarthritis, 44, 49
Osteoma, 57
Osteomalacia, and rickets, 49
Osteomyelitis, 48
Osteoporosis, 48
Osteosarcoma, 51
Otitis externa, 267
Otitis media, medical term, 259, 267
Otorhinolaryngologic services, 392
Ovary, 97, 213, 368, 372
  carcinoma of, 114
Ovulation, 98

P

PAC. See Premature atrial contraction
Pacemakers, and cardioverter-defibrillators, 351
Paget's disease, 49
Pain
  category, A-23
  chronic, A-25
  control, admission/encounter for, A-20
  devices, implants and grafts, A-24
  neoplasm related, A-25
Pain syndrome, chronic, A-25
Pancreas, 212, 372
  disorders of, 182
Pancreatic cancer, 187
Pancreatic cells, 164
Pancreatitis, 186
Pantothenic acid, 238
Papule
  illustration, 10f
  lesions, pathophysiology, 9
Papulosquamous disorders
  conditions associated with, 15
  types of, 16
Paranasal sinuses, 55
Paraphimosis
  phimosis and, 133
  symptom, 134
  treatment, 134
Parathyroid disorders, 223
Parathyroid glands, 212
Parathyroid hormone (PTH), 223
Parkinsonism, 238
Parkinson's disease, 238–239
Paronychium, 2
Paroxysmal atrial tachycardia (PAT), 79
Paroxysmal nocturnal dyspnea (PND), 60
Paroxysmal supraventricular tachycardia (PSVT), 79
Part A, hospital inpatient, 280
Part B, supplemental, 281
Past, family, and social history (PFSH), 305
PAT. See Paroxysmal atrial tachycardia
Patent ductus arteriosus (PDA), 93
Patient-controlled analgesia (PCA), 321
Patient(s)
  established, 313
  final status of, 315
  new, 313
PAWP. See Pulmonary artery wedge pressure
PCWP. See Pulmonary capillary wedge pressure
PEAP. See Positive end-airway pressure
Pediatric critical care, inpatient, 319–320

Index

PEEP. See Positive end-expiratory pressure
Peptic ulcers
   symptoms, 175
   treatment, 176
Percutaneous endoscopic gastrostomy, 167
Percutaneous transluminal coronary angioplasty, 79
Pericardial cavity, 76
Pericardial effusion, 93
Pericarditis
   acute, 92
   constrictive, 93
   restrictive, 93
   types of, 91
Pericardium, 76
Perimetrium, 97
Perinatal morbidity, maternal causes of, A-39
Peripheral arterial disease (PAD), 89
   rehabilitation, 359
Peripheral nervous system (PNS), 231, 233
Peritoneal dialysis, 391
Peritoneum, 164
Peritonitis
   symptoms, 179
   treatment, 179
   types, 178
PERL. See Pupils equal and reactive to light
Pernicious anemia, 201–202
Peyronie's disease, 134
PFT. See Pulmonary function test
Pharynx, 55, 163
Phimosis, 133
   and paraphimosis, 133
   symptoms, 133
   treatment, 134
Phlebitis, 88
Photodynamic therapy, 397
Physician status, types of, 314
Pilonidal abscess, 332
Pilonidal cyst, 332
Pineal, 213, 249
Pineal tumors, 249
Pink eye, 264
Pituitary glands, 211
   anterior, 220
   disorders, 220
   and pineal, 372
   posterior, 221
Pituitary tumor, 250
Pityriasis rosea, 17
Placenta forms, within uterine wall, 99
Placenta previa, 117f
   types of, 116
Plaque
   illustration, 10f
   lesions, pathophysiology, 9
Plethysmography, medical term, 125, 359
Pleural effusion-fluid, in pleural space, 67
Pleural space, pleural effusion-fluid in, 67
Pleurisy, 67
Pleuritis, 67
PND. See Paroxysmal nocturnal dyspnea
Pneumoconiosis, 67
Pneumonectomy, 349
Pneumonia, 68
Pneumothorax, 67

PNS. See Peripheral nervous system
POA examples, A-81
Point of service (POS), 286
   reimbursement terminology, 288
Poisoning, A-44
Poliomyelitis, 240
Polycystic kidney, 156
Polymenorrhea, 108
Polymyositis, 51
Positive end-airway pressure (PEAP), 60
Positive end-expiratory pressure (PEEP), 60
Posterior pituitary glands, 221
Postpartum, and peripartum periods, A-34
Postpartum care, 370
Postpolio syndrome (PPS), 240
Preferred Provider Organization
   reimbursement terminology, 288
Pregnancy, 99, 116
   anatomy and terminology, 97–99
   combining forms, 99
   current conditions complicating, A-33
   diabetes mellitus in, A-33
   ectopic, 118
   menstruation and, 98
   pathophysiology, 107
   prefixes, 100
   suffixes, 101
Premature atrial contraction (PAC), 79
Premature rupture of membranes (PROM), 102
Premature ventricular contraction (PVC), 79
Premenstrual syndrome (PMS), 108
Premenstrual tension (PMT), 108
Premenstruation, 98
Presbyopia, 263
Presenting problem
   high-severity, 312
   low-severity, 312
   minimal, 311
   nature of, 311
   self-limiting or minor, 311
Pressure ulcer, 337
   locations, 11
   stage I, II, III, and IV of, 12
   staging or classification system, 11
Preventive medicine services, 318
Prior authorization, reimbursement terminology, 289
PRO reviews, 282
Problem focused examination, 307
Proctosigmoidoscopy, 362
Proliferation phase, 98
Prolonged services, 317
PROM. See Premature rupture of membranes
Proprioceptors, 256
Prostate gland, disorders of, 135
Prostate-specific antigen (PSA), 124, 135
Prostatitis
   acute, 136
   causes, 135
   chronic, 136
   symptoms, 136
   treatment, 136
Proteus, 152
Provider Identification Number, reimbursement terminology, 289
Pruritus, 19
PSA. See Prostate-specific antigen

Pseudomonas, 152
Psoralens and ultraviolet A light therapy, 16
Psoriasis, 16
Psuedoaneurysm, 87
PSVT. *See* Paroxysmal supraventricular tachycardia
Psychiatry, 390
PTH. *See* Parathyroid hormone
Pubis, 34
Pubis symphysis, 34
Pulmonale, cor, 67
Pulmonary, 76
Pulmonary artery stenosis, 76, 94
Pulmonary artery wedge pressure (PAWP), 60
Pulmonary capillary wedge pressure (PCWP), 60
Pulmonary diseases, 65
Pulmonary disorders, signs and symptoms of, 65
Pulmonary function test (PFT), 60
Pulmonary valve, 91
Pulmonary veins, 76
Pulmonic regurgitation (PR), 92
Pupils equal and reactive to light (PERL), 258
Pupils equal, round, and reactive to light (PERRL), 258
Pupils equal, round, and reactive to light and accommodation (PERRLA), 258
Purkinje fibers, 77
Pustule
   illustration, 10f
   lesions, pathophysiology, 9
PVC. *See* Premature ventricular contraction
Pyelonephritis
   acute, 151–152
   chronic, 152
Pyloric stenosis, 176
   treatment, 177

Q

QIO. *See* Quality improvement organizations
Qualifying circumstances codes, 322
Quality improvement organizations (QIO), 282

R

RA. *See* Remittance advice; Rheumatoid arthritis
Radiation, Kaposi's sarcoma and, 25
Radiation oncology, subsection, 380
Radiation therapy, A-19
Radiotherapy, squamous cell carcinoma and, 25
Rapid eye movement (REM), 258
Raynaud's disease, 89
RBBB. *See* Right bundle branch block
RDS. *See* Respiratory distress syndrome
Real-time scan, 379
Red blood cells, 73
Regional enteritis, 177
Regular sinus rhythm (RSR), 79
Regurgitation, of the heart, 92
Reimbursement issues, 277–281
Reimbursement terminology, 286
Rejection/denial, reimbursement terminology, 289
Relative value units (RVUS), 284
REM. *See* Rapid eye movement
Remittance advice (RA), 43
Renal calculi, 154
Renal cancer, tumor staging for, 155
Renal failure, 149
Replantation, 342

Reproductive system, male, 123f
   procedures, 365
Resource-based relative value scale, 282
   reimbursement terminology, 289
Respiration, 40, 57
Respiratory acidosis, 66
Respiratory distress syndrome (RDS), 60
Respiratory system
   anatomy and terminology, 55–57
   combining forms, 57
   pathophysiology, 65
   prefixes, 58
   subsection, 345
   suffixes, 58
   upper and lower, 56f
Respiratory volume, 60
Restrictive pericarditis, 93
Retina, 254
   detached, 265
Retinopathy, 219
Review of systems (ROS), 305
Reye's syndrome, 245–246
Rheumatic fever, 91
Rheumatic heart disease, 91
Rheumatoid arthritis (RA), 50
Rickets, osteomalacia and, 49
Right bundle branch block (RBBB), 79
Right lower quadrant, 167, 178
Right upper quadrant, 167, 186
Right ventricular hypertrophy (RVH), 80
Ringworm, 23
Risk factor reduction, counseling, 318
ROS. *See* Review of systems
RSR. *See* Regular sinus rhythm
Rule of Nines, to calculate burn area, 338
RVH. *See* Right ventricular hypertrophy

S

Salivary glands, 161
   illustration, 162f
Scales
   illustration, 10f
   lesions, pathophysiology, 11
Scar
   illustration, 10f
   lesions, pathophysiology, 11
Schizophrenia, 241
   symptoms, 242
   treatment, 243
Scleroderma, 172
Scrotum, disorders of, 129
Sebaceous glands, 2
Seborrheic dermatitis, 15
Seborrheic keratosis, 24
Secretory phase, 98
"See" codes, A-9
"See Also" codes, A-9
Segmental bronchi, 55
Segmentectomy, 349
Seizures, 246
Senses
   anatomy and terminology, 253
   combining forms, 256
   pathophysiology, 263
   prefixes, 257
   suffixes, 257

Index

Sensorineural hearing, 268
Sepsis, A-14
   and severe sepsis
      with non-infectious process, A-17
      as principal diagnosis, A-15
      as secondary diagnosis, A-15
      sequencing, A-15
   SIRS with localized infection, A-15
Septa, 75
Septic arthritis, 50
Septic shock, A-16
   sepsis and, A-17
   sequencing of, A-16
   of severe sepsis, A-16
Septicaemia, A-14
   and bacterial sepsis, A27
Service codes, levels of, 296
Sexually transmitted disease (STD), 109
Shaving of lesions, 332
Shingles, 22
Sickle cell anemia, 202
Sigmoidoscopy, 362
Sinuses, paranasal/accessory, 55
SIRS, external cause of injury codes with, A-17
Skeletal divisions, 30
Skeletal muscle, 36
Skeletal system, 29, 35f
Skeletal traction, 47f
Skeleton
   appendicular, 34
   axial, 30
Skin
   epidermis and dermis, 2
   infections, 19
   lesions of, 10
   tumors of, 24
Skin grafts, split-thickness and full-thickness, 336
Skin replacement surgery, 335
Skin tag removal, 332
Skin traction, 48f
Skull, 30
   base, surgery of, 372
   frontal view of, 32
   lateral view of, 31f
   meninges, and brain, 372
Small intestine, 164, 177
Smell, 255
Smooth muscle, 37
Sonohysterogram, 102
Sores, cold, 21
Specific gravity, 144
Spina bifida occulta, 49, 241, 242f
Spinal cord, 231
   brain and, 230f
   injury, 248
   tumors of, 249–250
Spinal curvatures, 49
Spinal instrumentation, types of, 344
Spine, 32
Spontaneous rupture of membranes (SROM), 5, 102
Squamous cell carcinoma, 24
Standby service, 317
Staphylococci, 130
Stasis dermatitis, 14
State license number, reimbursement terminology, 289

STD. *See* Sexually transmitted disease
Stenosis, 92. *See also* Aortic valve; Mitral valve
Sternum, 34f
Stomach, 163
   disorders, 174
   malignant tumor of, 176
Strains, sprains and, 48
Strapping, 48
   and casting, 344
Streptococcal sepsis, A-16
Streptococcal septicaemia, A-16
Streptococci, 130
Stress urinary incontinence (SUI), 102
Stroke, 244, A-28
Sudoriferous glands, 2
SUI. *See* Stress urinary incontinence
Summing up formula, 322
Supraventricular tachycardia (SVT), 80
Surgery section, 329
SVT. *See* Supraventricular tachycardia
Synarthrosis, 36
Syphilis
   cause, 110
   symptoms, 110
   treatment, 111
Systemic inflammatory response syndrome (SIRS), A-14, A-63

T

T. pallidum, 129
T. vaginalis, 129
TAH. *See* Total abdominal hysterectomy
Tamoxifen, 112
Taste, 256
TEE. *See* Transesophageal echocardiography
Teeth, 161
Temporomandibular joint (TMJ), 43
Tendons, 37
   disorders of, 50
TENS. *See* Transcutaneous electrical nerve stimulation
Terminology, 97
Terrorism guidelines, A-66
Testes, 123, 213
   disorders of, 129
Tetralogy of fallot, 94
Text resources, further, A-124
Therapeutic services, 357
Thermograms, 359
Thermoreceptors, 256
Thighbone, 34
Third-party-payer, consultations, 315
Thoracic aorta, endovascular repair of descending, 353
Thoracic cage, 34f
Thoracic vertebrae, 43
Thorax, 33
Throat, 163
Thromboangiitis obliterans, 89
Thrombophlebitis, 88
Thrombus, 87–88
Thymus, 213
Thyroid, 212
   disorders, 221
Thyroidectomy, 372
Thyrotoxicosis, 221
TIA. *See* Transient ischemic attack

Index

Tibialis anterior, 40
Time, 322
Tinea pedis, 23
Tinea unguium, 23
Tissue
  subcutaneous, 2
  transfer, adjacent, 335
TLC. *See* Total lung capacity
TLV. *See* Total lung volume
TM. *See* Tympanic membrane
TMJ. *See* Temporomandibular joint
TNM stages, 138
Tongue, dorsum of, 162f
Torsion of testes, 131
Torsion of testis, 131
Total abdominal hysterectomy (TAH), 102
Total lung capacity (TLC), 60
Total lung volume (TLV), 60
Touch, 256
Tourette syndrome, 240
Toxic effects, A-44
Trachea
  and bronchi, 348
  opening to, 55
Transcatheter procedures, 356
Transcutaneous electrical nerve stimulation (TENS), 233
Transesophageal echocardiography (TEE), 80
Transfusion, 183
Transfusion medicine, 385
Transient ischemia, 85
Transient ischemic attack (TIA), 233, 243
  symptoms, 243
Transluminal angioplasty, 355
Transluminal atherectomy, 355
Transmission, 182, 204
Transurethral resection of bladder tumor (TURBT), 124
Transurethral resection of prostate (TURP), 124
Trauma, 247–248
Traumatic brain injury, 247
Traumatic cataract, 266f
Treadmill stress test (TST), 80
Trichomoniasis, 111, 133
Tricuspid, 76
Tricuspid regurgitation, 92
Tricuspid valve, 91
Trimesters, 369
Trunk, 40
TST. *See* Treadmill stress test
Tubular bones, 29
Tumors
  benign, 24
  of brain and spinal cord, 249
  categories, 114
  cranial nerve, 250
  epithelial, 115
  germ cell, 114
  gonadal stromal, 115
  illustration, 10f
  lesions, pathophysiology, 9
  of muscles, 52
  pituitary, 250
  spinal cord, 250
Turbinates, 55
TURBT. *See* Transurethral resection of bladder tumor
TURP. *See* Transurethral resection of prostate
Tympanic membrane (TM), 258

U

U. urealyticum, 132
UA. *See* Urinalysis
Ulcer
  decubitis, 11
  illustration, 10f
  lesions, pathophysiology, 11
  peptic, 175
  pressure, 11
Ulceration, 171
Ulcerative colitis, 180, 180f
  symptoms, 181
  treatment, 181
Ultrasound services, locations for, 379
Unbundling, 281
"Unspecified" codes, A-8
UPIN, reimbursement terminology, 289
UPJ. *See* Ureteropelvic junction
Upper respiratory infection (URI), 55, 60
Ureter, 142, 363
Ureteropelvic junction (UPJ), 144
Urethra, 143
  disorders of, 132
Urethritis
  symptoms, 132
  treatment, 133
URI. *See* Upper respiratory infection
Urinalysis (UA), 55, 144
Urinary bladder, 142
Urinary system, 141
  anatomy and terminology, 141–143
  combining forms, 143
  illustration, 141f
  pathophysiology, 149
  prefixes, 144
  subsection, 362
  suffixes, 144
Urinary tract infection (UTI), 144, 150, 154
Urodynamics, 364
URT. *See* Upper respiratory tract
Usual, customary, and reasonable, reimbursement terminology, 289
Uterine fibroids, 111
Uterine tubes, 97
Utero surgery, A-33
Uterus, 97
UTI. *See* Urinary tract infection

V

V codes, 409
  categories of, A-46
  miscellaneous, A-54
  nonspecific, A-55
  uses of, 409
V27.0, A-34
Vagina, carcinoma of, 97, 366
  symptoms, 116
  treatment, 116
Vaginal birth after cesarean (VBAC), 102
Vaginal delivery, 118
Valves, 76
Valvular heart disease, 91

Index

Valvular regurgitation, 92
Variable growth rate, 249
Varicella-zoster virus (VZV), 22
Varicocele, 130–131
Varicose veins, 89
Vas deferens, 123
Vascular access, guidance for, 356
Vascular dementia, 237
Vascular disorder, 85, 156, 243
Vascular injection procedures, 355
VBAC. *See* Vaginal birth after cesarean
Veins, 74
Venous reconstruction, 354
Ventilation/perfusion scan, 60
Ventricular fibrillation, 90
Verruca vulgaris, 22
Verrucae, 22
Vertebra injury, 248
Vertebral column, 231
   anterior view of, 33f
Vertex, 119
Vesical neck and prostate, 364
Vesicle
   illustration, 10f
   lesions, pathophysiology, 9
Vessels, 73
Viral hepatitis, 182

Viral herpes simplex, 21
Visceral muscle, 37
Visual disturbances, 263
Vitamin D analogs, 16
Voice box, 55
Vulva, 97, 116
   perineum, and introitus, 365

W

Warts, 22
   treatment for, 23
WBC. *See* White blood (cell) count
Wheal
   illustration, 10f
   lesions, pathophysiology, 9
White blood (cell) count (WBC), 73
Whitmore-Jewett stages, 137
Wilms' tumor, 157
Windpipe, 55
"With" codes, A-9
Womb, 97
Wound exploration, 341
Wound repair, 334

X

Xenograft, 336

TRUST CAROL J. BUCK
for your certification review needs!

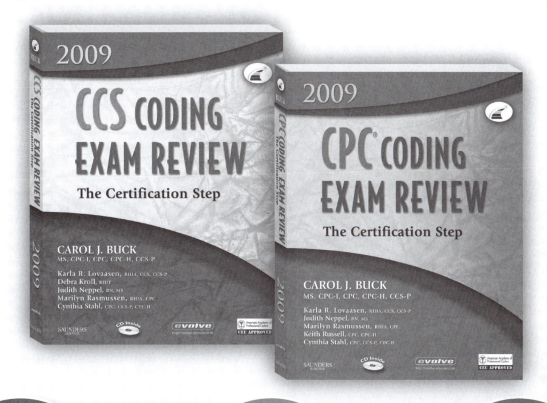

Everything you need to prepare for certification exams.

Study key topics with concentrated reviews.

Practice CDs with tests that mimic the real certification exams.

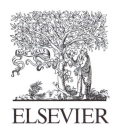

ELSEVIER

Get your copies today!

- Order securely at **www.elsevierhealth.com**
- Call toll-free **1-800-545-2522**
- Visit your **local bookstore**

Make the most of your CPC® certification exam review:

1. Assess! Take the Pre-Exam!
Use the **Pre-Exam** on the enclosed CD to get a feeling of your strengths and weaknesses, develop a plan for focused study, and gain a better understanding of the testing process!

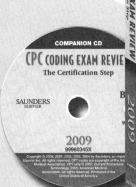
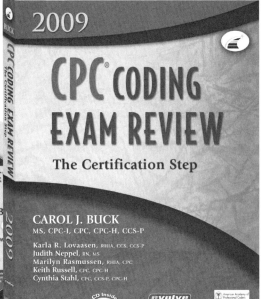

2. Study!
Use the quizzes in this book to sharpen your skills and build competency.

3. Apply! Take the Post-Exam!
After studying, apply your knowledge to the **Post-Exam** located on the CD. When finished, you'll receive scores for both exams and a breakdown of incorrect answers to help you identify areas in need of more detailed study and review.

4. Test! Take the Final Exam!
Gauge your readiness for the actual CPC® exam with the **Final Exam**, located in unit IV, to boost your test-taking confidence and ensure certification success.

Perfect your understanding and prepare for certification – start your review now!

Trust Carol J. Buck and Elsevier for the resources you need at *each step* of your coding career!

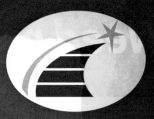

Track your progress toward complete coding success!

Step 1: Learn

- ☐ Step-by-Step Medical Coding 2009 Edition • ISBN: 978-1-4160-4566-3
- ☐ Workbook for Step-by-Step Medical Coding 2009 Edition • ISBN: 978-1-4160-4565-6
- ☐ Medical Coding Online for Step-by-Step Medical Coding 2009 • ISBN: 978-1-4160-6042-0
- ☐ Virtual Medical Office for Step-by-Step Medical Coding 2009 Edition

Step 2: Practice

- ☐ The Next Step: Advanced Medical Coding 2009 Edition • ISBN: 978-1-4160-5679-9
- ☐ Workbook for The Next Step: Advanced Medical Coding 2009 Edition • ISBN: 978-1-4160-5677-5
- ☐ Advanced Medical Coding Online for The Next Step: Advanced Medical Coding 2009 Edition • ISBN: 978-1-4160-6043-7

Step 3: Certify

- ☐ CPC®Coding Exam Review 2009: The Certification Step • ISBN: 978-1-4160-3713-2
- ☐ CCS Coding Exam Review 2009: The Certification Step • ISBN: 978-1-4160-3686-9
- ☐ The Extra Step: Facility-Based Coding Practice • ISBN: 978-1-4160-3450-6
- ☐ The Extra Step: Physician-Based Coding Practice 2009 Edition • ISBN: 978-1-4160-6162-5

Step 4: Specialize

- ☐ Evaluation and Management Step: An Auditing Tool 2009 Edition • ISBN: 978-1-4160-6724-5

Coding References

- ☐ 2009 ICD-9-CM, Volumes 1 & 2, Professional Edition • ISBN: 978-1-4160-4448-2
- ☐ 2009 ICD-9-CM, Volumes 1, 2, & 3, Professional Edition • ISBN: 978-1-4160-4450-5
- ☐ 2009 ICD-9-CM, Volumes 1 & 2, Standard Edition • ISBN: 978-1-4160-4449-9
- ☐ 2009 ICD-9-CM, Volumes 1, 2, & 3, Standard Edition • ISBN: 978-1-4160-4447-5
- ☐ 2009 HCPCS Level II Professional Edition • ISBN: 978-1-4160-5203-6
- ☐ 2009 HCPCS Level II Standard Edition • ISBN: 978-1-4160-5204-3

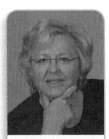

Author and Educator
Carol J. Buck,
MS, CPC-I, CPC,
CPC-H, CCS-P

Get the next resources on your list today!

- Order securely at **www.elsevierhealth.com**
- Call toll-free **1-800-545-2522**
- Visit your local bookstore

Need more ICD-9 study resources?

This clear, easy-to-use textbook is **your key to ICD-9-CM coding success,** offering **everything you need to understand and apply the official codes of the ICD-9-CM.** You'll find **detailed background information** on the evolution and importance of medical coding, as well as **reliable, straightforward guidelines** for each of the coding classifications you'll use in practice.

Master the ICD-9-CM concepts needed to ensure proper reimbursement with features like…

- **ICD-9-CM guidelines** that open each coding chapter, with examples that clearly demonstrate their real-world applications.
- A **full-color design** that makes anatomy and physiology stand out and provides visual reinforcement of key content.
- **Illustrations and overviews of anatomy, physiology, and related disease conditions** in each coding chapter that help you better visualize and understand what the codes represent.
- **Problem-solving exercises** throughout each chapter that provide valuable practice using key coding principles as you learn them.
- **Also available as a paperless eBook!** Visit http://evolveebookstore.elsevier.com to find out more!

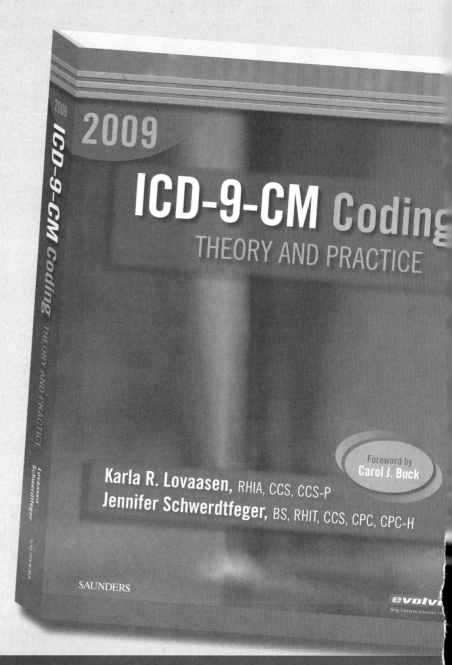

ICD-9-CM Coding: Theory and Practice, 2009 Edition
Karla R. Lovaasen, RHIA, CCS, CCS-P a[nd]
Jennifer Schwerdtfeger, BS, RHIT, CCS, CPC, CPC-[H]
2009 • 768 pp., 400 illus. • ISBN: 978-1-4160-5881-